**Systems
and
Medical Care**

The MIT Press Cambridge,
Massachusetts,

and
London,
England

Systems and Medical Care

Edited by
Alan Sheldon

Frank Baker

and
Curtis P. McLaughlin

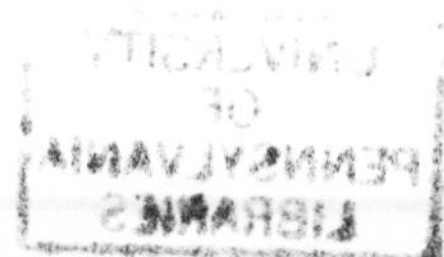

Set in Linotype Caledonia
Printed by The Book Press
Bound in the United States of America by The Book Press

ISBN 0 262 19077 X (hardcover)

Library of Congress catalog card number: *74-118353*

Contributors

Frank Baker is head of the Program Research Unit of the Laboratory of Community Psychiatry and Lecturer in Psychology in the Department of Psychiatry at Harvard Medical School. Dr. Baker received his M.A. and Ph.D. in social psychology from Northwestern University. Before joining the faculty at Harvard Medical School in 1965, he was Assistant Professor of Social Psychology at Lehigh University. Dr. Baker is the author of numerous journal articles and editor of a number of books. He is vice-chairman of the Health Systems Committee of the Society for General Systems Research.

Louis B. Barnes is Professor of Organizational Behavior at the Harvard University Graduate School of Business Administration, where he was formerly Assistant Professor of Business Administration and Associate Professor of Organizational Behavior. He holds the B.A. degree from Amherst College and the M.B.A. and D.B.A. degrees from Harvard University. Dr. Barnes has done considerable research in the area of organizational development and organization change and is a consultant to many industrial and community organizations. He has published numerous articles and books on organizational research and theory.

Robert Chin is Professor of Psychology at Boston University and Research Associate at the University's Human Relations Center. Dr. Chin received his Ph.D. degree from Columbia University. He has served as general editor of *Journal of Social Issues* and in various other capacities in Division 9 of the American Psychological Association and the Society for the Psychological Study of Social Issues, of which he is currently president. Dr. Chin has authored and edited numerous publications in the field of psychology and applied behavioral sciences.

Mark G. Field, Professor of Sociology at Boston University, Associate of the Russian Research Center at Harvard University, and Assistant Sociologist in the Department of Psychiatry at the Massachusetts General Hospital, holds the A.B., A.M., and Ph.D. degrees from Harvard University. In 1967–1968 he also was a research associate in the Program on Technology and Society at Harvard. Dr. Field's main areas of interest are the sociology of the professions, with particular stress on the medical profession in the Soviet Union; Soviet social institutions; medical sociology; the comparative study of medical systems; and the sociology of science; and he has written extensively on these subjects. He is a member of the editorial board of the *Review of Soviet Medical Science* and of *Soviet Sociology* as well as an editorial consultant to the *International Journal of Psychiatry*, and he has served as a member of the Advisory Committee on the Study of Medical Education in the Developing Countries carried out by the Association of American Medical Colleges for the Agency for International Development. A consultant to Arthur D. Little, Inc., he also served as a consultant to the World Health Organization in Geneva in the summer of 1969.

Daniel Howland is currently Professor of Management at the College of Administrative Science, Ohio State University, where he has held a number of appointments. He obtained his Sc.B. in Engineering from Brown University and subsequently the M.A. in Psychology and Ph.D. in Psychology and Industrial Engineering from Ohio State. He is a member of numerous research, industrial, and administrative committees, both academic and national, many of which deal with systems and/or health issues, and also of several professional organizations in the health, systems, and engineering fields. His current interests lie in developing systems models in the health area.

Sidney S. Lee, M.D., Dr. P.H., is the Associate Dean for Hospital Programs of the Harvard Medical School and Clinical Professor of Hospital and Medical Care Administration at the Harvard School of Public Health. Prior to his present appointment, he was general director of Boston's Beth Israel Hospital. From 1950 to 1954, he served as a commissioned officer in the U.S. Public Health Service with experience in local and state health departments.

Curtis P. McLaughlin is Associate Professor of Business Administration at the University of North Carolina, Chapel Hill, and Visiting Lecturer on Health Systems Analysis at the Harvard School of Public Health. After taking a B.A. in chemistry at Wesleyan and an M.B.A. from Harvard Business School, he worked in industry for some years before returning to Harvard Business School for his doctorate and subsequent appointments leading to an assistant professorship. He has been a consultant to RAND and numerous health agencies. He has written and lectured widely on systems analysis in the health field, and his interests lie in the area of the production of information and professional services, especially in medicine and engineering. His current work includes a major project on program design for family planning in developing countries.

Dr. James G. Miller received the A.B., A.M., M.D., and Ph.D. degrees from Harvard University. He had an internship in medicine and residency in psychiatry at the Massachusetts General Hospital. He was a Junior Fellow of the Harvard Society of Fellows and served briefly as Assistant Professor of Social Relations at Harvard. He was chief of the Clinical Psychology Section of the Veterans Administration after World War II, and then became chairman of the Department of Psychology at the University of Chicago, where he was also chairman of the Committee on Behavioral Science. Founder and first director of the Mental Health Research Institute and Professor of Psychiatry and Psychology at the University of Michigan from 1955 to 1967, he is presently Vice President for Academic Affairs at Cleveland State University and Vice President and Principal Scientist of EDUCOM (The Interuniversity Communications Council).

Gregory M. St. L. O'Brien, who received his Ph.D. from Boston University, is an Associate in Psychiatry (Psychology) in the Laboratory of Community Psychiatry, Department of Psychiatry, Harvard Medical School. At Boston University, Dr. O'Brien was a predoctoral NIMH Fellow in Community Psychology at the Department of Psychology and Human Relations Center. He is currently engaged in research on the changing roles of, and relationships among, voluntary human service organizations. He acts as evaluation research consultant for programs in education and social welfare.

Gerald Rosenthal is currently Associate Professor at Brandeis University, where he teaches in the Department of Economics and at the Florence Heller Graduate School of Social Welfare. He is actively interested in the economic aspects of medical care: the economic role of physicians, the structure of health manpower, the social and economic consequences of alternative methods of payment, and the role of government in the medical-care market. He has lectured and written widely on these subjects as well as on the general issues of planning and evaluation. He has also been a member of various committees dealing with medical care problems, including Budget Bureau Renal Disease Study Committee; Ad Hoc Committee on Medical Care Facilities (USPHS); Committee on Health Services Research, Medical Care Section (APHA); and Chairman, Legislative Committee, Massachusetts Public Health Association. He is Senior Associate, Organization for Social and Technical Innovation, Cambridge, Massachusetts.

Herbert C. Schulberg, Ph.D., S.M.(Hyg.) is Associate Director for Planning and Resources at United Community Services of Metropolitan Boston, and Assistant Clinical Professor of Psychology at Harvard Medical School. Trained in clinical psychology at Columbia University and in community mental health at the Harvard School of Public Health, Dr. Schulberg's interests include program planning and evaluation as well as research on the changing nature of comprehensive health programs. Dr. Schulberg's publications have covered a wide variety of programmatic developments, and he has served as a consultant to many state and local agencies.

Alan Sheldon is Assistant Professor of Psychiatry at Harvard Medical School and Lecturer in Business Administration at Harvard Business School. Educated at Cambridge University and Westminster Hospital Medical School, he trained in psychiatry and later engaged in several sociological studies of health-related topics. More recently, his interest in systems, in futures work, and in the theory and management of organizations especially as applied to health systems management and planning has led him to study, consult, and write extensively on health and organizational topics as well as to engage in program innovations in these areas. He is chairman of the Health Systems Committee of the Society for General Systems Research, and associate editor of *Social Science and Medicine.*

Acknowledgements

The editors would like to express their grateful thanks to the sponsors of the Symposium on Systems and Medical Care: Sandoz Pharmaceuticals, E. R. Squibb & Sons, Smith Kline and French Laboratories, and Dr. Gerald Caplan, Director of the Laboratory of Community Psychiatry, Harvard Medical School; and to the National Institute of Mental Health, whose Public Health Service special grant MH–02914 supported much of the work of Dr. Baker and Dr. Sheldon. They would also like to thank the discussants, whose enthusiastic response and stimulating ideas were particularly appreciated: Professor Odin W. Anderson, Dr. Edgar H. Auerswald, Professor Gerald Caplan, Mr. Robert Colbourne, Professor Paul M. Densen, Dr. Frederick J. Duhl, Dr. John R. Finch, Dr. Arnold Golodetz, Dr. Harold P. Halpert, Dr. Joseph J. Harrington, Dr. Kenneth J. Jones, Dr. Melvin J. Krant, Dr. Samuel Levey, Dr. Gilbert Levin, Mr. Steven Lorch, Professor Edward B. Roberts, Professor William B. Schwartz, Dr. Victor W. Sidel, Dr. John D. Stoeckle, Professor Renato Tagiuri, and Dr. Henry Wechsler.

Members of the staff of the Laboratory of Community Psychiatry whose help was essential included Miss Marie Killilea, Mrs. Joyce Brinton, Miss Tonia Aminoff, Miss Marjorie Lewis, Mrs. Rose Marie Toon, Mrs. Shelley Vickery, and Miss Sandra Weintraub.

Finally, the authors of the papers deserve a special vote of appreciation for their diligence and patience in reworking their material so that this book was possible.

Preface

In early 1968 the editors of this volume, aware of the increasing interest of diverse individuals in the application of systems concepts and techniques to health issues and problems, decided that this emergent field needed considerable definition and clarification, and that the beginner in this field could benefit from an explication of the various theories, concepts, and techniques currently in vogue.

We therefore proposed to hold a short symposium, focused around a limited set of draft chapters especially written with this book in mind. The editors suggested a range of subjects and invited authors to write on these topics. The resulting drafts were circulated to all participants in the symposium in advance. The number of participants was limited to a small group so that each topic could receive attention in depth.

This book represents the final outcome of this experience. The chapters have been revised several times in the light of the discussion at the conference. A further concluding essay has been prepared by the editors, in an attempt to distill the wisdom of the discussants and focus the reader's attention on some of the problems and issues with which this new and exciting field is struggling.

The first three chapters represent an overview of the concepts and of the recent literature most relevant to health care systems in the linked subjects of general systems (Baker), systems analysis (McLaughlin) and cybernetics (Sheldon).

Two chapters follow (Miller, Sheldon) which discuss basic systems models of disease and medical care, and a further two chapters (Lee and McLaughlin, Field) which examine the recent evolution of the medical care system. Baker and Schulberg, and Chin and O'Brien develop more specific interorganizational systems models. McLaughlin and Howland then each demonstrate the utility and application of systems analysis techniques and concepts in health. Finally, Rosenthal discusses health systems planning, and Barnes explores the processes of change in systems. The editors, in the concluding chapter, attempt to sum up with an overview of the state of the field, building on the symposium discussion.

The editors feel strongly that despite all the deficits, errors, and exaggerations of a struggling adolescent, systems concepts and techniques hold much promise for the health field. This field, bedeviled as it is by its hierarchical nature, disciplinary splitting, and fragmentation of care can benefit greatly from systems approaches, particularly as the latter offer the hope of integration. The eventual success of this dialectic, however, will not be without some pain. It is probably true that systems theory is antidisciplinary rather than interdisciplinary, and the relinquishment of cherished affiliations, however necessary, is still a loss.

To our knowledge, this book is the first attempt to bring together in one volume the variety of systems theories and techniques and to explore their applications to the health system. We hope that it will provide an introduction for the health professionals who are unfamiliar with these approaches, and also that it will supply a review of the state of the art for those already engaged in systems work.

A. S.
F. B.
C. P. McL.

Preface
x

Frank Baker — **1. General Systems Theory, Research, and Medical Care**
1

Curtis P. McLaughlin — **2. Health Operations Research and Systems Analysis Literature**
27

Alan Sheldon — **3. Cybernetics and Medical Care**
49
Some Recent Literature

James G. Miller — **4. A General Systems Approach to the Patient and His Environment**
62

Alan Sheldon — **5. Toward a General Theory of Disease and Medical Care**
84

Sidney S. Lee and Curtis P. McLaughlin — **6. Changing Views of Public Health Services as a System**
126

Mark G. Field — **7. The Medical System and Industrial Society**
143
Structural Changes and Internal Differentiation in American Medicine

Frank Baker and Herbert C. Schulberg
8. Community Health Care-Giving Systems
182
Integration of Interorganizational Networks

Robert Chin and Gregory M. St. L. O'Brien
9. General Intersystem Theory
207
The Model and a Case of Practitioner Application

Curtis P. McLaughlin
10. Systems Analysis for Health
230

Daniel Howland
11. Toward a Community Health System Model
268

Gerald Rosenthal
12. Planning in the Health Care System
290
The Choice of Policies

Louis B. Barnes
13. Designing Change in Organizational Systems and Structures
314

Alan Sheldon, Frank Baker, and Curtis P. McLaughlin
14. Current Issues in Systems and Medical Care
329

Index
349

Figures

Chapter 3
Figure 1 56
Figure 2 57

Chapter 5
Diagram 1 100
Diagram 2 104
Diagram 3 104

Chapter 7
Figure 1. Exchange of medical and nonmedical time. 150
Figure 2. The social system and the medical system. 153
Figure 3. Generalists and specialists in medicine in the United States, 1900–1976. 158
Figure 4. Generalists and specialists in medicine in the United States, 1984. 158
Figure 5. Health personnel. 162

Chapter 8
Figure 1. Functional overlap of three models of providing comprehensive health and related community services. 201

Chapter 10
Figure 1. One conceptualization o systems analysis. 234
Figure 2. Preliminary model of a state kidney disease control program. 241

Chapter 11
Figure 1. Trends in costs and demands for hospital service. 269
Figure 2. The functional levels of a health system. 274
Figure 3. The research process. 281
Figure 4. Cybernetic models of adaptive systems. 282
Figure 5. Data log sheet. 284
Figure 6. Data coding sheet. 285
Figure 7. Patient demand for resources as a function of time. 285
Figure 8. Patient response to resource utilization in surgery. 286

Tables

Chapter 4

Table 1. The Critical Subsystems. 70

Chapter 6

Table 1. Comparative Organizational Units, U.S. Public Health Service, 1948 and 1957. 129-130

Chapter 7

Table 1. Persons Employed in Selected Health Professions in the United States, by Decades, 1900–1960. 160

Table 2. Estimated Number of Physicians, Dentists, Professional Nurses, and Other Health Workers in the United States, 1960. 161

Chapter 10

Table 1. Time-Cost Evaluation of Operating Room Personnel Skills. 258

Table 2. Linear Programming Matrix for Surgical Suite Staffing Model. 259

Table 3. Concepts Applied to the Health Area—Examples. 263

Systems
and
Medical Care

Frank Baker

1. General Systems Theory, Research, and Medical Care

In recent years, the term *system* has become so extremely popular that it may even be in serious danger of becoming merely a meaningless fad word. Of course this word, unlike the related popular technical term *cybernetics*, is not a recently coined word, and through long and extensive use it has acquired a number of unfortunate colloquial meanings. The concept of system as a conglomeration of parts has been employed for hundreds of years; what is new, as Ackoff (1959, p. 6) has pointed out, is "the tendency to study systems as an entity."

Ashby (1958) describes the change from an emphasis on the analysis of complex structures into component simple units to an emphasis on the study of the whole system—the units in combined action—as an important new scientific movement. The "systems movement" began to grow in size and influence shortly after World War II, although its roots can be traced back several centuries (Bertalanffy 1968).

To many people, the "systems movement" suggests only the military and industrial applications of systems concepts in such new applied technologies as systems engineering, systems analysis, and systems design. However, there is a broader aspect of systems development in science related to the renewed quest for a "general" theory. In a time of ever increasing specialization, the appeal of a "general" theory has drawn together individuals from a variety of widely differing disciplines who seek to bridge the gaps among disciplines and who feel the need for a *general systems theory*, that is, a body of organized theoretical constructs which can be employed to discuss the general relationships of the empirical world. Boulding (1956, p. 198) has identified two objectives of general systems theory: "At a low level of ambition but with a high degree of confidence it aims to point out similarities in the theoretical constructions of different disciplines, where these exist, and to develop theoretical models of study. At a higher level of ambition, but with perhaps a lower degree of confidence it hopes to develop something like a 'spectrum' of theories—a system of systems which may perform the function of a 'gestalt' in theoretical construction." As Boulding observes, one of the greatest values of such a "system of systems" or "gestalt" is its potential for directing researchers and theorists to gaps in theoretical models.

A key figure in the development of general systems theory, who is usually given credit for originating the idea, is Ludwig von Bertalanffy. Bertalanffy, a theoretical biologist who pioneered in promoting an organismic view in biology, first developed his "general systems theory" in the thirties, but he did not publish his ideas until the conclusion of World War II. He first presented his general systems theory in 1937 in a seminar at the University of Chicago, explaining his delay in publication by noting that "at the time theory was in bad repute in biology" and that he was afraid of the reception such abstract generalization might receive (Bertalanffy 1968, p. 90).

By the late forties and early fifties the intellectual climate had changed, model building had come back into fashion, and Bertalanffy not only found good reception for his ideas, but also found that a number of scientists were independently evolving similar approaches. In 1954 Bertalanffy, with a multidisciplinary group at the Center for Advanced Study in the Behavioral Sciences at Stanford, discussed the formation of a scientific society centering around general systems. In 1955, Bertalanffy and his colleagues from Stanford organized the Society for the Advancement of General Systems Theory at the annual meeting of the American Association for the Advancement of Science in Berkeley, California. The multidisciplinary organizing committee, in addition to Bertalanffy, included Kenneth E. Boulding, economist; Ralph W. Gerard, biologist; and Anatol Rapaport, mathematician. In 1956 the Society began publication of the *General Systems Yearbook*, and through the ensuing years it has been one of the key publication outlets for papers which develop, modify, and apply the general systems theory described by Bertalanffy and other key investigators, including Boulding (1956), Ashby (1958), and Rapaport and Horvath (1959). The parallel development of Wiener's cybernetics (1948), Shannon and Weaver's (1949) information theory, and von Neumann and Morgenstern's (1947) game theory produced important cybernetic feedback, including information concepts that enriched the general systems formulations arising out of biology and the economic and social sciences.

Two other multidisciplinary groups should be mentioned before concluding this brief review of the history and development of general systems theory. During the period from 1951 to 1956, a group of biologists, psychologists, psychiatrists, and social scientists met for twelve biannual conferences in Chicago. Roy R. Grinker edited a volume based on the transcript of discussions at the early meetings. This symposium volume, entitled *Toward a Unified Theory of Human Behavior*, was published in 1956 and contains a number of important early attempts to integrate different disciplines using systems concepts.

Another multidisciplinary group of importance in the development of general systems research and theory was formed by James G. Miller at the University of Chicago in 1949. Miller, a psychiatrist and psychologist, with his associates sought to develop what he called a "general systems behavior theory." Later in 1955, Miller moved to the University of Michigan Medical School, where he started the Mental Health Research Institute. In 1956 the journal *Behavioral Science*, the official publication of the Institute, was started, and over the years the structural and behavioral properties of many different systems have been analyzed in articles published in it. In 1965 Miller published in this journal three related articles summarizing the results of the work done by him and his associates over the years to clarify and elaborate the assumptions, definitions, and propositions of general systems theory (Miller, 1965b, 1965c, 1965d).

The literature dealing with systems has continued to expand at an accelerated pace in the last few years. Recent books making valuable applications of general systems theory in the social sciences include the work of David Easton (1965) in political science, Walter Buckley (1967) in sociology, and F. K. Berrien (1968) in social psychology. Buckley (1968) has edited a volume reprinting many of the best articles from the *General Systems Yearbook*.

Before proceeding to discuss the relation of general systems theory to research, and medical care, it seems important to ask the question: Is general systems theory really a theory? It is significant that the founders of the Society for General Systems Theory later changed the name to the less pretentious Society for General Systems Research. The term "theory" has been thought to be overused in recent years, and scientists have become increasingly reluctant to apply it (Caws 1968). While general systems theory may not yet meet the purist's definition of a theory, it is at least a set of useful concepts and working hypotheses and is a vigorous approach to the basic similarities believed to exist between certain properties of all systems. Care should be taken, therefore, to distinguish it from the "systems orientation." The latter approach attempts to encompass the complexity of relationships among disparate events without a predetermination of singularity or direction. At its best, it is an original and creative attempt to deal with complicated phenomena in a simple fashion while still attempting to be inclusive. However, upon examination it often becomes the application of a new jargon to an old set of unsolved problems in the hope that they will seem more amenable to solution.

Basic General Systems Concepts

In an earlier attempt to survey the work that had been done in the field of general systems theory, Young (1964, p. 61) observed. "The basic key to general systems theory lies in the types of concepts and polarities of concepts that have been elaborated to describe, explain, and predict the behavior of a general system. These concepts form the basis of all work done to date in the field and it is to these concepts that one must turn in thinking about applications of general systems theory to any specific discipline or problem." This seems wise advice to follow in reviewing the application of the conceptual framework to the field of medical care, and accordingly the next section of this chapter will present some of these basic concepts.

DEFINITION OF "SYSTEM" A system has been defined as the totality of elements in interaction with each other (Bertalanffy 1956), the totality of objects together with their mutual interactions (Hall and Fagen 1956), unity consisting in mutually interacting parts (Ackoff 1960) and a recognizably delimited aggregate of dynamic elements that are in some way interconnected and interdependent and that continue to operate together according to certain laws and in such a way as to produce some characteristic total effect (Boguslaw 1965). Other similar definitions have been given, and it seems that each writer in discussing systems must answer the question, "What is a system?" before feeling that he can assume such knowledge on the part of his reader. These definitions in essence agree that a system is a set of units or elements that are actively interrelated and that operate in some sense as a bounded unit.

General systems theory is, then, primarily concerned with problems of relationships, of structure, and of interdependence rather than with the constant attributes of objects. Older formulations of systems constructs had dealt with the closed systems of the physical sciences, in which relatively self-contained structures could be treated successfully as if they were independent of external forces. As a biologist, Bertalanffy was more interested in living systems that are open to, and acutely dependent upon, an external environment.

SYSTEMS LEVELS The concept of hierarchical levels of systems is basic in the writing of Bertalanffy (1968), Miller (1965a), and other general systems theorists. Boulding (1956) has offered a classification of systems levels: (1) static structures—the level of frameworks, for example, the anatomy of the universe; (2) simple dynamic systems—the level of clockworks, systems with predetermined necessary motions; (3) cybernetic systems—the level of the thermostat, the system of self-regulating in moving to maintain equilibrium; (4) open-systems—the level of self-maintaining systems, life as differentiated from nonlife, includes living organisms, the level of the cell; (5) genetic-societal systems—the level of cell society, characterized by a division of labor among cells; (6) animal systems—the level of increased mobility, evidence of goal-directed behavior, and self-awareness; (7) human systems—the level of the individual human, ability to interpret symbols and communicate ideas; (8) social systems—the level of human organization; and (9) transcendental systems—level of ultimates and absolutes that exhibit systematic structures and relationships, but that are inescapable and unknowable in essence.

Theoretical models are best developed at the first two levels. Work at the cybernetic and open systems levels has been receiving increasing attention in recent years, and progress is beginning to be made at these levels. Beyond these levels, systems theory is only beginning to be developed, although some progress is occurring. The use of analogies between lower and higher levels and the attempt to find universals that cut across all levels help to develop the understanding of higher levels.

Bertalanffy, while attempting to point to the isomorphies

cutting across systems levels, has emphasized that part of general systems theory which he calls "open systems." As he points out, living systems differ from nonliving systems in being open to their environments as opposed to the relatively closed nature of nonliving systems. Miller (1965b, 1965c, 1965d), in presenting his thorough and well-developed exposition of a general systems behavior theory, limits his concern to the subset of living systems: cells, organs, organisms, groups, organizations, societies, and supranational systems.

In the analysis of medical care systems, each of the systems levels identified by Miller is of concern. However, it is important to take cognizance of the level of system that is being dealt with at a particular time. At the most microscopic level one focuses on the normal and abnormal functioning of the cells, on the organs of the human organism, and in particular on the response of the human system to particular disease processes and degenerative malfunctionings. At higher levels of systems the individual as a gestalt is of primary concern, and that focus is on individual physical and psychological adaptation to the environment. At still more molar levels one is concerned with social systems such as the small group, particularly the family and work group; the variety of organizational systems, particularly the medical care organizations; and also the larger society.

CLOSED AND OPEN SYSTEMS An ideal closed system would be one into which no energy is received from an outside source, and from which no energy is expended to its surroundings. This is a special case in which the system has impermeable boundaries through which no matter, energy, or information transmissions of any sort can occur. No real, naturally occurring system is ever in fact completely closed; systems, therefore, are only relatively closed. Equilibrium is a state of a closed system, independent of time, in which all macroscopic variables remain constant and all macroscopic processes cease. According to the second law of thermodynamics, every closed system finally attains a state of equilibrium with maximum entropy and minimum free energy. Bertalanffy rejected the second law of thermodynamics in his description of living systems as open systems (Gray 1969).

In contrast with such relatively closed systems are the "open systems" that characterize living cells and organisms (though organisms too may have some equilibrium systems of the closed sort). Open systems are those through which there is a continuing flow of component materials from the environment, and a continuous output of products of the system's action back to the environment. To survive, open systems must move against the tendency toward entropy (maximum disorganization or disorder); open systems must acquire negative entropy. Open systems acquire a steady state of "negentropy" even though entropic changes occur in them as they do everywhere else; they do this by taking in inputs higher in complexity of organization, i.e., lower in entropy than their outputs. Thus they restore their own energy and repair breakdowns in their own organization. There is then a general trend in an open system to maximize this ratio of imported to expended energy. Open systems typically seek to improve their survival position and to acquire in their reserves a comfortable margin in operation.

INPUT, TRANSFORMATION, OUTPUT The pattern of activities of the energy exchange of an open system has a cyclic character. Open systems take in input, i.e., they import some form of energy from the external environment, and then transform or reorganize it through the application of *throughput* processes. The body converts starch and sugar into heat and action. The personality converts chemical and electrical forms of stimulation into sensory qualities, and information into thought patterns. The organization creates a new product, processes materials, trains people, or provides a service. Open systems export some products into the environment, i.e., they produce outputs. The outputs of one system become available for use as inputs for another system. This basic conception of an open system as a cycle of input—conversion—output facilitates the analysis of living systems at a variety of levels from the cell to the society.

SUBSYSTEMS In every system it is possible to identify an element or functional component of the larger system that fulfills the conditions of a system in itself, but that also plays a specialized role in the operation of a larger system. Taking a particular living system as the focus, one can define the totality of all the structures in the system that carry out a particular process as a *subsystem*. Thus, at least three types of subsystems can be identified for an open system: an input subsystem, a conversion or operating subsystem, and an output subsystem. There is not necessarily a one-to-one relationship between process and structure, and one or more processes may be carried on by two or more subsystems. Miller (1965b, 1965c, 1965d) makes a distinction between subsystems, which he calls *process units*, and *components*, which he calls *structural units.* Guest (1962) observed that the survival of any living organism is dependent upon the ongoing interaction of its parts. As Miller explains, relationships among subsystems or components involve either structures or processes; the structural relationships are spatial in character, and the process relationships are either purely temporal or involve spatial changes in time.

SUPRASYSTEM AND ENVIRONMENT "The suprasystem of any living system is the next highest system in which it is a component or subsystem (Miller 1965b, p. 218). As an example, the suprasystem of a cell or tissue is the organ containing it; the suprasystem of an individual is the group of which he is a member. The suprasystem, however, is not to be confused with the *environment.* The immediate environment of a system is the suprasystem of which it is a part minus the system itself. The entire environment includes this immediate environment plus the suprasuprasystem and the systems at all the higher levels which contain it. Hall and Fagen (1956, p. 20) define the environment of a given system as "the set of all objects a change in whose attributes affect the system and also those objects whose attributes are changed by the behavior of the system." As was previously noted, in order to survive, a system must interact with and somehow adjust to its environment, the other parts of the suprasystem. Characteristically living systems adapt to their environments, but they also in turn affect their environments and change them.

DIFFERENTIATION AND INTEGRATION There is movement in open systems in the direction of differentiation and elaboration. Specialized functions replace diffuse global patterns. Primitive nervous tissue evolves into highly differentiated structures of sense organs and the rest of the nervous system. The personality grows from crude, rather primitive organizations of mental functions into hierarchically structured and well-differentiated systems of beliefs and feelings. Organizations move in the direction of multiplication and elaboration of roles with greater specialization of functions.

For example, in this country today there are more medical specialists than general practitioners. The reintegration of differentiated parts is crucial at the level of the organism. Angyal (1941, pp. 273–275) has discussed this issue in the following manner:

> The organism tends to be economical with respect to differentiation. Diffuse functions become differentiated only when there is a pronounced need for individualized, specific functions. . . . The parts of a system may be differentiated in various degrees according to functional requirements. . . . In a highly differentiated whole, the parts are more individualized and have a greater relative autonomy, a greater independence from the whole. Thus, in the process of differentiation, there is a distinct tendency towards the breaking up of the unity of the whole, that is, the danger of disintegration. This tendency is normally counter-balanced by the whole through its integrating function. In this case the whole exerts its influence not by opposing differentiation but by coordination of the differentiated part functions under the general system principles. When this latter phase is successfully accomplished, the whole reaches a higher degree of efficiency and becomes capable of more adequately differentiated functioning. The evolution of wholes is itself accomplished in steps of successive differentiation and systematic reintegration.

EQUIFINALITY AND EQUICAUSALITY As early as 1940 Bertalanffy suggested the principle of equifinality (Gray 1969). According to this principle, a system can reach the same final state from differing initial conditions and by a variety of paths. An example of a living organism reaching a final state from different initial conditions in different ways is that of a normal sea urchin, which can develop either from a complete egg or from a half egg. The amount of equifinality in an open system may be reduced as the system moves toward regulatory mechanisms to control its operations. It is also true that the same cause may produce a wide variety of manifestations under differing conditions, and this phenomenon is called equicausality.

FEEDBACK Miller (1965b, p. 227) asserts that cybernetics, the study of methods of feedback control, is an important part of systems theory. "It has led to the recognition of certain formal identities among various sorts of living and nonliving systems." Feedback describes the situation in which a portion of the output (e.g., behavior) is returned to the input so as to modify succeeding outputs of the system. Miller views a living system as self-regulating because in it input not only affects output, but output often adjusts input. *Negative feedback* is a situation in which information comes back to the system as input in such a way as to decrease the deviation of output from a steady state. *Positive feedback* occurs when signals are fed back over the feedback channel in such a manner that they increase the deviation of the output from a steady state. Miller (1965b) emphasizes the critical nature of negative feedback in his proposition that when a system's negative feedback discontinues, its steady state vanishes, and at the same time its boundaries disappear and the system ceases to survive. If there is no corrective device to get the system back on its course it will expend too much energy or it will ingest too much energetic input and no longer continue as a system. Feedback will be discussed further in Chapter 3, on cybernetics.

MONITORING AND BOUNDARY CONTROL ACTIVITIES Miller and Rice (1967) point out the importance of regulation in preserving the boundary of a system, and they discuss two types of regulatory activity: monitoring and boundary control. Monitoring is an intrasystem regulatory activity and involves checking an operating activity or taking action to institute a new or modified operating activity. Boundary regulation is a regulatory activity external to the operating activities of a system and consists of activities that relate a system to its environment by controlling the input and output transitions across the system's boundary. Miller and Rice argue that this implies that the boundary around a system is not a line but a region. They call this region "boundary control function" and describe it as existing between the operating activities of the system and the environment; there are two boundaries involved, "one between the internal activities of the system and the region of regulation, and a second between the region of regulation and the environment" (p. 9).

MORPHOSTASIS AND MORPHOGENESIS Buckley (1967) has asserted that the actions of complex open systems are not simply and directly a function of forces impinging on them from the environment. As open systems increase in complexity, mediating processes develop within them that intervene between external forces and behavior.

Buckley suggests the term *morphogenesis* to describe processes in complex system-environment exchanges that tend to elaborate or change a system's organization, state, or form. *Morphostasis* describes those processes which tend to preserve or maintain a given system's form, structure, or state. Biological evolution, learning, and societal development are examples of morphogenesis; homeostatic processes in organisms and ritual in sociocultural systems are examples of morphostasis. Systems on the phylogenetic, higher psychological, and sociocultural levels typically display morphogenic or structure-elaborating characteristics that are related to their capabilities in remaining viable, on-going systems.

THEORETICAL CONCEPTUAL SYSTEMS AND REAL OR CONCRETE SYSTEMS Systems may be classified as analytical or real. An *analytical system* is the same as a model, or theoretical conceptual system. A *real, concrete*, or *veridical system* can be either man-made or natural (Miller 1965 a–d). The focus in this paper is on the study of real, open systems, and this study has been approached through the use of an analytical or theoretical conceptual system. Science advances as a formal identity or isomorphism increases between a theoretical conceptual system and objective findings about concrete systems.

The Individual as a System

Relatively little work has been done on conceptualizing the individual as a system. However, studies of the individual human organism as an information-processing system have begun to emerge in the last decade and a half. Miller (1960, 1963) has described work at the Mental Health Research Institute of the University of Michigan which employs a general systems orientation. The group has been testing propositions about information-processing channels at five levels of systems: cell, organ, individual, group, and organization. Miller suggests that if information-input overload causes similar performance curves and mobilization of comparable defenses at all levels of behaving systems, then it can be applied to the psychopathology of everyday life and clinical practice.

In a paper on general systems and psychiatry, published in the third volume of *The American Handbook of Psychi-*

atry, Bertalanffy (1959) also suggests that mental disturbance may be looked at as a system dysfunction, rather than the loss of a single function as in the traditional mechanistic viewpoint. He argues against what he calls the previously held "robot" model of personality which he sees most psychologists as continuing to support. He says that this view should be replaced by the model of an "active personality system" (p. 2) considered as a dynamic ordering of parts and processes.

As early as 1960, Gordon Allport, the esteemed personality psychologist, repudiated the static view of personality and argued for a view of personality as an open system (1965). He saw psychology as moving away from "disorganized complexity" and toward an interest in systems theory. This new interest grew out of the organismic conception reflected in the work of Bertalanffy and Goldstein, and also out of certain aspects of gestalt psychology. Allport asserted that "Most current theories of personality take full account of two of the requirements of an open system. They allow interchange of matter and energy, and they recognize the tendency of organisms to maintain an orderly arrangement of elements in a steady state" (p. 234). However, two additional criteria of open systems neglected by much of current personality theory express the view that at least at the human level there is more than mere intake and output of matter and energy and there is extensive transactional commerce with the environment.

There were not as many personality theories when Allport wrote his article over a decade ago as there are today. But even then, theories recognized the tendency of the human personality to go beyond steady states, to enhance their degree of order, and to grow even at the cost of considerable disequilibrium. Many personality theories, however still took an integumented view of personality. Parsons (1951) and F. H. Allport (1955), recognizing the validity of both approaches, attempted to harmonize the integumented personality system with systems of social interaction.

One of the most widely discussed systems theories in social science is that elaborated by Parsons (1951) and his associates (Parsons, Bales, and Shils, 1953; Parsons and Smelser, 1956; Parsons, 1959). Combining his early social behavioralist conceptualizations with the systems problems of a small group as identified by Bales, Parsons developed a functionalistic formulation which he has applied to a number of social system levels. In this scheme, systems problems are linked to the individual in society by means of the concept "role," with the solution of social systems problems dependent upon the adequate functioning of specific individuals occupying positions in the social system.

Parsons (1959) discusses the interpenetration of four systems levels: (1) the organism, (2) the personality or psychological system, (3) the social system, and (4) the cultural system. This differs from his earlier formulations in that the organism is added to the other three primary subsystems of his general theory of action. He continues to rely on the four primary systems functions: goal attainment, adaptation, integration, and pattern maintenance, which he considers as major systems problems at all four systems levels. Parsons makes an analytical distinction between the personality system and the organism, and emphasizes that the individual actor is not of concern. What is important to him is the personality system acting in relation to another system, considered as environment. There are many critiques of the Parsonian framework because of its looseness, however. As Buckley (1967, p. 24) has pointed out, "the critical analyst of Parsonianism soon learns that statements can be found in the work which seemingly refute almost any critical point made against it."

Boundary phenomena are of particular importance in considerations of the individual as a system. Ruesch (1956) distinguished four crucial boundaries that delineate the individual: (1) physical boundaries such as the skin and meninges, (2) the boundaries of organ systems, (3) the biochemical boundaries as exemplified by the selective absorption of the intestinal tract, and (4) the psychological boundary.

Research has shown that in regard to psychological boundaries, individuals differ in the degree to which they experience their boundaries as clearly demarcating them from their environment. Fisher and Cleveland (1958) developed an index derived from an analysis of inkblot responses, the Barrier score, which they used in a series of studies to measure body-boundary definitions. They proposed a theory about the role of the perceived firmness of the body image boundary in the location of psychosomatic symptoms, and they have obtained a number of differences between high and low Barrier scores. These differences support the validity of the Barrier score as a measure of the firmness of body image boundaries.

Fisher and Cleveland hypothesized that a firm body image boundary would lead to a location of psychosomatic symptoms in exterior sites. As predicted, they found high Barrier scores among arthritis, dermatitis, and conversion symptom patients, and low Barrier scores among patients with colitis and stomach disorders. These authors extended their assumptions about the firmness of a body image boundary in the production of disease in their studies of cancer patients, and found that individual patients with cancer at exterior body sites had firmer body image boundaries than did patients with cancer at interior body sites. Although the findings using the Fisher and Cleveland measures of psychological boundaries are not without contradictions, they do provide evidence of the possible importance to medical care of further theory and research on the relations of psychological boundaries to individual system impairment.

Individual-Environment Fit

Clearly the individual, as does any living system, depends upon the environment for survival; he must interact with it and adjust to it. Although much of the history of psychology has revolved around the often acrimonious debate as to whether individual or environment is more important, open systems theory emphasizes that the individual and the environment (both social and physical) mutually influence one another. Pervin (1968) assumes that for each individual there are interpersonal and noninterpersonal environments which more or less match or "fit" that individual's personality. In those cases where there seems to be a "fit" between individual and environment, Pervin sees as an outcome of the resulting interactions "high performance, satisfaction, and little stress in the system whereas a 'lack of fit' is viewed as resulting in decreased performance, dissatisfaction, and stress in the system" (p. 56). One of the outcomes of viewing human effectiveness as specific to a particular individual in a particular environmental setting is that pathology is redefined by this ecological conception of behavior. Kelley (1966, p. 538), one of the most active proponents of ecological analysis in the provision of mental health services, summarizes this position: "Behavior is not viewed as sick or well but is defined as transactional—an outcome of reciprocal interactions between specific social situations and the individual. Adaptive behavior then can be expressed by any individual in a restricted number of social settings or in a variety of environments and can vary from time to time as well as from place to place."

Maelzer (1965) observes that ecologists have two concepts of environment: the environment of the individual and the environment of the population. General ecology or bioecology is concerned with supraorganismic systems and includes (1) *populations*, the term originally coined to denote a group of people and broadened by biologists to include individuals of any one kind of organism; (2) *communities*, which in the ecological sense includes all of the populations occupying a given area; and (3) *ecosystems*, which includes the community and the nonliving environment which function together as an ecological system, e.g., pond or lake. The ecosystem is the basic functional unit in ecology since it includes both the entire living populations of a given territory and the related inorganic environment (Duncan 1964). Psychologists until recently have paid little attention to developments in bioecology, but they are now beginning to be attentive to this area; increased concern is being given to psychological ecology, which views life not only as an aggregate but also as an individual phenomenon (Barker 1965, Kelley 1966, Sommer 1965).

Ecology, the study of organisms in their environment, is in turn just recently beginning to make use of systems concepts, and Odum (1964) has spoken of a "new ecology," which he defines as a "systems ecology."

As medical care shifts its attention to primary prevention, as dysfunctional human behavior gets defined in terms of "ill health" behavior rather than in disease terms, and as the work load of mental health researchers and practitioners increases, more importance and greater attention to human beings as open systems seems to be urgently required.

Groups as Systems

Social scientists have found that systems models are particularly useful in attempting to deal with the complex interrelationships of social phenomena in natural settings. A vast literature has developed on the sociology and social psychology of small face-to-face groups, and much research has also developed dealing with large complex formal organizations. As contrasted with research in organizations, small-group research has not made use of systems models. The reason may lie in the fact that much of the research on social groups has occurred in the controlled environment of the laboratory, where at least the attempt can be made to deal with a restricted set of variables while holding others constant. The limitations of theoretical and conceptual models based on bivariate as opposed to multivariate thinking are probably more apparent in studies of organizations in the complex nonlaboratory environment.

Berrien's attempt in a recent book, *General and Social Systems* (1968), to fit social groups into the framework of general systems theory is therefore a major contribution to the development of useful models of the complex interrelationships which characterize these entities in their natural environment. Berrien emphasizes the preliminary nature of his effort and the need to develop new methodologies to study the small group and larger social systems as sets of components in continuous interaction.

While theorists and researchers have been slow to utilize general system concepts, clinicians have begun to try to apply these ideas to such face-to-face groups as families or psychotherapy groups. At recent meetings of the American Psychiatric Association, several papers have been presented by psychiatrists seeking to apply general systems theory. For example, Laqueur (1967, p. 10) in discussing multiple family therapy, observes that groups are usefully considered as systems: "In the same way as the human organism can be described as an integration of subsystems, efficiently working together for the common goal of survival, dyadic, triadic, and larger groups of human organisms can be seen as systems that partly submerge individual needs in order to create jointly a new larger system for ensuing survival in cooperation and competition with, or even in battle against other similar systems."

Bolman (1967), while discussing the potential usefulness of general systems theory to psychiatry, has argued against the inclusion of "family" as a type of group. Bolman suggests that family be treated as a separate system level between group and organization. His rationale is that even though the family system is a group, to treat it as a type of group results in a reduction of theoretical power; and that the family as a system has "sufficiently unique structural and functional characteristics to warrant separate treatment" (p. 21).

In a paper on psychotherapy, Zweber and Miller (1968) have described a therapeutic and teaching technique which they call "systems games." The technique, which consists of group participants role-playing four specific modes of interaction, is, as they describe it, "an outgrowth of the basic notion that a symptom in an individual is a product of the entire family system" (p. 73). Such application of the basic definition of interpersonal groups as a type of system have begun to appear frequently in the psychiatric literature.

Organizational Systems

The concept of the "organizational system" is a commonplace in organization theory today, and Scott (1961) argues that modern organization theory differs from classical and neoclassical organization theory in its acceptance of "the premise that the only meaningful way to study organization is to study it as a system" (p. 15). In the 1930's, Henderson (1935, p. 86), writing about Pareto's sociology observed, "The interdependence of variables in a system is one of the widest inductions from experience that we possess; or we may alternatively regard it as the definition of a system." Roethlisberger and Dickson (1939) in the classic Hawthorne studies integrated Pareto's idea of the social system into their study of behavior in organizations. Scott (1961) observes that although the concept of a social system guided the work of Hawthorne researchers, this insight was apparently lost in the development of the human relations school of organization that followed. In the sixties the consideration of organizations as systems began to be widely used.

Katz and Kahn (1966) have published a book which takes an open-system approach to the study of the social psychology of organizations. They attempt to spell out open-system concepts which can be used as a framework for organizing the research on complex organizations, even though much of that research was generated from either a closed-system approach or a fragmented or nonsystem approach.

Members of the Organizational Behavior Group at Harvard

Business School have been active in research and theory that views the organization as an open system. Seiler (1967) has published a book which focuses on systems concepts of organizational behavior at a level useful to the administrator. He describes systems analysis as a natural response to organizational problems. Lawrence and Lorsch (1967) from the same group review some of the literature treating an organization as a system, and describe an empirical study of industrial firms in which they focus on the processes of differentiation and integration as they take place within these organizational systems. Their findings suggest that the degree of differentiation and integration differs in effective organizations in relation to the demands of their particular environment. Effective organizations in more stable and less diverse environments, like the container industry when contrasted with the plastics industry, a more diverse and dynamic field, are less highly differentiated. Intregration in a high degree must still be achieved in the container industry.

States of differentiation and integration tend to be inversely related, and it is necesary that an effective organization have integrating devices which are consistent with the degree of differentiation of the organization and diversity of the environment. These findings in industrial organizations should be tested for their generalizability to medical care organizations. They suggest that organizational adaptations are necessary for effective medical service organization in a highly complex urban environment, but that this may not be the case in rural or suburban environments.

In England, workers at the Tavistock Institute of Human Relations, who have been active in developing organizational systems concepts, have been influenced considerably by Bertalanffy's work, which first revealed the importance of a system's being either open or closed to the environment. The open-system model of the Tavistock group assumes that (1) organizations are defined by their primary task; (2) organizations are open systems, i.e., an organization admits inputs from the environment, converts them, and sends outputs back into the environment; and (3) organizations encounter boundary conditions that rapidly change the characteristics of the organization.

Rice (1963) used systems terms in writing up his work at the Ahmedabad Calico Mills and elaborated Trist and

Bamforth's (1951) concept of a production system as a sociotechnical system. Rice (1958) first introduced the concept of "primary task" to discriminate between the varied goals of industrial enterprises. He defined the primary task as the task that an institution had been created to perform. In his later book, Rice (1963) recognized the difficulty of treating the organization as if it had a single goal or task, and he cited the teaching hospital, the prison, and mental health services in particular as examples of institutions which carry out many tasks at the same time.

Trist and his associates (1963) described the "long wall" coal-mining study they made in systems terms and further developed the sociotechnical approach, with emphasis on the multiple channels of interaction of individuals, groups, and organization with the environment. Miller (1959) defined the three dimensions, (1) territory, (2) technology, and (3) time, which he views as intrinsic to the structure of the task of any production system. Emery and Trist (1965, p. 22) described the "causal texture of the environment."

Hutton (1962 a and b) in two papers published in *Human Relations* applied the concept of the primary task, and the system theory of organization developed by his colleagues at the Tavistock Institute to the problems of hospital administration. He picks up and elaborates some of the differences found by Sofer (1955) in his comparison of staff relations in three British hospitals. Hutton's study demonstrates that an organization can be used for purposes for which it is not designed. The changing mental hospital studied by Hutton worked in spite of its formal system, and his organizational analysis demonstrates how such an analysis can lessen the difficulties that occur in changing a medical care organization.

As organizational systems theory continues to develop, it promises to be extremely useful in defining the problems of management, of changing medical care organizations, and particularly of organization-environment interaction and interorganizational relations. Because it provides a more complete technique of evaluation, it supplements traditional final outcome analysis of organizational performance with an emphasis on system process variables which will allow greater generalizability of findings and analysis of program failure. By recognizing Bertalanffy's (1968) principle of equifinality, i.e., that identical final states may be reached from different initial starting positions and by different routes, the examination of operating systems can determine which system is more efficient to produce the same outcome.

Bauer (1966) has edited a book devoted to the topic of social indicators that might provide evidence of where the nation stands with respect to its values and goals, and in particular that would allow the evaluation of a variety of specific programs, including health and welfare programs. In the various papers which comprise this book, social indicators are discussed in the framework of general systems concepts. Of particular interest as an application of general systems concepts is Gross's (1966) chapter, in which he presents a model of a social system at the national level.

Beginning with the example of national economic accounting utilizing a set of economic indicators, Gross (1965) broadens these concepts in his model for the assessment of the state of the nation through the use of social indicators and a process of "social systems accounting." He claims: "According to this model, the state of any nation at any period of time—past, present, future can be analyzed in terms of two interrelated, multidimensional elements: system structure and system performance. The elements of system structure deal with the internal relations among the system's parts, the elements of system performance with the acquiring of inputs and their transformation into outputs. Both involve relations with the external environment" (p. 155). He builds on his earlier work in applying system concepts to single organizations.

Applications of Systems Concepts to Medical Care Organizations

Although, as has been previously noted, organizational system theory holds much promise for useful application to medical care organizations, there have been relatively few studies of such organizations based on general systems models or even on classical organizational models. Reviewing the contents of *Public Health Reports* and the *American Journal of Public Health* between 1950 and 1965, Blum (1966, p. 59) found only a "handful of significant, specifically organizational research projects."

While, as Blum indicated, technology has received a great

deal of research interest, and while there has been an increase in the last few years in the amount of research on social planning and on the legislative process of forming policy, there has been relatively little research into the organization of health service organizations. Blum calls for increased organizational research on health agencies, arguing, "Organizational processes, the means whereby technology can be applied, and at the same time the vehicle upon which policy makers can place new social programs cannot be allowed to continue relatively unresearched" (p. 52).

Organizational research is especially relevant in the evaluation of programs of medical care. Health programs are usually carried out within a formal organization and as such constitute an organizational process within specific units of organizational structure. Application of open-systems concepts to large hospital organizations has been shown to have distinct advantages over traditional nonsystems approaches (Rice, 1961; Howland, 1964a–c; Baker, 1968).

Hospitals, Communities, and Larger Systems

At a time when sociologists inform us that American society has lost its sense of community (Stein 1960), mental health professionals have rediscovered the community, and a persuasive mental health ideology is on the ascendancy that makes an orientation to the community one of its fundamental tenets (Baker and Schulberg, 1967; Schulberg and Baker, 1969a and b). However, an informal content analysis of community mental health documents reveals that the subtleties of the sociological meanings of community are conspicuously absent from most writings in this rapidly developing field. Despite this lack, there seems to be a growing commitment to orient all mental health services to specific populations, and to encourage coordination of all health and welfare services within specific territorial entities.

What are the implications of such reorganization of services around a territorial community focus? One clear implication is that as a mental health organization becomes more open to influence from a specific geographical community, the nature of that ecological system and its subsystems become of heightened importance in the mix of environmental forces. These forces affect the action of the organizational system in both a direct and an indirect causal fashion. As an agent of exchange with the environment, the mental health organization is subject to constraints functionally related to the changing character of its primary environmental systems. Since organizations reflect the characteristics of the publics they serve, as an organization limits its publics, the power of the remaining clients is likely to be increased.

To plan adequately for an organizational system, it is necessary to consider not only its internal functioning but also its place in larger, more inclusive systems. In an earlier paper, the author presented a framework for the study of the changing mental hospital organizational system and its relations to the community based on the concepts of open-systems theory (Baker, 1968). With H. C. Schulberg, the author is applying this open-systems conceptual model in studying the transition of a state mental hospital to a community mental health center. Chapter 9 in this book elaborates this initial hospital system model and conceptualizes the community organizational network as a suprasystem.

At a suprasuprasystems level, the national medical care system has, as Horvath (1966, p. B391) described it, "evolved through a series of trial and error modifications rather than by deliberate design." Mullendorfer and Attinger (1968), using a model based on the concept of adaptive feedback systems, have discussed the relations of health, education, and economy at the supranational systems level and describe "global systems dynamics." At whatever level or system one focuses, from the individual to the supranational entity, it is clear that general systems concepts, while as yet limited in application, offer extremely useful tools for analysis, synthesis, and design of medical care.

References

Ackoff, R. L.
(1959), "Games, Decisions and Organizations." *General Systems Yearbook, 4*, 145–150.
——— (1960), "Systems, Organizations and Interdisciplinary Research." *General Systems Yearbook, 5*, 1–8.
Allport, F. H.
(1955), *Theories of Personality and the Concept of Structure*. New York: Wiley.
Allport, G. W.
(1965), "An Open System Model for Personality." In G. Linzey and C. S. Hall (eds.), *Theories of Personality: Primary Sources in Research*. New York: Wiley.

Angyal, A.
(1941), *Foundations of a Science of Personality.* Cambridge: Harvard University Press.
Ashby, W. R.
(1958), "General Systems Theory as a New Discipline." *General Systems Yearbook, 3,* 1–G.
Baker, F.
(1968), "The Changing Hospital Organizational System: A Model for Evaluation." Read at General Systems Session of AAAS Annual Meeting, Dallas, Texas. To be published in *Man in Systems: Proceedings of the 14th Annual Meeting of the Society for General Systems Research.*
———, **and H. C. Schulberg**
(1967), "The Development of a Community Mental Health Ideology Scale." *Community Mental Health Journal, 3,* 216–225.
Barker, R. G.
(1965), "Explorations in Ecological Psychology." *American Psychologist, 20,* 1–14.
Bauer, R. A.
(1966), *Social Indicators.* Cambridge: M.I.T. Press.
Berrien, F. K.
(1968), *General and Social Systems.* New Brunswick: University Press.
Bertalanffy, L. von
(1956), "General Systems Theory." *General Systems Yearbook, 1,* 1–10.
——— (1959), "General Systems Theory and Psychiatry." *American Handbook of Psychiatry, 3,* 705–721.
——— (1968), *General Systems Theory,* New York: Brazillier.
Blum, H. L.
(1966), "Research into the Organization of Community Health Service Agencies: An Administrator's Review." *The Milbank Memorial Fund Quarterly, 44,* 52–91.
Boguslaw, W.
(1965), *The New Utopians.* Englewood Cliffs: Prentice-Hall.
Bolman, W. M.
(1967), "Theoretical and Empirical Bases of Community Mental Health." *Community Psychiatry,* Supplement to the *American Journal of Psychiatry, 124,* 4, 8–13.
Boulding, K. E.
(1956), "General Systems Theory—The Skeleton of Science." *General Systems Yearbook, 1,* 11–17.
Buckley, W.
(1967), *Sociology and Modern Systems Theory.* Englewood Cliffs: Prentice-Hall.
———, **(ed.)**
(1968), *Modern Systems Research for the Behavioral Scientist. A Source Book.* Chicago: Aldine.
Caws, P.
(1968), "Science and System: On the Unity and Diversity of Scientific Theory." *General Systems Yearbook, 13,* 3–12.
Duncan, O. P.
(1964), "Social Organization and the Ecosystem." In R. E. L. Farris (ed.), *Handbook of Modern Sociology.* Chicago: Rand McNally.
Easton, D.
(1965), *A Systems Analysis of Political Life.* New York: Wiley.
Emery, F. E., and E. L. Trist
(1965), "The Causal Texture of Organizational Environments." *Human Relations, 18,* 21–32.

Fisher, S., and S. L. Cleveland
(1958), *Body Image and Personality.* Princeton: Van Nostrand.
Gray, W.
(1969), "History and Development of General Systems Theory." In W. Gray, F. J. Duhl, and N. D. Rizzo (eds.), *Psychiatry and General Systems Theory.* Boston: Little, Brown.
Grinker, R. R. (ed.)
(1956), *Toward a Unified Theory of Human Behavior.* New York: Basic Books.
Gross, B. M.
(1964), *The Managing of Organizations.* Glencoe: Free Press.
——— (1965), "What are Your Organization's Objectives: A General Systems Approach to Planning." *Human Relations, 18,* 195–216.
——— (1966), "The State of the Nation: Social Systems Accounting." In R. A. Bauer (ed.), *Social Indicators.* Cambridge: MIT Press.
Guest, R. M.
(1962), *Organizational Change: The Study of Effective Leadership.* Homewood, Ill.: Irwin-Dorsey.
Hall, A. D., and R. E. Fagen
(1956), "Definitions of System." *General Systems Yearbook, 1,* 18–28.
Henderson, L. J.
(1935), *Pareto's General Sociology.* Cambridge: Harvard University Press.
Horvath, W. J.
(1966), "The Systems Approach to the National Health Problem." *Management Science, 12,* B391–B395.
Howland, D.
(1964a), "Approaches to the Systems Model." *General Systems Yearbook, 9,* 283–286.
——— (1964b), "A Hospital Systems Model." *General Systems Yearbook,* 9, 287–292.
——— (1964c), "The Measurement of Patient Care: A Conceptual Framework." *General Systems Yearbook,* 9, 293–196.
Hutton, G.
(1962a), "Management in a Changing Mental Hospital." *Human Relations, 15,* 283–310.
——— (1962b), "Managing Systems in Hospitals." *Human Relations, 15,* 311–333.
Katz, D., and R. L. Kahn
(1966), *The Social Psychology of Organizations.* New York: Wiley.
Kelley, J. G.
(1966), "Ecological Constraints on Mental Health Services." *American Psychologist, 6,* 535–539.
Laqueur, H. P.
(1967), "General System Theory and Multiple Family Therapy." Read at Annual Meeting of the American Psychiatric Association, Detroit (May 12).
Lawrence, P., and J. Lorsch
(1967), *Organization and Environment.* Cambridge: Harvard University Press.
Maelzer, D. A.
(1965), "Environment, Semantics and Systems Theory in Ecology." *Journal of Theoretical Biology, 8,* 395–402.
Miller, E. J.
(1959), "Technology, Territory and Time: The Internal Differentiation of Complex Production Systems." *Human Relations, 12,* 243–272.
———, and A. K. Rice
(1967), *Systems of Organizations.* London: Tavistock.

Miller, J. G.
(1960), "Information Input, Overload, and Psychopathology." *American Journal of Psychiatry, 116,* 695–704.
——— (1963), "The Individual as an Information Processing System." In W. S. Fields and W. Abbott (eds.), *Information Storage and Neutral Control.* Springfield: Thomas.
——— (1965a), "The Organization of Life." *Perspectives in Biology and Medicine,* 9, 107–125.
——— (1965b), "Living Systems: Basic Concepts." *Behavioral Science, 10,* 3, 193–237.
——— (1965c), "Living Systems: Structure and Process." *Behavioral Science, 10,* 4, 337–379.
——— (1965d), "Living Systems: Cross-Level Hypotheses." *Behavioral Science, 10,* 4, 380–411.
Mullendorfer, H., and E. O. Attinger
(1968), "Global Systems Dynamics." *Medical Care,* 6, 467–489.
Odum, E. P.
(1964), "The New Ecology." *Biological Science, 14,* 14–16.
Parsons, T.
(1951), *The Social System.* Glencoe: Free Press.
——— (1959), "An Approach to Psychological Theory in Terms of the Theory of Action." In S. Koch (ed.), *Psychology: A Study of a Science.* New York: McGraw-Hill. Vol. 3.
———, R. F. Bales, and E. A. Shils
(1953), *Working Papers in the Theory of Action.* Glencoe: Free Press.
———, and N. J. Smelser
(1956), *Economy and Society.* Glencoe: Free Press.
Pervin, L. A.
(1968), "Performance and Satisfaction as a Function of Individual-Environment Fit." *Psychological Bulletin, 69,* 56–68.
Rapaport, A., and W. J. Horvath
(1959), "Thoughts on Organization Theory and a Review of Two Conferences." *General Systems Yearbook, 4,* 87–94.
Rice, A. K.
(1958), *Productivity and Social Organization: The Ahmedabad Experiment.* London: Tavistock.
——— (1963), *The Enterprise and Its Environment.* London: Tavistock.
Rice, C. E.
(1961), "A Model for the Empirical Study of a Large Scale Organization." *General Systems Yearbook, 6,* 101–106.
Roethlisberger, F. J., and W. J. Dickson
(1939), *Management and the Worker.* Cambridge: Harvard University Press.
Ruesch, J.
(1956), "Epilogue." In R. R. Grinker (ed.), *Toward a United Theory of Human Behavior.* New York: Basic Books.
Schulberg, H. C., and F. Baker
(1969a), "Community Mental Health: The Belief System of the 1960's." *Psychiatric Opinion, 6,* 14–27.
——— (1969b), "Is the Mental Hospital Really Changing?" *Hospital Community Psychiatry 20,* 159–165.
Scott, W. S.
(1961), "Organization Theory: An Overview and an Appraisal." *Journal of Academic Management, 4,* 1, 7–26.

Seiler, J. A.
(1967), *Systems Analysis in Organization Behavior.* Homewood, Ill.: Irwin-Dorsey.
Shannon, C., and W. Weaver
(1949), *The Mathematical Theory of Communication.* Urbana: University of Illinois Press.
Sofer, C.
(1955), "Reactions to Administrative Change: A Study of Staff Relations in Three British Hospitals." *Human Relations, 8,* 291–316.
Sommer, R.
(1965), "Small Group Ecology." *Psychological Bulletin, 67,* 145–152.
Stein, M. R.
(1960), *The Eclipse of Community.* Princeton: Princeton University Press.
Trist, E. H., and K. W. Bamforth
(1951), "Some Social and Psychological Consequences of the Longwall Method of Goal-Getting." *Human Relations, 1,* 4, 3–38.
Trist, E. L., et al.
(1963), *Organizational Choice.* London: Tavistock.
von Neumann, J., and O. Morgenstern
(1947), *Theory of Games and Economic Behavior.* Princeton: University Press.
Wiener, N.
(1948), *Cybernetics.* New York: Wiley.
Young, O. R.
(1964), "A Survey of General Systems Theory." *General Systems Yearbook, 9,* 61–80.
Zweber, J. E., and R. L. Miller
(1968), "The Systems Games: Teaching, Training, and Psychotherapy." *Psychotherapy: Theory, Research and Practice, 5,* 73–76.

Curtis P. McLaughlin

2. Health Operations Research and Systems Analysis Literature

The individual, his health, and the mechanisms influencing his health are readily perceived as natural systems. Today, when any perceived system is a target for systematic scrutiny, numerous health system perceptions have been defined, structured, analyzed, and occasionally manipulated by individuals with such diverse backgrounds as electrical engineering, economics, and medicine. Each such researcher provides a fresh insight, makes a contribution to the literature, usually that of his own profession, and then frequently moves on to study some other system. These efforts show the way in which analytical methods developed elsewhere can diffuse into medical care activities, but their cumulative effect has tended to be small because of their low visibility and use of highly specialized terms.

Meanwhile, the rising costs and high political visibility of health services have led to a widely held view that there must be a better way to organize and provide them. Consequently, less transient groups of professionals are emerging and are maintained by society as medical care economists, health planners, health systems analysts, hospital-industrial engineers, etc. If nothing else, these new compound citizens may concentrate the literature in a few places, probably under the rubrics of operations research and systems analysis.

At the risk of being charged with flippancy and oversimplification, we might distinguish among systems people by saying that general systems types generalize about systems, operations researchers research operands, and systems analysts analyze systems. By and large the latter two groups bring to the health and medical field an application orientation, taking on the goals of a specific project or attacking the problems that are most evident or most tractable. Their contributions to the literature, therefore, are innovations rather than inventions. Their work tends to be simple conceptually, but couched in the jargon, often mathematically symbolized, of their own professions. Hence it often seems unintelligible to medical practitioners and administrators, who then extend the professional courtesy of assuming that this is due to complexity and intellectual subtlety.

Ackoff and Rivett (1963) suggest three essential attributes of operations research: a systems viewpoint; the use of interdisciplinary team; and the application of formal, often mathematical, models. A fourth attribute that is added by some, especially those who call themselves systems analysts, is commitment to the solution of an empirical problem. These practitioners do not have a discipline; they believe that a commitment to the use of any and all disciplines to attack highly complex problems is a sine qua non of professionally competent work. Journals and academic departments notwithstanding, Harrington's observation that "Operations Research really lacks a subject matter" is a relevant one (1966, p. 1342). In a highly readable article, Affel goes even further: "First, I must skirt the semantic quicksands into which almost all discussions of systems engineering seem to be drawn. . . . Almost any short anwer that I have been able to come up with sounds suspiciously like ordinary *good* engineering. . . . So let me now define a system in terms of what the system engineer in the real world devlops in practice: A system is a set of operations organized to satisfy a definable user requirement" (1964, p. 19).[1]

Because operations research has not developed a disciplinary structure, a study of the literature can be organized around either techniques or applications. This book focuses on an application area, health, so the present chapter will be organized around applications—national planning and resource allocation, basic medical science, diagnosis, treatment and epidemiology, hospitals, other medical care services, and community health planning. These application categories are not mutually exclusive. Because this literature review is limited primarily to American sources, hospital applications are the largest segment of the literature. The hospital is the most obvious and most highly structured component of care. If we were looking at literature from European countries, we would find more emphasis on the

[1] The reader who wishes to gain a broad cultural appreciation of systems analysis without special reference to health might do well to look first at Ackoff and Rivett (1963), Flagle, Huggins and Roy (1960), Goode and Machol (1957), and Hall (1962).

comprehensive health-care systems with the hospitals viewed as a community care center.

National Planning and Resource Allocation

National health care planning activities have attracted much attention. National planning is a recognized necessity, is highly visible and large in scale. Kissick (1967) offers a useful description of his activities in the Office of the Surgeon General, and numerous economists have given the rationale behind these efforts.[2] Most studies proceed as if we are on firm ground in the area of measurement and evaluation. Yet it is obvious that we are not.[3] For bad or good, however, quantitative analysis of health systems has become institutionalized at the national level.

One of the most hotly debated issues is the role to be played by benefit-cost analysis. Dorfman (1965) summarizes the resource allocator's dilemma quite succinctly in his introduction to a Brookings Institution symposium volume. He points out that theoretically the pricing mechanism and private initiative motivated by prices should combine to allocate scarce resources in our society. Where the results are socially worthwhile, but unprofitable, public bodies step in to provide a collective good. Yet these public bodies must still allocate resources in a portion of the environment where the pricing mechanisms are a priori inoperative. The frequently suggested alternative is the benefit-cost ratio, the ratio of the social benefits derived from an expenditure to that expenditure, a ratio hopefully greater than one. Dorfman gives a well-known health example of social benefits: "When a man is treated for a communicable disease, the relief afforded him is only part of the social value; every resident of his community benefits from the reduced danger of infection. . . . In other words the consumer of a good or service is not the sole beneficiary, and the amount he is willing to pay does not measure the entire value of the good to society. The act of consumption, in effect, creates a collective good" (1965, p. 5).

[2] For examples, see Blumberg (1967); M. S. Feldstein (1964); Harris (1964); Klarman (1965 a and b); Long (1964); and Wiseman (1963).

[3] Evaluation problems are discussed in M. S. Feldstein (1967); Klarman (1965b); Roemer, Moustafa, and Hopkins (1968); Saunders (1964); Sullivan (1966); and Weisbrod (1961).

The problems of applying the benefit-cost ratio, however, have proved virtually insurmountable in health. Klarman (1965b) points out some of them. What is the value of a life saved, of pain avoided, of medical treatment not required, of earning power not lost? There has been a continuous debate, documented in Klarman's paper, on what benefits might legitimately be included and how they should be valued over time. The economist and the systems analyst still consider benefit-cost ratios to be a basic professional tool. Studies by Arrow (1963) and McKean (1959) give the basic structure of welfare and social benefit-cost analysis. At a less theoretical level, Rice's *Estimating the Cost of Illness* (1966) already seems destined to be a classic. Klarman (1965b) describes the application of this analytic approach to syphilis control, Lechat and Flagle (1965) to leprosy control, and Rice (1965) to cardiovascular disease and cancer.

Because of the conceptual problems involved in developing a universally accepted and politically acceptable benefit structure, those who must make the decisions have shied away from formal application of the benefit-cost concept. They have adopted a "cost-effectiveness" approach instead, which seeks the most effective (usually lowest cost) method of achieving a given set of benefits. The present state of this art is described by Crystal and Brewster (1966) and W. F. Smith (1968). Cost-effectiveness studies are turned out regularly by the Offices of the Surgeon General and of the Secretary of Health, Education, and Welfare. These studies draw upon the skills of epidemiologists, treatment specialists, researchers, and economists to map out and evaluate the alternative for future actions in order to arrive at a reasonably attractive set of final alternatives for the decision-maker.

It is not well understood that the objective of the systems analyst, at least as exemplified in health fields by cost-effectiveness studies, is not to provide a single, final, best recommendation. On the contrary, one intent of health operations research studies has been to move decision-makers away from the action-document approach. A major objective is to bring to light all of the alternatives, including those not recommended, and to state clearly the assumptions underlying the recommendations. Otherwise the decision-maker may learn later to his dismay that his staff has led him into a box by making improper assumptions or by failing to consider the full logical consequences.

Even when systems analysts are content to serve in their roles as advisers and presenters of alternatives, they face a fundamental criticism based on the analysts' bent for quantification. Not all goals and all aspects of a system can be treated numerically, and the critics fear a more rapid development of tangible goals oriented toward the quantifiable aspects. Warner and Havens (1968) show that intangible goals are displaced by tangible ones and that this process frequently results in the bureaucratization of the organization. Perrow (1965) comments on this as a problem of health organizations. The real task, then, is to keep the unimportant goals from becoming more tangible than the important ones.

Here at least two tactical factors present problems. First, the higher we go in level of system aggregation, the greater are the limitations on numerical analysis; and second, if the systems analyst is an efficient design engineer, he tends to work first on those areas which are most tractable. Price (1965, p. 126) observes that "operations analysts, in manufacturing operations as well as in government service, repeatedly observe that their scientific techniques work with greater power and precision at lower levels of the administrative hierarchy. They observe that the higher the rank of the official needing answers to policy questions, the less exact and less reliable are the answers that scientific techniques can provide." Asimow (1962) points out that a design engineer should select among his alternatives for development on the basis of their cost *and* tractability. In the freer-form health environment, it is extremely tempting to select first those problems that are most tractable (and occasionally most trivial). After all, analysis takes place over time, and evidence of interim output may have considerable survival value. Thus Smalley and Freeman (1966) can write a whole book on *Hospital Industrial Engineering* which, while technically competent, fails to deal with most of the pressing problems of that environment.

The systems analyst always has to keep in mind the question of relevance. Wohlstetter (quoted in Price 1965, p. 127) suggests that in many areas we have "studies which try to determine the exact best way to perform an operation which shouldn't be performed at all." Dorfman (1965, p. 2) summarizes part of this debate in his preface to a symposium volume on *Measuring Benefits of Government Investment* as follows: "The practitioners were very skeptical and inclined to doubt whether the most important social effects of government investments could ever be appraised quantitatively by cost-benefit analysis or any other formalized method. One of them likened the problem to appraising the quality of a horse-and-rabbit stew, the rabbit being cast as the consequences that can be measured and evaluated numerically, and the horse as the amalgam of external effects, social, emotional, psychological impacts, and historical and aesthetic considerations that can be adjudged only roughly and subjectively. Since the horse was bound to dominate the flavor of the stew, meticulous evaluation of the rabbit would hardly seem worthwhile."

Professor Dorfman's summary remarks pertained to only one technique of quantitatively oriented analysis of health and other public welfare activities, but the horse-and-rabbit stew analogy can be applied to all aspects of the field of health. Dorfman, however, also presents the counterargument, that "the process of political decision can be sharpened significantly by removing as many aspects as possible from the realm of unsupported opinion and emotive rhetoric. . . . At the very least, such a process enables attention to be focused on the question of whether the unmeasurable benefits are deemed impressive enough to justify sustaining the measureable costs that they entail."

Health systems decisions are political decisions, but as Lee and McLaughlin point out in Chapter 6 of this book, even the politically oriented decision-maker can benefit from rigorous analysis of the system, its facilities, its control mechanisms, its decision rules, and its modes of operation. Such systems studies serve an educational purpose by dispelling myths and misguided intuition. They can serve that educational purpose of considerable value, even when the models used or the calculations developed are not directly applicable. For example, mathematical models of clinic waiting lines and patient and physician idleness are unlikely to tell the clinic administrator exactly how to schedule any but the largest volume facilities, but they do show that our inituitive decision rules are among the poorest choices (Fry 1964). Although the behavior of waiting lines are intuitively perceived to be linear, analysis of the mathematics shows that they are decidedly nonlinear (Morse 1965). Once a man begins to understand the behavior of waiting lines, he is in a much better position to accept or reject the way things are presently done in clinic settings even though he cannot forecast the results accurately.

A related benefit is that analysis and argument should, if properly conducted, "force the consideration of alternatives and more detailed analysis of objectives; it can direct decision-makers to think in terms of systems and so avoid the temptation to consider segments only" (Eddison 1966, p. 299). This is the optimistic view. Others would argue that it might also limit consideration primarily to the quantifiable.

With respect to these criticisms that tangible goals drive out intangible ones, and that the bias of the systems approach may be toward the trivial, one can mutter and complain; but one must choose a variant of three representative stances: forego any analysis, select the subsystems to analyze in a sequence planned to minimize these tendencies, or attempt to quantify all goals. Even Warner and Havens (1968) in their article, which emphasizes the displacement of intangible goals, argue that "More effective ways must be developed for changing organizational goals from unanalyzable abstractions into meaningful descriptions of the desired states of affairs." This is a utopian view, but it is worth moving toward. In the interim, anyone who is actively involved in systems analysis and concerned about these problems should review his strategy to make sure that the sequence of activities and evaluations will minimize these effects.

The weaknesses of systems analysis that are highlighted in the criticisms of its benefit-cost activities point out one great short-run potential payoff to the application of general systems theory. Merely by its existence and persistence it serves to counterbalance the analyst's penchant for dealing with small, closed systems. On the other hand, there must be a corresponding questioning of the view that holistic approaches are intrinsically good, that figuratively they wear white hats or imply that a hierarchy of system levels implies an ordering of importance. What we are after are decision-makers and planners who seek the most appropriate level of aggregation, make their analyses, and then check the implications, if not the reality, of their conclusions at other levels before they accept them as relevant or seek to impose them on the nation as a whole.

Basic Medical Science

Because of its reliance on logic and the scientific method, virtually all medical research can be classified as systems analysis. Certainly ecology and epidemiology are systems sciences in their breadth, complexity, and interdisciplinary approach. Almost any highly regarded effort in these fields can provide insights for students of systems analysis. The beginner can gain a comprehensive overview of mathematical approaches to medicine from N. T. J. Bailey's *The Mathematical Approach to Biology and Medicine* (1967).

Looming below the surface, however, are many new approaches based on mathematical models and on complex interactions evaluated through computer simulations. In his editorial for the August 1968 issue of *Computers and Biomedical Research*, Garfinkel notes that although the computer simulation of biomedical systems is an approach already twenty-five years old, it is not yet widely seen in biomedical articles. Several of the eight articles in that special issue involve simulation of endocrine functions and their feedback responses.

Sheldon's review of the cybernetics literature in Chapter 3 of the present volume outlines the concept of feedback mechanisms, while his Chapter 5 on a new view of the disease process applies this approach to a specific subject. That the feedback mechanism already is a basic concept of endocrinology is exemplified by Gann's (1963) fine article and by its consideration in elementary textbooks (Turner, 1966). Harvey's (1965) and Machin's (1964) review articles suggest a wider application in medicine in the future. In endocrinology the systems viewpoint does not appear to be an electromechanical analogue to cybernetic systems, but these concepts still apply directly to the chemical-neurological systems, just as Forrester (1961) has shown how they apply to the administrative environment, where human decision-makers replace the circuits and black boxes.

Other approaches frequently encountered in operations research should prove increasingly useful in medical science. In other health application areas we frequently encounter Monte Carlo simulation, probability theory, and linear programming. Harrington (1966) has reviewed their potential for environmental science and engineering. Watt (1968) has summarized the methods available for *Ecology and Resource Management.* Once the reader has progressed through the basic texts cited in the first footnote of this chapter, Watt probably ought to be his next stop. Bartlett (1961) and Kendall (1945) describe a number of ways in which mathematical models can be applied to epidemiology.[4] Waaler, Gesser, and Anderson (1962) explore the use of several models to study the spread of tuberculosis. Epidemiological and ecological studies also use classical statistics heavily to design experiments and analyze results, further illustrating the interdisciplinary nature of all health systems study.

Diagnosis

In recent years the diagnosis of disease has become the focus of investigation by decision theorists and model builders. It is a process in which a discrimination must be made and acted upon in short order; on rare occasions that discrimination may be a life or death matter. The extensive effort to develop computer programs for diagnosis has not been an attempt to outdo the physician, but rather to develop a supportive logical structure to assist him. The process that most responsible investigators envisage would be much like the military command and control system in which the available data are entered, manipulated by computers, and then presented to the human decision-maker for evaluation and action. Unfortunately some articles give the impression that the objective is for the computer to best the physician. In some cases this is poor judgment, but mostly it seems to reflect the necessity of showing that the new system is at least comparable to the old.[5]

[4] Bartlett's article concentrates on Monte Carlo simulation. The term "simulation" can be applied to many activities from scale models to play therapy. Monte Carlo simulations involve the incorporation of elements which are probabilistic, or "random" events, into the model. Thus the exact outcome of a simulation run is not reproducible, but the set (distribution) of outcomes from a series of runs should be.

[5] To those who feel ill at ease with this rapid intrusion of the computer and

Early and basic articles concerning the logic of diagnosis were prepared by Ledley and Lusted (1959) and by Warner, Toronto, *et al.* (1961). Specific computer programs have been reported for diagnosis of cardiovascular disorders, hematologic disorders, liver diseases, thyroid disorders, gynecological disorders, etc.[6] Such supportive programs can be proliferated infinitely according to well-established procedures. The next step, however, must be to develop similar computer methods for treatment selection and evaluation. Although differential diagnosis establishes the most likely patient problem or problems, there are still alternatives to be considered for treatment, and there is a need to develop more efficient and economically feasible routines for both diagnosis and treatment evaluation.

Gorry (1967) has reported an effort to develop strategies for solving diagnosis problems with less computer time. Even with efficient programs, however, systems must be developed to evaluate the consequences of information errors, treatment risk, and treatment cost. Yerushalmy (1955) and Scheff (1963) outline the error problem. Tsao (1967) offers a mathematical approach to allow revision of weightings in a Bayesian analysis for risks due to diagnostic error or treatment effects in order to achieve the best net outcome. Flagle (1965) and Lechat and Flagle (1963) also deal with the broad problem of selecting screening and therapeutic strategies on a large scale. Rubel (no date) goes even further by attempting to incorporate into the analysis the values placed on the outcome by the patient rather than by the physician. The point of evaluating the results from the correct viewpoint has been emphasized strongly by Schlaifer

---

mathematical logic into medicine, we would recommend two acculturating books: H. A. Simon (1960) *The New Science of Management Decision* and R. Schlaifer (1959) *Probability and Statistics for Business Decisions.* Schlaifer deals with the technology at an introductory level. Simon gives a penetrating analysis of human intellectual functions and their relative adaptability to computerization. He leaves a great deal of the important work to us humans, but we can expect the jurisdictional disputes to go on for some time. A hint of the outcome may be Tufts University Medical School's 1968 decision to introduce a course in statistical decision theory into its regular curriculum.

[6] Regarding cardiovascular disorders, see Bruce and Yarnall (1966), Caceres and Rilke (1961), and Toronto, 1963. Regarding hematological disorders, see Lipkin, Engle, *et al.* (1961); liver disease, Lincoln and Parker (1967); thyroid disorders, Overall and Williams (1962) and Wayne (1960); and gynecological disorders, Peterson *et al.*, 1966.

(1959). This is one aspect of the problem that has been forgotten or totally beclouded in the current rush to apply decision theory to medical decisions, but it must be faced squarely before a truly rational system can be established.

Treatment and Epidemiology

The use of a systems approach in treatment and epidemiology has already been cited. It is important to recognize, however, that systems analysis concepts can be introduced to ask not only how to treat, but whether and when. In a world of scarce resources, and especially today when health care may not be a high priority item in politically sensitive areas, such analyses are extremely important. The conceptual approach to such analyses is the same as the benefit-cost and cost-effectiveness studies at the national level. Personal goals and values are substituted entirely or in part for national welfare functions.

Very little has been written about the extension of computer-aided techniques to treatment decisions for the individual patient, involving his opportunity costs for his time, his attitude toward illness, and his utility for the resources he has to put into acquiring treatment. Tsao's matrix could be adapted to take into account individual desires, and Rubel's approach is specifically aimed at selecting the strategy for treatment best suited to the patient's, not the physician's, values. Presumably, the reason why this area has received little attention is that there is an economics of return, if not of scale, to the application of a national benefit-cost study that makes it far more attractive to the analyst. I suspect that his bias also is supported by the fact that one need develop but one value function for a nation; but to apply these techniques to the individual would require developing a function for each separate case, and one man's life may be too short for that.

Hospitals

The hospital has been the subject of many of the published systems studies. Hospitals are large, relatively self-contained health care units; they have imbedded in their several hierarchies an administrative function which has undergone a partial professionalization. As is usual, the professionalization process (Vollmer and Mills 1966) has included an attempt to establish a body of knowledge which would legitimate the hospital administrator's status.

Portions of a hospital's activities can be treated in the same manner as corresponding commercial activities. The laundry, the kitchens, the pharmacy, the maintenance shop, and the central stores all have counterparts on the outside, and they can be studied in the same fashion. Smalley and Freeman (1966) have argued that the large hospital should employ a full-time industrial engineer to improve its efficiency. Their book outlines standard industrial engineering concepts that could apply, and gives illustrative studies. In California many hospitals participate in a cooperative organization, CASH, which performs industrial engineering studies (Edgecumbe 1965). The hospital journals are full of reports of such activities.

On the other hand, hospitals and other health service organizations do offer a number of challenges that warrant special attention and that are relatively unusual, if not unique. These involve the scheduling of patients, facilities, and personnel; the utilization of specialized facilities; the evaluation of the quality of care; and information storage and retrieval. The hospital has been likened to a job shop manufacturing establishment in which many different demands are processed in small lots using a wide variety of processes. This is a good analogy, except that it is much more difficult for the hospital to gain in advance a concrete definition of demand (the patients) and to define specifically the available work stations. More importantly, the average hospital has less control over the orders it books or the delivery times that it promises. But the flow of events in the hospital can be described by small discrete distributions of events that call for probabilistic methods of analysis. Consequently, the literature of hospitals (and job shops too) emphasizes queuing theory, Monte Carlo simulation, and Markov chains. Much of the analysis centers on the outpatient clinics, maternity services, surgical suites, and patient census.[7]

[7] Articles on outpatient clinic schedules include Bailey (1952); Blanco-White and Pike (1964); Fetter and Thompson (1966); Welch and Bailey (1966); and Williams, Covert, and Steele (1967). Those on maternity services include M. S. Feldstein (1965) and Thompson, Fetter *et al.* (1963). Surgery scheduling systems are reported in Kavet (1967) and Whitson (1965). Methods pertaining to forecasting and controlling the patient census are discussed in Balintfy (1960) and (1966); Handyside and Morris (1967); Thomas (1968); and Young (1963).

If there is any one property set that these studies share, it is a large amount of data and machine output, a lack of experimental hypotheses, and a lack of interpretation of the results to yield useful rules of thumb for decision-makers. This is especially true of the currently popular simulation approach, which often seems to produce results that are readily evident to anyone who understands the properties of distributions and the behavior of queues. Moreover, simulation studies do not offer much assistance with basic problems of the hospital, such as divided responsibility (H. L. Smith 1958), haphazard evaluation of the quality of care (Donabedian 1966; Howland and McDowell 1964), and lack of a workable concept of the role the hospital should play in medical care (Horvath 1967; Long and Feldstein, 1967; Reidel and Fitzpatrick 1964).

The basic problems of medical care do not relate solely to the hospital. The hospital is but one element in the overall system. Thus the broader systems approaches, even if they lack models and quantification, are of prime importance to understanding the hospital. Fortunately, legislative activists have been willing to go ahead without studies and induce regional planning and new methods of organizing medical care (Lee and McLaughlin, Chapter 6 of this volume).

Within the hospital, personnel assignment problems, especially nursing assignments (Connor 1960, 1961; Young with Wolfe 1965a and b) are a critical area for study. The typical hospital employs two or more people per active bed, so that any increased labor efficiency is significant. Linear programming techniques are applicable to the assignment problem, but their practical application awaits suitable work classification and prediction methods. Connor, Wolfe, and Young of the Johns Hopkins group have struggled manfully with this problem, but more research and evaluation are needed.

Certainly effective allocation of hospital manpower is dependent upon our ability to predict patient workloads a few days in advance. This in turn requires good data on current caseloads and a means of predicting the status of these patients a day or two ahead. Both variables might be available once the large digital computer becomes a standard accessory of most general hospitals. The computer-based information system could easily compile aggregate figures on current and anticipated caseloads. Then it is conceivable that forecasts could be attempted of the patients' progress over a brief interval. Balintfy (1966) has observed that a patient with a relatively common diagnosis has specific chances or probabilities of making a transition from one state to another. These transition probabilities are typical inputs for Markov chain analysis to predict mathematically the status of a set of patients over time. Thomas (1968) rigorously applied Balintfy's general Markovian approach to the recovery of coronary patients. For large hospitals with groups of patients large enough and homogeneous enough to provide a statistically significant sample, this method may have real merit. Unfortunately, separate analyses will have to be made for each set of common diagnoses.

The computer-based hospital information system is one of the most talked about areas for future development. Information about the patient, medical science, and the institution all are indispensible to good care, and it represents a major cost (Gross and Jydstrup 1966). The digital computer obviously offers a future assist to the administration of care as well as to diagnosis and treatment selection. Wolfe (1967) illustrates how the computer might assist the utilization review committee by preselecting cases. The literature also is full of applications of the computer for systems modeling, patient scheduling, and patient records.[8] But the early wave of optimism may have passed. While many rosy predictions ultimately will come true, we must recognize that on a practical scale the information output of a hospital swamps the storage capacity of second-generation and third-generation computers.

Other Services

There is almost universal agreement that the hospital alone provides too limited a conceptual basis for systems analysis in medical care. Yet it is so compact and so well defined that it alone seems to attract would-be analysts, at the expense of all other organizations. Fortunately, our national policymakers have not been taken in by this attraction and they have emphasized primary patient and long-term care facilities.

[8] For examples concerning systems modeling see Flagle (1967); Le Tourneau, 1960; and Souder, Clark, *et al.*, 1964. Concerning patient scheduling see Barnett and Castleman (1967) and Rossiter and Reynolds (1963); for patient records, see Allen, Barnett and Castleman (1966); and Baruch and Barnett (1966).

A few studies of medical services independent of the hospital are worthy of mention. John Fry's work on the appointment system for general practice is especially interesting in that it suggests simple rules of behavior that do not appear to be in use today (Fry 1964). Other articles can be found dealing with long-term care facilities (Flagle 1964a), dental care (Soricelli 1966), and emergency transport of the sick and injured (Jacobs and McLaughlin 1967). But the number of good studies is quite limited.

The Community

It is at a community or multicommunity level that the outlook for effective systems analysis appears most promising, despite nagging questions about the opportunities and mechanisms for implementation at any level. For years there has been talk about regionalization, but the heightened interest of quantitatively trained economists and systems analysts will have added impact in the future. Packer (1968) and Densen, James, and Cohart (1966) offer good discussions of the rational planning process at the local level. Interesting techniques for using the graphics storage and analytical capabilities of the computer to do detailed analysis of community activities and spatial relationships are described in the literature[9], but they have been omitted here for the sake of brevity.

Regional and community planning is one area where our decision to concentrate this review on American health problems and American literature is most costly. The interested reader should not overlook the extensive efforts of foreign investigators. He should become familiar with and follow the work and publications of the Nuffield Provincial Hospitals Trust in England (Davies *et al.* 1962; McLachlin 1964, 1966). These contain good descriptive data and outline several attempts to apply operations research techniques at a practical level.

Overviews and Future Sources

A review of the literature is obsolete as soon as its author publishes it. One way to lessen this problem is to suggest to the reader how he might stay current in the future. For

[9] An overview of this field can be acquired from the following references: Drossness, Reed, and Lubin (1965); Greenes and Sidel (1967); Lubin, Drossness and Wylie (1965); Lubin, Reed, Worstell, and Drossness (1966); and Schneider (1967).

that purpose he may find it useful to rely on a series of listening posts. Several observers of the applications of operations research to the health field are worthy of continuous surveillance, for example Horvath (1966, 1967, 1968), Flagle (1960, 1962, 1964, 1967), and Thompson (Fetter and Thompson 1966; Thompson, Avant and Spiker 1960; Thompson, Fetter, *et al.* 1963). One can also count on a spate of economists to incorporate the latest advances into their writings—Fein, Klarman, the Feldsteins, and Rosenthal. For journals to follow we would recommend *Medical Care, Public Health Research, Journal of American Public Health Association, Hospitals, Management Science*, and *Inquiry*. *Hospital Administration* does not often contain technical articles, but it does occasionally publish primers and survey articles, such as Greenwood and Kendrick (1968) on simulation and Paul Feldstein (1968) on concepts of economics relevant to hospitals.

References

Ackoff, R. L., and P. Rivett
(1963), *A Manager's Guide to Operations Research.* New York: Wiley.

Affel, H. A., Jr.
(1964), "System Engineering." *International Science and Technology, 35,* 18–26.

Allen, S. I., G. O. Barnett, and P. A. Castleman
(1966), "Use of Time-Sharing General-Purpose File-Handling System in Hospital Research." *Proceedings of the IEEE, 54,* 1641–1648.

Arrow, K. J.
(1963), "Uncertainty and the Welfare Economics of Medical Care." *American Economic Review, 53,* 941–973.

Asimow, M.
(1962), *Introduction to Design.* Englewood Cliffs: Prentice-Hall.

Bailey, N. T. J.
(1952), "Studies of Queues and Appointment Systems in Hospital Outpatient Departments with Special Reference to Waiting Times." *Journal of the Royal Statistical Society* (*Series B*), *41,* 185–198.

——— (1967), *The Mathematical Approach to Biology and Medicine.* New York: Wiley.

Balintfy, J. L.
(1960), "A Stochastic Model for the Analysis and Prediction of Admissions and Discharges in Hospitals." In C. W. Churchman and M. Verhulst (eds.), *Management Sciences: Models and Techniques.* New York: Pergamon. Vol. 2, pp. 288–299.

——— (1966), "A Hospital Census Predictor Model." In Smalley and Freeman (1966).

Barnett, G. O., and P. A. Castleman
(1967), "A Time-Sharing Computer System for Patient Care Activities." *Computers and Biomedical Research, 1,* 41–51.

Bartlett, M. S.
(1961), "Monte Carlo Studies in Ecology and Epidemiology. *IV, Proceedings of the 4th Berkeley Symposium on Mathematics, Statistics and Probability*. Vol. IV, pp. 39–55.
Baruch, J. J., and G. O. Barnett
(1966), "Real-Time Shared On-Line Digital Computer Operations." *Journal of Chronic Diseases, 19,* 377–386.
Blanco-White, M. J., and M. C. Pike
(1964), "Appointment Systems in Outpatients' Clinics and the Effect of Patients' Unpunctuality," *Medical Care, 2,* 133–145.
Blumberg, M. S.
(1967), "Systems Analysis and Health Manpower: Medical Manpower—Continuing Crisis," *Journal of the American Medical Association, 201,* 856–860.
Bruce, R. A., and S. R. Yarnall
(1966), "Computer-Aided Diagnosis and Diagnosis of Cardiovascular Disorder," *Journal of Chronic Disease, 19,* 473–484.
Caceres, C. A., and A. E. Rilke
(1961), "The Digital Computer as an Aid in the Diagnosis of Cardiovascular Disease." *Transactions of the New York Academy of Science, 23* (January), 240–244.
Connor, R. J.
(1960), "A Hospital Inpatient Classication System." Doctoral dissertation, The Johns Hopkins University, Industrial Engineering Department.
———, et al.
(1961), "Effective Use of Nursing Resources: A Research Report." *Hospitals, 35* (May 1), 30–39.
Crystal, R. A., and A. W. Brewster
(1966), "Cost Benefit and Cost Effectiveness Analysis in the Health Field." *Inquiry, 3,* 3–13.
Davies, J. O. F., et al.
(1962), *Towards a Measure of Medical Care*. London: Published for the Nuffield Provincial Hospitals Trust by the Oxford University Press.
Densen, P. M., G. James, and E. Cohart
(1966), "Research Program Planning and Evaluation." *Public Health Reports, 81,* 49–56.
Donabedian, A.
(1966), "Evaluating the Quality of Medical Care." *Health Services Research I, Milbank Memorial Fund Quarterly, 44,* Part 2, 166–206.
Dorfman, R. (ed.)
(1965), *Measuring Benefits of Governmental Investments*. Washington, D.C: The Brookings Institution.
Drossness, D. L., I. M. Reed, and J. W. Lubin
(1965), "The Application of Computer Graphics to Patient Origin Study Techniques." *Public Health Reports, 80,* 33–39.
Eddison, R. T.
(1966), "Introduction and Commentary" to "Part III: Social Effects of Politics and Their Measurements." In J. R. Lawrence (ed.), *Operational Research and the Social Sciences,* London: Tavistock. Pp. 297–304.
Edgecumbe, R. H.
(1965), "The CASH Approach to Hospital Management Engineering." *Hospitals, 39* (March 16), 70–74.
Feldstein, M. S.
(1964), "Net Social Benefit Calculations and the Public Investment Decision." *Oxford Economic Papers, 16,* 114–131.

——— (1965), "Improving the Use of Hospital Maternity Beds." *Operational Research Quarterly, 16,* 65–76.

——— (1967), *Economic Analysis for Health Service Efficiency.* Amsterdam: North Holland.

Feldstein, P. J.

(1968), "Applying Economic Concepts to Hospital Care." *Hospital Administration, 13,* 68–79.

Fetter, R. B., and J. D. Thompson

(1966), "Patients' Waiting Time and Doctors' Idle Time in the Outpatient Setting." *Health Services Research, 1* (Summer), 66–90.

Flagle, C. D.

(1960), "Operations Research in a Hospital." Chapter 25 in C. D. Flagle, W. H. Huggins, and R. H. Roy (eds.), *Operations Research and Systems Engineering.* Baltimore: Johns Hopkins University Press.

——— (1962), "Operations Research in the Health Services." *Operations Research, 10,* 591–603.

——— (1964a), "Prospects for Research in Long Term Care." *The Gerontologist, 4,* 2 (Part II), 38–40.

——— (1964b), "Operations Research in Community Services." Chapter 13 in D. B. Hertz and R. T. Eddison (eds.), *Progress in Operations Research,* New York: Wiley. Vol. 2.

——— (1965), "A Decision Theoretical Comparison of Three Methods of Screening for a Single Disease." *Proceedings of the 5th Berkeley Symposium on Mathematics, Statistics and Probability.* Vol. 5, pp. 887–898.

——— (1967), "A Decade of Operations Research in Health." In F. Zwicky and A. G. Wilson, *New Methods of Thought and Procedure.* New York: Springer-Verlag. Pp. 33–45.

———, W. H. Huggins, and R. H. Roy (eds.)

(1960), *Operations Research and Systems Analysis,* Baltimore: John Hopkins University Press.

Forrester, J. W.

(1961), *Industrial Dynamics.* New York: Wiley.

Fry, J.

(1964), "Appointments in General Practice." *Operational Research Quarterly, 15,* 233–237.

Gann, D. S.

(1963), "Systems Analysis in the Study of Homeostasis with Special Reference to Cortisol Secretion." *American Journal of Surgery, 114,* 95–102.

Garfinkel, D.

(1968), "Editorial," *Computers and Biomedical Research. 2,* i.

Goode, H. H., and R. E. Machol

(1957), *System Engineering.* New York: Wiley.

Gorry, G. A.

(1967), "Problem Solving Strategies in a System for Computer-Aid Diagnosis." Cambridge: M.I.T. Sloan School Working Paper No. 267–68.

Greenes, R. A., and V. W. Sidel

(1967), "The Use of Computer Mapping in Health Research." *Health Services Research, 2,* 243–258.

Greenwood, F., and C. R. Kendrick

(1968), "Computer Technology: A Challenge for Hospital Administrators." *Hospital Administration, 13,* 62–67.

Gross, M., and R. A. Jydstrup

(1966), "Cost of Information Handling in Hospitals." *Health Services Research, 1,* 235–271.

Hall, A. D.

(1962), *A Methodology for Systems Engineering,* Princeton: Van Nostrand.

Handyside, A. J., and D. Morris
(1967), "Simulation of Emergency Bed Occupancy," *Health Services Research, 2,* 287–297.
Harrington, J. J.
(1966), "Operations Research—A Relatively New Approach to Managing Man's Environment." *New England Journal of Medicine, 275,* 1342–1350.
Harris, S. E.
(1964), *The Economics of American Medicine.* New York: Macmillan.
Harvey, N. A.
(1965), "Cybernetic Applications in Medicine." *New York State Journal of Medicine, 65,* 765–772, 871–875, 995–1002.
Horvath, W. J.
(1966), "The Systems Approach to the National Health Problem." *Management Science, 12,* B–391—392.
——— (1967), "Operations Research in Medical and Hospital Practice." In P. M. Morse and L. W. Bacons (eds.), *Operations Research for Public Systems.* Cambridge: M.I.T. Press.
——— (1968), "Organizational and Management Problems in the Delivery of Medical Care." *Management Science, 14,* B–275–279.
Howland, D., and W. McDowell
(1964), "The Measurement of Patient Care: A Conceptual Framework." *Nursing Research, 13* (Winter), 4–7.
Jacobs, A. R., and C. P. McLaughlin
(1967), "Analyzing the Role of the Helicopter in Emergency Medical Care for a Community." *Medical Care, 5,* 343–350.
Kavet, J.
(1967), "The Application of Computer Simulation Techniques to the Surgical Subsystem." Unpublished Master's Essay, Yale University School of Medicine.
Kendall, D. G.
(1945), "Mathematical Models of the Spread of Infection." In Mathematics Research Council, *Mathematics and Computer Science in Biology and Medicine,* London, pp. 213–225.
Kissick, W. L.
(1967),"Planning, Programming and Budgeting in Health." *Medical Care, V,* 201–207.
Klarman, H. E.
(1964), "Some Technical Problems in Areawide Planning for Hospital Care." *Journal of Chronic Disease, 17,* 735–747.
——— (1965a), *The Economics of Health.* New York: Columbia University Press.
——— (1965b), "Syphilis Control Programs." In Dorfman (1965), 367–410.
Lechat, M. F., and C. D. Flagle
(1963), "Statistical Decision Theory and the Selection of Diagnostic and Therapeutic Strategies in Public Health." *Proceedings of the Third International Conference on Operational Research,* Oslo.
——— (1965), "Allocation of Medical and Associated Resources to the Control of Leprosy." Chapter 9 in N.N. Barish and M. Verhulst (eds.), *Management Sciences in the Emerging Countries.* Oxford: Pergamon Press.
Ledley, R. S., and L. B. Lusted
(1959), "Reasoning Foundations of Medical Diagnosis." *Science, 130,* 9–21.
Le Tourneau, C. U.
(1960), "The Influence of Cybernetics on Hospital Development." *Hospital Management, 89,* 44–46.

Lincoln, T. L., and R. D. Parker
(1967), "Medical Diagnosis Using Bayes' Theorem." *Health Services Research, 2,* 34–45.
Lipkin, M., R. L. Engle, Jr., et al.
(1961), "Digital Computer as an Aid to Differential Diagnosis. Use in Hematological Diagnosis." *Archives of Internal Medicine, 108,* 57–72.
Long, M. F.
(1964), "Efficient Use of Hospitals." In S. J. Axelrod (ed.), *The Economics of Health and Medical Care,* Ann Arbor: University of Michigan Press.
Long, M., and P. J. Feldstein
(1967), "The Economics of Hospital Systems: Peak Loads and Regional Coordination." *American Economic Review, b–2,* 119–128.
Lubin, J. W., D. L. Drossness, and L. G. Wylie
(1965), "Highway Network Minimum Path Selection Applied to Health Facility Planning." *Public Health Reports, 80,* 771–777.
———, **I. M. Reed, G. L. Worsteli, and D. L. Drossness**
(1966), "How Distance Affects Physician Activity." *Modern Hospital, 107,* 80–82ff.
Machin, K. E.
(1964), "Feedback Theory and Its Application to Biological Systems." *Symposia on Social and Experimental Biology, 18,* 421–445.
McKean, R. N.
(1959), *Efficiency in Government through Systems Analysis.* New York: Wiley.
McLachlin, G. (ed.)
(1964), *Problems and Progress in Medical Care: Essays on Current Research.* London: Published for the Nuffield Provincial Hospitals Trust by the Oxford University Press.
——— (1966), *Problems and Progress in Medical Care: Essays on Current Research,* second series. London: Published for the Nuffield Provincial Hospitals Trust by the Oxford University Press.
Morse, P. M.
(1965), *Queues, Inventories and Maintenance.* New York: Wiley. 5th ed.
Overall, J. E., and E. M. Williams
(1962), "A Computer Procedure for Diagnosis of Thyroid Function." In K. Enslein (ed.), *Data Acquisition and Processing in Biology and Medicine.* London: Pergamon Press. Vol. 2.
Packer, A. H.
(1968), "Applying Cost-Effectiveness Concepts to the Community Health System." *ORSA Journal, 16,* 343–350.
Perrow, C.
(1965), "Hospitals: Technology, Structure and Goals." In J. G. March, *Handbook of Organizations,* Chicago: Rand-McNally. Pp. 910–966.
Peterson, O. L., et al.
(1966), "A Study of Diagnostic Performance: A Preliminary Report." *Journal of Medical Education, 41,* 797–803.
Price, D. K.
(1965), *The Scientific Estate.* Cambridge: Belknap Press of Harvard University Press.
Reidel, D. C., and T. B. Fitzpatrick
(1964), *Patterns of Patient Care.* Ann Arbor: University of Michigan Press.
Rice, D. P.
(1965), *Economic Cost of Cardiovascular Diseases and Cancer, 1962.* USPHS Health Economics Series No. 5, Washington, D.C.: Government Printing Office.

——— (1966), *Estimating the Cost of Illness,* USPHS Health Economics Series No. 6, Washington, D.C.: Government Printing Office.

Roemer, M. I., A. T. Moustafa, and C. E. Hopkins
(1968), "A Proposed Hospital Quality Index: Hospital Death Rates Adjusted for Case Severity." *Health Services Research, 3,* 96–118.

Rossiter, C. E., and J. A. Reynolds
(1963), "Automatic Monitoring of the Time Waited in Out-Patient Departments." *Medical Care, 1,* 218–225.

Rubel, R. A.
(no date), "Decision Analysis and the Treatment of a Sore Throat." Boston: Harvard University Graduate School of Business Administration. Mimeographed.

Saunders, B. S.
(1964), "Measuring Community Health Levels." *American Journal of Public Health, 54,* 1063–1070.

Scheff, T. J.
(1963), "Decision Rules, Types of Errors and Their Consequences for Medical Diagnosis." *Behavioral Science, 8,* 97–107.

Schlaifer, R.
(1959), *Probability and Statistics for Business Decisions.* New York: McGraw-Hill.

Schneider, J. B.
(1967), "Measuring the Locational Efficiency of the Urban Hospital." *Health Services Research, 2,* 154–169.

Simon, H. A.
(1960), *The New Science of Management Decision.* New York: Harper.

Smalley, H., and J. Freeman
(1966), *Hospital Industrial Engineering.* New York: Wiley.

Smith, H. L.
(1958), "Two Lines of Authority: The Hospital's Dilemma." In E. G. Jaco (ed.), *Patients, Physicians and Illness.* Glencoe: Free Press. Pp. 468–477.

Smith, W. F.
(1968), "Cost-Effectiveness and Cost-Benefit Analysis for Public Health Programs." *Public Health Reports, 83,* 899–906.

Soricelli, D. A.
(1966), "Methods of Administrative Control for the Promotion of Quality in Dental Programs." Paper presented at the 94th Annual Meeting of the American Public Health Association, San Francisco.

Souder, J. J., W. E. Clark, et al.
(1964), "Planning for Hospitals: A Systems Approach Using Computer-Aided Techniques." *Hospitals, 38* (February 16), 59–61.

Sullivan, D. F.
(1966), *Conceptual Problems in Developing an Index of Health.* Washington, D.C.: National Center for Health Statistics. Series 2.

Thomas, W. H.
(1968), "A Model for Predicting Recovery Progress of Coronary Patients." *Health Services Research, 3,* 185–213.

Thompson, J. D., O. W. Avant, and E. D. Spiker
(1960), "How Queuing Theory Works for the Hospital." *Modern Hospital, 94* (March), 75–78.

———, **R. B. Fetter, et al.**
(1963), "Predicting Requirements for Maternity Facilities." *Hospitals, 37* (February 16), 45–49 ff.

Toronto, A. F.
(1933), "Evaluation of Computer Program for Diagnosing Heart Disease." *Progress in Cardiovascular Disease, 5,* 362–377.

Tsao, R. F.
(1967), "A Second Order Exponential Model for Multidimentional dichotomous Contingency Tables, with Applications in Medical Diagnosis." IBM Cambridge (Mass.) Scientific Center Report, 320–2014.
Turner, C. D.
(1966), *General Endocrinology,* Philadelphia: Saunders. 4th ed.
Vollmer, H. M., and D. L. Mills
(1966), *Professionalization.* Englewood Cliffs: Prentice-Hall.
Waaler, H., A. Gesser, and S. Anderson
(1962), "The Use of Mathematical Models in the Study of the Epidemiology of Tuberculosis." *American Journal of Public Health, 52,* 1002–1013.
Warner, H. R., A. F. Toronto, et al.
(1961), "A Mathematical Approach to Medcal Diagnosis." *Journal of the American Medical Association, 177,* 75–81.
Warner, W. K., and A. E. Havens
(1968), "Goal Displacement and the Intangibility of Organizational Goals." *Administrative Science Quarterly, 12,* 539–555.
Watt, K. E. F.
(1968), *Ecology and Resource Management.* New York: McGraw-Hill.
Wayne, E. J.
(1960), "Clinical and Metabolic Disease in Thyroid Disease." *British Medical Journal 1,* 1–11, 78–90.
Weisbrod, B. A.
(1961), *Economics of Public Health: Measuring the Economic Impact of Diseases.* Philadelphia: University of Pennsylvania Press.
Welch, J. D.
(1964), "Appointment Systems in Hospital Outpatient Departments." *Operational Research Quarterly,* 15, 224–232.
———, and N. T. J. Bailey
(1966), "Appointment Systems in Hospital Outpatient Departments." *Lancet, 1,* 1107–1952.
Whitson, C. W.
(1965), "An Analysis of the Problems of Scheduling Surgery." *Hospital Management,* 99 (April) 58–66, and (May) 45–49.
Williams, N. J., R. P. Covert, and J. D. Steele
(1967), "Simulation Modeling of a Teaching Hospital Outpatient Clinic." *Hospital, 41* (November), 71–75.
Wiseman, J.
(1963), "Cost-Benefit Analysis and Health Service Policy." In A. T. Peacock and D. J. Robertson (eds.), *Public Expenditure: Appraisal and Control.* Edinburgh: Oliver & Boyd, 128–145.
Wolfe, H.
(1967), "Computerized Screening Device for Selecting Cases for Utilization Review." *Medical Care, 5,* 44–51.
Yerushalmy, J.
(1955), "Reliability of Chest Radiography in the Diagnosis of Pulmonary Lesions." *American Journal of Surgery, 89,* 231–240.
Young, J. P.
(1963), "A Queuing Theory Approach to the Control of Hospital Inpatient Census." (Abstract), *Operations Research, 2,* 1 (January-February).
———, with H. Wolfe
(1965a), "Staffing the Nursing Unit. Part I: Controlled Variable Staffing." *Nursing Research, 14,* 3, 236–243.
———, with H. Wolfe
(1965b), "Staffing the Nursing Unit. Part II: The Multiple Assignment Technique." *Nursing Research, 14,* 4, 299–303.

Alan Sheldon

3. Cybernetics and Medical Care

Some Recent Literature

Cybernetics has been defined as the science of control (Arbib, 1966) or, more specifically, as "the entire field of communication theory control, whether by machine or in the animal" (Maron, 1965). Of the many reviews of the field (Apter 1966, Ashby 1963, George 1965, Lange 1965, Stanley-Jones 1960, Wiener 1948, Yovits and Cameron 1960), Apter (1966) presents an excellent discussion of the history and development of cybernetic theory. This he regards as providing a conceptual framework which allows the behavior of a system to be described both in terms of the system as a whole and in terms of its dynamic processes. From cybernetic theory, generalizations may be made to any purposeful or control system, and this results in the development of dynamic models which allow the prediction of behavior.

Apter discusses the use of cybernetic models as they apply to hardware, but he also makes the point that they may lead to a resolution of the mechanism-vitalism controversy. Rapoport (1965 pp. 148 and 153) echoes this point in an essay on cybernetics and biology: ". . . the philosophical import of the cybernetic approach is the link it has established between the concept of mechanism and that of organism. . . . Cybernetics also provides the psychologist and the social scientist with a deeper understanding about the continuity between the non-human and the human world, namely that the transition between instinct and intelligence is only a quantitative one, involving the amount of conditionality in the way an organism's responses are determined by the impact of the external world and by its own internal organization."

The major area of application of cybernetics in the biological sciences is to biology itself and to the understanding of normal processes. Kment (1966) reviews this field, while Grodins (1963) provides a more comprehensive mathematical treatment. Arbib (1966) notes that much of the current work is at the microscopic level, especially in its applications to brain function (Zeman 1965, and Wiener 1965) and to the understanding of motor activity (Chase 1965), in terms of information systems and flow. This field is generally seen as exotic, so Chapman (1965) has proposed an educational program which would make it less restricted.

This preoccupation with the microscopic is emphasized by David (1964, pp. 181–182) who defines cybernetic medicine as "a medicine using cybernetic attainments for diagnosis and treatment or for simply understanding the process of illness. . . . Cybernetic workers show an unmistakable preference for those functions that seem the most obscure. . . . Work on artificial organs exerts an attraction proportionate to their degree of complexity. . . . We should remember M. Louis de Broglie's profound remark that cybernetics will not give the entire explanation because of its macroscopic approach, when all explanations must belong to the microphysical order. Undoubtedly cybernetics will not account for everything, and they cannot give anything without the assistance of the natural sciences. But their prediction for what is macroscopic, simple, explainable, throws a light on the cybernetic spirit." But the broader implications of cybernetic principles applied to large systems are indicated by Muses (1965, p. 220): "Cybernetic psychiatry—the study of psychiatry and the sociology of psychopathology from the viewpoint of systemic balances, feedback controls, and the standards that direct the interacting feedback and feedforward loops in the individual-societal network."

The major problems with cybernetic modeling are not only the potential lack of humanism suggested by David, but the usual difficulty of applying a half-digested set of new ideas to an old field without rethinking basic preconceptions. Thus when Menninger (1957) describes the ego as a control mechanism maintaining homeostasis between the Nirvana principle and the life principle, he is merely dressing up psychoanalytic constructs in new terminology. Similarly, Laqueur (1967) adds little to his discussion of family therapy by invoking systems terms.

In addition to modeling in the abstract, cybernetics theory extends to the concretization of models in the form of automata, that is, models of organisms and automation. Rappoport (1967) and LeTourneau (1960) describe the application of automation to various aspects of hospital systems, from research and laboratory procedures to housekeeping. The ultimate application of cybernetics is discussed by Siebold (1966), who proposes the development of a man-machine symbiosis which would optimize the capabilities of machines and men's minds.

Cybernetic Medicine

Probably the most relevant review of the potentialities of cybernetics in the area of medicine are three articles by Harvey (1965a, b, c). Harvey suggests that "complexity remains the central problem of the biologic sciences," and that "the essential problem in modeling is combining simplicity with validity so that neither objective is seriously compromised." He defines cybernetics as essentially "a theory of living and non-living systems that is concerned not with purely physical aspects but with their behavior." Feedback is "the process of transferring energy or information from the output of a circuit to its input, the generally accepted control mechanism in all types of self-regulating systems that use closed loop negative feedback networks." This corrective device can be seen in the regulation of many body functions.

The concept of homeostasis is central to control functions, as Horvath (1959, p. 204) notes: ". . . homeostatic mechanisms maintain within a limited range factors in the internal environment which are crucial to the life processes of an organism. The organism is stressed when its homeostatic mechanisms are unable to maintain these factors in a state of dynamic equilibrium." He criticizes the local nature of much research, which emphasizes certain stressors or situations only. He provides a definition of stress that invokes homeostatic mechanisms as relevant to psychology: "Psychological stress is a state which occurs when an individual is subjected to conditions which disturb or threaten to disturb crucial psychological variables from within their normal limits. (1) threat to continued existence. (2) threat to some aspect of personality structure or ego " (p. 208). However, homeostasis is not necessarily beneficial in the area of controlling variation in output. Vickers (1959) reminds us that conflict is by no means always stressful, although it is a function of the increasing complexity of our social organizations. This point is well taken by Katz and Kahn (1966), who find that many managers who are in high stress situations have a high capacity for handling stress as well.

There are at least two forms of feedback mechanism. In addition to the feedback of output to input, whether negative or positive, Maruyama (1968) has described what he calls mutual causal processes. These are linked systems or elements which influence each other, either simultaneously or alternately. He notes that there has been an overemphasis on the deviation-counteracting aspect of mutual causal networks, that is, on self-regulating and equilibrating systems. Examples of amplifying mutual causal systems are the evolution of living organisms, the rise of cultures, international conflicts, and all so-called vicious circles, where processes "amplify an insignificant or accidental initial kick, build up deviation and diverge from the initial condition" (p. 304). This he calls the "second cybernetics" (p. 304), and it represents morphogenesis, not morphostasis. He adds that "the law of causality is now revised to state that similar conditions may result in dissimilar products" (p. 306).

The mechanism of amplifying mutual causal processes provides an understanding of how unlike effects may result from like causes, or vice versa, since a small deviation of high probability can result in a large deviation of low probability via these networks. This is a major advance over the unicausal and unidimensional organismic theory of disease. Harvey invokes this newer model as an explanation of the placebo effect and other suggestible phenomena; a suggestion resulting in an effect may have this effect amplified by a positive feedback loop, thus rendering the original suggestion more effective. Finding psychiatry a fruitful area for the application of such concepts, he describes models explaining drug addiction and neurosis. He also feels that asthma can be explained by such a positive feedback model and describes a number of the possible loops involved.

This approach is taken up in more detail by Falliers (1966), who questions why we do not all have asthma, and also points out that control mechanisms employing negative feedback have a spontaneous tendency to go into oscillatory states. Falliers notes the importance of having several feedback loops,[1] both positive and negative, in a state of dynamic equilibrium where too little negative or too much positive feedback may disrupt the balance and result in disease. Harvey suggests that the utility of this model lies not only in providing an explanation, but in indicating a therapy: the cause of the disease may be much less important to correct than a therapy directed toward one of the elements in the loop network (Whatmore and Kohli 1968).

[1] See also Priban (1968).

In addition, Harvey feels such models have an application in the teaching of medicine.

In his second paper, Harvey (1965b) turns to a discussion of more general issues. He states that organismic disease theory is outmoded and that complex constitutional factors may amplify or nullify the effects of pathogenic agents. For those subsets of disease which are internally generated, such as the autoimmune, degenerative, neoplastic, and congenital, the classic causality model is clearly inadequate, and concepts such as sequential probability and efficient cause (that cause of several which is most easily controlled) are more germane.

Discussing the role that cybernetics may play in resolving the heredity environment conflict, Harvey claims that cybernetics is the only model which considers the various sources of information contributing to the design of an individual, namely, genetic as well as environmental, as well as random sources of information and the mechanism of deviation amplification. Cybernetic theory thus makes clearer what is meant by the interaction of heredity and environment.

Cybernetics has corrected many misconceptions about the functioning of the brain. The brain functions as a regulator and is remarkably suited to achieving the goals of survival in this environment. But since the brain is adaptive only in relation to defined goals, general adaptation is lacking. Diseases of adaptation are examples of the failure of the process of general adaptation. Much work on the brain and its functioning derives from Shannon and Weaver's (1949) work on communication and information theory. Shannon and Weaver posit a law stating that the amount of appropriate selection that the brain can accomplish is limited by the amount of information it has received and processed.

Jacobs (1964, p. 726) reiterates the modern concept of disease as "the clinical manifestation of the response in the body of secondary compensatory mechanisms when an initial system decompensates." He explains Ashby's ultrastable model, or homeostat, which is a network containing two feedback loops which respond to the environment—one directly between the environment and the systems it reacts to, and the other from the environment to these systems through a sensing element, or receptor, and a mediator. The first feedback occurs on the reaction of the organism to the environment, and the second regulates that reaction. The first varies continuously, whereas the second varies discretely and intermittently as the detector samples the environment. Jacobs states that ultrastability lies in the interrelation of two feedbacks,[2] and discusses the application of this model to a number of specific diseases.

Other authors have invoked similar models to explain particular diseases. Potter (1962) reviews biochemical studies on certain cancers and suggests that feedback deletion may be an important mechanism in explaining the functional ineffectiveness of certain enzyme mechanisms that may in part account for the production of some tumors. Iversen (1965, p. 76), commenting on this theory, defines malignancy as "a cell, or a population of cells, that does not react normally to the physiological growth-regulation mechanism." Stanley-Jones (1965) attempts to explain the disease cyclothymia, a relatively rare psychiatric condition in which mania and depression alternate, by suggesting that this is a periodic psychosis, a species of abnormal oscillation. Since all oscillations involve negative feedback, and since such negative feedback is controlled by the autonomic system, and particularly by the parasympathetic nervous system, cyclothymia may therefore be a cybernetic dysfunction of the parasympathetic system. Similar mechanisms are invoked in the control of emotion in general; changing levels from the cell through physiological to mental processes, Stanley-Jones (1966) suggests that the subject matter of psychoanalysis is nothing more than the regulation and control processes which govern the behavior of the human organism.

In addition to cybernetics providing powerful models of normal and pathological function as related to disease process, two recent authors have developed cybernetic models for the process of aging. Samis (1968) proposes that aging is the progressive loss of coordination among many independent oscillating systems. Coordination is the linking of rhythmic biological functions with oscillations of the environment at various levels of biological organization. Loss of coordination, that is, of temporal organization, results in the dissociation of cyclic processes, which then respond independently

[2] See also Cowan (1965).

to compensate for insults, in turn reducing the capacity of the organism to respond to subsequent insults.

Goldman (1968) elaborates a more detailed theory. He suggests that control systems in living organisms become increasingly subject to certain types of random errors with the passage of time. In terms of information theory, this refers to an increase in the noise level. These errors represent disorganization in the system, since perfect function implies complete organization and available choice diminishes as the system disorganizes.

Since control systems function to diagnose and correct errors, they slow the rate of disorganization. But to some extent and in some respects such disorganization is irreversible; and this loss of available choice is characteristic of the aging process. Goldman notes various types of thresholds of dynamic stability, the borders between regions of stability and of instability in dynamic, stable organisms. These unstable regions are where the internal forces of the organism tend to disorganize and produce irreversible damage. One of these thresholds is the feedback stability threshold, where negative feedback changes to positive feedback and increases error in a spiraling cycle. Although the effect of each single error involved in the aging process is insignificant, the cumulative effect of many errors occurring over time produces the degeneration known as aging. It can thus be hypothesized that aging is the result of the slowing down of homeostatic controls.

The Cybernetics of Large Systems: The Health System

In his third paper Harvey (1965c) attempts to apply cybernetic regulation theory to medical practice. Harvey presents the law of requisite variety, which he feels is central to the understanding of the functioning of large systems. This law states that in a regulator, only more variety or complexity can overcome more variety or complexity in the disturbance. The problem of regulation may be stated as follows: A disturbance threatens to drive a single variable or set of variables in a system beyond the desired range. The solution lies in forming another system or another regulator so that when the new formation is coupled with the original system, they act jointly to keep the variable or variables

(a) D → R → T → E	D prevented by R from reaching T	D = Disturbance R = Regulator
(b) D → F → E ■ ↑ R → T	R redesigns T to form F blocks D	T = System E = Variable F = Redesign of T by R
(c) D → T → E ↘ ↑ R	R receives information of D as soon as D acts on T and transmits correction to T	

Figure 1.

within certain limits. Harvey suggests three models of regulation by blocking, as shown in Figure 1. In this figure, (a) might be the model for preventive medicine, as seen in accident prevention, where the disturbance is prevented from ever reaching the system. In (b) the physician causes some alteration in the patient so that in his new state he resists the disturbance, such as in active or passive immunization. An example of (c) might be the news of an outbreak of polio reaching a public health official, who institutes a mass oral vaccination program to prevent further spread and the possibility of a major epidemic.

In feedback regulation, the regulator reacts not to the original disturbance but only to variations in the function of the system. An example would be patient monitoring during anesthesia and surgery. Such regulators, which do not strive for complete control, allow an elasticity of regulation. Trial-and-error regulation is another important type. As described in cybernetics, Markov chains, which are a mathematical method of describing the alteration of states within a system according to a matrix of transition probabilities, illustrate trial-and-error regulation. A concrete example is the use of medical therapy as the only recourse left to the physician for gathering new information about a patient.

A major question for a large system is, How much regulation is actually desirable? This might alternatively be phrased, Cannot the physician do better by lowering or redefining his standards of regulation? One problem to be faced by medical care organizations is that high degrees of control appear to discourage innovation (Rosner, 1968). If small deviations are allowed to occur, more information about the underlying disturbance reaches the physician. An instance of too great concern with regulation is the early administration of antibiotics and subsequent creation of a situation where the offending organism can no longer be identified. In many areas, particularly oncology, iatrogenic disorders become common and the regulatory device—therapy—produces more problems than the original disease.

An alternative to redefining regulatory standards is to increase the power of the regulator. An application of this is the role of the physician as general medical regulator who should have as much primary regulatory power as possible. It is absurd for him to act only as a signaling device directing the patient to the proper specialist. The use of constraint-information patterns, for example from personal histories, which assist the physician in reducing the set of diagnostic possibilities is an example of a function of a primary regulator.

From a medical view, however, perhaps the most useful aspect of the cybernetic regulation of large systems is the principle of amplification. Amplification involves the design of secondary regulators to assist the physician in his efforts. Secondary regulators include the instrumental, the chemical, the biologic, and the human varieties. Figure 2 illustrates the use of human secondary regulators. Amplification of regulation occurs where disturbances contain more variety than R_1 can control directly. Here R_1, a generalist, employs R_2, an internist who calls in R_3, a psychiatrist, for definite regulation. The secondary regulator is often the patient himself, and effective regulation of the patient can take place only if blocks to communication have been overcome.

While organization theorists (Scott 1967, Beer 1959) have increasingly turned to cybernetics, only recently have such concepts been applied to health and welfare systems. Eicker and Burgess (1968) note that such large systems interact

D

↓

T → E

↓ ↘

$R_3 \leftarrow R_2 \leftarrow R_1$

Figure 2.

in a complex fashion, and the effects of change in one often have unforeseen ramifications. Thus the reduction of mortality rates in India created a crisis in housing. They describe an evaluative research program with the goals of designing new health and welfare systems using systems analysis, modeling, computer simulation, and systems design. Such simulation models take note of fragmentation—the lack of links and feedbacks—and attempt to design the necessary interrelations for the attainment of specified system requirements.

From the broadest point of view, Attinger and Millendorfer (1968) state that the societal guidance of technology is needed to solve major problems, and that the multidisciplinary approach of systems analysis and operations research holds promise. Biological systems are more complex than technological systems, and there is the need for a focus on the behavior of overall systems as well as on the interaction among their parts. The very concept of such systems belongs to the domain of cybernetics, since such behavior is pervasive and applies at any level: molecular, organismic, and societal. According to Attinger and Millendorfer, the object of living systems is systemic stability, and the number of states a system can adopt is called its variety. Control is exercised only by the controller's having at least as high variety as the system to be controlled. Such control is spread throughout the system.

While this general argument may be convincing in theory, its realization is difficult. The authors illustrate their argument as it applies to large systems such as the linked public health, education, and economic systems. Their basic contention is that improvement in health leads to productivity, which increases inputs to the economic system, increasing health expenditures and in turn, the demands on the public health system. They develop a model of the interconnections among these systems that is useful for the analysis of subsystem interrelations, as well as for the interrelations of the system and its components with those of other countries. From this model, they derive zones of equal health development. These zones carry the implication that among countries within them there is greater communication than among countries outside them. Other behavior is also believed to be similar within zones, for example, the relation between per capita income and caloric intake. Essentially, this cybernetic model, developed for the study of complex systems, uses parametric performance analysis to allow the effects of changes of various system parameters to be obtained.

Cybernetic concepts, developed from physical systems and increasingly applied to theories of biology and disease processes, are just beginning to be used in the understanding and design of large systems. Cybernetics offers considerable promise for clarifying some of the complexities inherent in the interrelationships of social and biological events, as well as in the functioning of large systems such as the health system itself.

References

Apter, M. J.
(1966), *Cybernetics and Development.* London: Pergamon.

Arbib, M.
(1966), "A Partial Survey of Cybernetics in Eastern Europe and the Soviet Union." *Behavioral Science, 11,* 3, 193–216.

Ashby, W. R.
(1963), *Cybernetics.* New York: Wiley.

Attinger, E. O., and H. Millendorfer
(1968), "Performance Control of Biological and Social Systems." *Perspectives in Biological Medicine, 12,* 1, 103–128.

Beer, S.
(1959), *Cybernetics and Management.* New York: Wiley.

Chapman, B. L.
(1965), "The Teaching of Cybernetics." *Progress in Biocybernetics, 2,* 200–210.

Chase, R. A.
(1965), "An Information Flow Model of the Organization of Motor Activity. I. Transduction, Transmission and Central Control of Sensory Information." *Journal of Nervous and Mental Diseases, 140* (April), 239–251.

Cowan, J. D.
(1965), "The Problem of Organismic Reliability." *Progress in Brain Research, 17,* 9–63.

David, A.
(1964), "Meeting with Machines." *Progress in Biocybernetics, 1,* 181–187.

Eicker, W., and J. Burgess
(1968), "Systems Technology Applied to the Social Symbiosis of Mental Health." Presented at Systems Science and Cybernetics Conference, San Francisco.

Falliers, C. J.
(1966), "Asthma and Cybernetics (or why doesn't everyone have asthma?)." *Journal of Allergies, 38* (November), 264–267.

George, F. H.
(1965), *Cybernetics and Biology.* Edinburgh and London: Oliver and Boyd.

Goldman, S.
(1968), "Aging, Noise and Choice." *Perspectives in Biological Medicine, 12,* 1 (Autumn), 12–30.

Grodins, F. S.
(1963), *Control Theory and Biological Systems.* New York: Columbia University Press.

Harvey, N. A.
(1965a), "Cybernetic Applications in Medicine. I. Medical Model Making." *New York Journal of Medicine, 65* (March 15), 765–772.
——— (1965b), "Cybernetic Applications in Medicine. II. Clarification of Current Concepts." *New York Journal of Medicine, 65* (April 1), 871–875.
——— (1965c), "Cybernetic Applications in Medicine. III. The Physician as Regulator of a Large System." *New York Journal of Medicine, 65* (April 15), 995–1002.

Horvath, F.
(1959), "Psychological Stress: A Review of Definitions and Experimental Research." *General Systems, 4,* 203–225.

Iversen, O. H.
(1965), "Cybernetic Aspects of the Cancer Problem." *Progress in Biocybernetics, 2,* 76–110.

Jacobs, G.
(1964), "Cybernetics, Homeostasis and a Model of Disease." *Aerospace Medicine, 35* (August), 726–731.

Katz, D., and R. L. Kahn
(1966), *The Social Psychology of Organizations.* New York: Wiley.

Kment, H.
(1966), "The Problem of Biological Regulation and Its Evolution in Medical View." *General Systems, 4,* 75–83.

Lange, O.
(1965), *Wholes and Parts.* London: Pergamon.

Laqueur, H. P.
(1967), "General System Theory and Multiple Family Therapy: An Attempt at System Analysis of MFT." Read at Annual Meeting of APA, Detroit.

LeTourneau, C. U.
(1960), "The Influence of Cybernetics on Hospital Development." *Hospital Management,* No. 89 (April), 44–46.

Maron, M. E.
(1965), "On Cybernetics, Information Processing and Thinking." *Progress in Brain Research, 17,* 118–138.

Maruyama, M.
(1968), "The Second Cybernetics: Deviation Amplifying Mutual Causal Processes." In W. Buckley (ed.), *Modern Systems Research for the Behavioral Scientist.* Chicago: Aldine.

Menninger, K. A.
(1957), "Psychological Aspects of the Organism Under Stress." *General Systems, 2,* 142–172.

Muses, C. A.
(1965), "Aspects of Some Crucial Problems in Biological and Medical Cybernetics." *Progress in Biocybernetics, 2,* 211–263.

Potter, V. R.
(1962), "Enzyme Studies on the Deletion Hypothesis of Carcinogenesis." In *The Molecular Basis of Neoplasia.* Austin: University of Texas.

Priban, E.
(1968), "Models in Medicine." *Scientific Journal, 4,* 6 (June).

Rapoport, A.
(1965), "The Impact of Cybernetics on the Philosophy of Biology." *Progress in Biocybernetics,* No. 2, 141–156.
Rappoport, A. E.
(1967), "Cybernetics Enters the Hospital Lab." *Modern Hospital, 108* (April), 107–111.
Rosner, M. M.
(1968), "Administrative Controls and Innovation." *Behavioral Science, 13,* 1 (January), 36–43.
Samis, H. V., Jr.
(1968), "Aging: The Loss of Temporal Organization." *Perspectives in Biological Medicine, 12,* 1 (Autumn), 95–102.
Scott, W. G.
(1967), *Organization Theory.* Homewood, Ill.: Irwin.
Shannon, C. E., and Weaver, W.
(1949), *The Mathematical Theory of Communication.* Urbana: University of Illinois.
Siebold, G.
(1966), "Science in the World of Widening Horizons, A Triology. I. The Cyborg." *New York Journal of Medicine, 66* (September 1), 2231–2233.
Stanley-Jones, D.
(1960), *The Cybernetics of Natural Systems.* London: Pergamon.
——— (1965), "The Cybernetics of Cyclothymia." *Progress in Brain Research, 17,* 151–168.
——— (1966), "The Thermostatic Theory of Emotion: A Study in Cybernetics." *Progress in Biocybernetics, 3,* 1–20.
Vickers, G.
(1959), "The Concept of Stress in Relation to the Disorganization of Human Behavior." *General Systems, 4,* 243–247.
Whatmore, G. B., and D. A. Kohli
(1968), "Dysponesis: A Neurophysiological Factor in Functional Disorders." *Behavioral Science, 12,* 2 (March), 102.
Wiener, N.
(1948), *Cybernetics.* Cambridge: M.I.T. Press.
——— (1965), "Perspectives in Cybernetics." *Progress in Brain Research, 17,* 399–408.
Yovits, M. C., and S. Cameron
(1960), *Self-Organizing Systems.* London:Pergamon.
Zeman, J.
(1965), "Information and Psychic Activity." *Progress in Brain Research, 17,* 151–168.

James G. Miller

4. A General Systems Approach to the Patient and His Environment

This chapter presents a framework in which to view current and future health care in any American community. It raises the issue of whether training for health professionals in the future should assume that they will be allocated according to the same roles that have been customary in the past. It brings up a number of related questions but answers none of them. It is meant, rather, to create a background for discussion of how a modern university should train personnel for all the different roles that will exist in the coming American health delivery system.

Sheldon, Baker, and McLaughlin conclude in the Preface to this volume that "systems theory is antidisciplinary rather than interdisciplinary." I agree, and I accept the implications of Russell Ackoff's statement that "it is fortunate that God created the universe exactly divided into the traditional academic disciplines." The health sciences are included in these disciplines.

Among the fundamental concepts of general systems behavior theory are *space, time, matter-energy*, and *information*. These are fundamental notions of natural science which apply also to the biological and social behavioral sciences and are indeed basic to all systems, nonliving or living.

Systems science has often been equated with information science alone. This is not accurate. Both matter-energy and information processing are essential in all living systems. Interactions between matter-energy and information processing are also of great importance. The reason there has been so much talk in recent years about information processing is because information science and cybernetics are novel. Before that the primary emphasis of science was on matter-energy processing, the energetics of systems. Systems science should certainly deal with both matter-energy and information.

It is important also to make a distinction among three fundamental sorts of systems—*conceptual, concrete*, and *abstracted systems.*

1. The conceptual system is in the mind of the observer

or scientist, or it may be presented by him in the form of a prose statement or a mathematical model. In recent years, it may also be presented in the form of a computer simulation of the system. It is in some way isomorphic to a system which can be studied as a subject of science—either a concrete system or an abstracted system. And indeed, what we mean by progress in science is the improvement of conceptual systems so that they gradually become more isomorphic to concrete or abstracted systems. Then they facilitate better understanding and more accurate prediction of the latter type of systems.

2. Concrete systems are the characteristic objects of natural science. To physicists and biologists, the atom, the molecule, the cell, and the organism are all concrete systems. Nouns are ordinarily used to describe them and the structures which make them up. Verbs are commonly used to describe their processes of change over time or the relationships among their parts or components.

3. The abstracted system is more characteristically used by social scientists, including those who study personality, psychoanalysts, and large-scale social scientists with the possible exception of some organization theorists and operations researchers. Abstracted systems are in some ways the reverse of concrete systems. The nouns in discourse about them characteristically refer to roles or relationships among the components, for example, "motherhood" or "the Presidency of the United States." The verbal forms concern the individuals, groups, or other units which are in these relationships. The Parsonian theory of systems is of this sort, viewing the society fundamentally as a set of roles or relationships which individuals, groups, or organizations step into at one time or out of at another.

It is important to distinguish among these three kinds of systems, and it should be clear at all times which sort of system is under discussion. Furthermore, I believe that the most effective form of science in the long run—which will, incidentally, unite the natural and the behavioral sciences—is that science which develops conceptual systems about concrete systems rather than about abstracted systems.

There are a number of reasons for this. It is easier to think in terms wherby we employ nouns to designate structures, as we ordinarily do from childhood on. We say, "the ball bounces" or "the boy runs," using verbs for the relationships. This is more like common practice than saying, "the Presidency has been occupied by Eisenhower," or "the mother of the home is Ann." Furthermore, one can more easily use quantification, space-time coordinates, and other aspects of natural science if we deal with concrete systems. Therefore using them is the best strategy for the social sciences. Difficult as it may be in some instances to obtain clarity, it is, however, possible to construct theories of behavioral science in terms of abstracted systems. In this chapter the word "system" refers to concrete systems unless the text states otherwise.

Concrete systems may be divided into two major categories: the nonliving and the living systems. The lowest level of complexity of nonliving systems is the particle. The next higher level is the atom made up of particles, then the molecule made up of these lower levels of systems. Then there is the crystal, made up of molecules. The level of the crystalizing virus is the first sort of system which has some of the characteristics of life. It is generally agreed that the virus is not a living system, but that the cell is the most permanent, least complex form of living system.

The subset of living systems begins at the cell level and goes on to the organ, made up of cells; the organism, made up of organs; the group (like a family or a herd of cattle) made up of organisms; the organization, made up of echelons of groups; the society, made up of these lower levels of systems; and finally the supranational system, as in the European Common Market, or the Warsaw Pact powers. Above that there are mixed living and nonliving systems, like the planet, the solar system, and the galaxy. The earth is a mixed living and nonliving system. Many other planets, solar systems, and galaxies may be only nonliving systems.

Every one of these systems, nonliving or living, has two characteristics: (1) *structure*, which is patterned arrangement in three-dimensional space, and (2) *process*, which is change in three-dimensional space over time. There are two kinds of process: (1) reversible process or *function*, and (2) irreversible process or *history*.

At each level individual living systems may be classified into a number of *types*, or species. There are, for instance, various sorts of white blood cells—neutrophils, eosinophils, and basophils, as well as fibroblasts, macrophages, and many others. As to organs, there are excretory systems, vascular systems, body coverings, and so forth. At the level of the organism, there are various typologies-species such as hydra, flea, platypus, rat, cat, gorilla, man being one, male and female being another, and black, white, and yellow being still another.

In science, generalizations from one individual to another are common and respectable. They are the first order of scientific generalization. A second order is generalization across types—for instance, cats in general are more intelligent than rats, monkeys more intelligent than cats, and human beings more intelligent than monkeys. Finally, there is a third order of generalization. Generalizations across levels include more variance than generalizations among individuals—variance among types as well as variance among individuals. But they are scientifically more powerful because they identify and deal with similarities in structure or process among all the individuals of all the types of multiple levels—perhaps all—from cell to society. This is the fundamental approach of general systems behavior theory. It does not look for poetic analogy, but for quantitative similarities (or formal identities) across levels. Far from denying the importance of differences among types or individuals, it asserts them, stating that both the similarities and the differences are integral to the development of a general theory of living systems.

Another basic concept in general systems behavior theory is the *echelon*, a concept in some ways like that of the level, but one which should be clearly distinguished from it. It refers to that part of living systems which carries out the process of deciding. In certain types of living systems, some decisions are made on a centralized basis while others are made on a decentralized basis. In cells, for instance, the nucleus makes certain overall cellular decisions and through the messenger RNA and the transfer RNA these decisions are implemented. Local organelles like ribosomes manufacture enzymes which make many separate local decisions about rates of chemical reactions within the cell. Comparable echelons of decision-making can be found at other levels of living systems. Of course echelons are commonly discussed in organization theory and in applied areas like military science.

All systems in a hierarchy such as living systems constitute, naturally, have *suprasystems* (the system at the next highest level which includes this system) and *subsystems* (systems at the next lower level which make up this system). There are also *components.* It is important to make the distinction between subsystems and components. Consider the difference between what an anatomist and a physiologist mean by the word "organ." To an anatomist the word organ is what we would call a component: a local collection of matter such as a liver or kidney, with parts which are contiguous and to some extent homogeneous in character, separated from other masses. To a physiologist, on the other hand, an organ is all of the masses in the body which carry out a comparable process or processes. For example, the reticuloendothelial system eliminates foreign matter from the body fluids. This system is made up of similar cells but is dispersed throughout the organism, located in many different components. This is essentially what we mean by a subsystem.

A component may have all of a single subsystem in it, or just part of it. A component would then share that subsystem with other components. Or conversely, there may be two or more subsystems in a single component. One of the most interesting classes of problems in biology, a sort of problem commonly dealt with by operations researchers but rarely by biologists, is why certain processes are allocated to certain specific components, why some of them are centralized in a single component while others are dispersed. What does any particular such arrangement mean in terms of the efficiency of the total system? Questions of this sort can be asked also of community health delivery systems.

Another fundamental concept of general systems behavior theory is that of the *critical subsystem,* any subsystem which is essential for the continuation of life. Unless the processes of such a subsystem continue to be carried out, the system cannot endure. The processes must be carried out either by that subsystem or by some other system with which it has a parasitic or symbiotic relationship. The latter system may be a nonliving artifact. The critical subsystems are listed in Table 1 and described in the following text.

In concrete systems there are three sorts of transmissions, *inputs, internal processes,* and *outputs.* They may be either *matter-energy* or *information.* All functions in open systems (those with significant inputs and outputs across their boundaries) serve to maintain steady states of certain variables. Each of these steady states is within a specific range, and if the system variables pass beyond these ranges, some adjustment must be made or a pathological state develops which may end in the termination of the system.

Whenever there is an inadequate rate of input of any sort of matter-energy or information into a system, it is referred to as a *lack stress*. When there is too much of a given sort of matter-energy or information input, this is an *excess stress*. If the stresses continue, they disturb steady states within the system, that is, they create *strains*. Signals that come to the organism which it has learned to interpret as indications of impending stresses are *threats*.

The processes by which a system diminishes strains are called *adjustment processes*. This notion is similar to the Freudian concept of the mechanism of defense. All these adjustment processes which maintain steady states, I believe, are controlled by negative feedbacks. In affirming this position the general systems approach incorporates cybernetic theory.

There are two kinds of *power*. One is energic power, such as electrical or steam power. There is also that power whereby one system, by power in processing information, controls or influences another. To control System B, System A must send a signal over a channel in physical space from A to B. Both A and B must be coded the same way, that is, speak the same language, so that B can understand the signal. It must be clear to B in some way that A is authorized by the suprasystem to send this command signal to B. Under these circumstances, if it is a legitimate command signal and is understood, B may or may not comply. If, for example, B receives several competing command signals at the same time, B may comply with another one. Under such circumstances if B rarely complies with A's commands, then the power of A over B is low. If, on the other hand, B almost always complies with signals from A, then A's power is high.

Conflict occurs when a receiving system like B gets two or more signals from inside or outside the system which tell it to operate in competing ways. If it is to act, B must make a decision resolving this conflict.

The *purpose* of a system is determined by the way it relates to its suprasystem. It is the role or function which it carries out in the larger system of which it is a part. Its *goal*, on the other hand, is a specific end to which the system works in order to accomplish its purpose. It may be, for instance, that the purpose of a particular system is to obtain stability in the suprasystem, and that one of its variables is temporarily out of equilibrium. Perhaps it is hungry, with low blood sugar. Then its immediate goal to accomplish its overall purpose is to find food in the environment which can restore its blood sugar back into the normal steady-state range.

The goal of a heat-seeking missile is to follow the course leading to the hottest signal coming to it. This is very comparable to the goal of a dog out hunting a rabbit. Fundamentally, a negative feedback directs the behavior of the system toward its target or goal in each case.

General systems behavior theory incorporates the economic notion that for every *benefit* to a system there is a *cost*. Everything that is achieved must be paid for. The cost may be an expenditure of matter-energy or of information. (Money is one sort of information.) Fundamentally a trade-off must occur between the system and its environment, or between one system and another, just as in the open market a certain utility or scarce and desired possession or service is traded from the system to its environment or to another system in return for some other utility which the system wishes to have. Cost-benefit analyses, evaluating the efficiency of such exchanges, can be made for living systems at all levels.

Systems Analysis of the Health Care Delivery System

So much for the fundamental concepts of general systems behavior theory. We shall now turn to a community's health care delivery system as an example of one sort of living system. First of all, what levels make it up? We begin with the level of the cell. In the health care delivery system, the cells of the patient are central concerns. Are they in a normal or an abnormal state? Since all the medical workers in the health delivery system are human beings, they are subject to illness. They also have cells which must be taken into consideration. Also the states of organs of patients and of health workers in the system are fundamental considerations.

The organisms on which the health care delivery system concentrates are the patients, the workers in the health delivery system, and certain other organisms, such as animals used in laboratory tests.

At the level of the group, we are concerned with the physical and mental health of groups like the family or the office working group. The ward in the hospital, where several patients are found together with those who care for them, is also a group. It is an essential component of the health care delivery system.

The most obvious health organizations in a community are clinics and hospitals, but industrial medicine is concerned with firms, the companies in which the health program is carried out. And of course military health programs serve military organizations. Different echelons of societies are involved in states, regional, or national medical programs. And at the level of the supranational system we find the World Health Organization, which is developing more and more overall, coordinating, and decision-making functions which influence practices in communities throughout the world. In discussing health care we must deal with all these levels, moving in discourse from one of them to another. In order to prevent confusion, it is essential that we keep the levels clearly distinguished, so that the reader understands to which levels the writer is referring when he mentions the system, the subsystem, and the suprasystem.

The patient is a cameo, as it were, sticking out in three dimensions into his environment, fitting it as a cameo might fit an exactly matching intaglio. Each of them, the patient as a system and the environmental system, mirrors the other. Together they constitute the suprasystem. It is an essential of the systems approach, therefore, that we study both the system and its environment in comparable terms and dimensions.

Environmental medicine, psychiatry, social psychiatry, and epidemiology have long emphasized the importance of the environment to health. And today we are thinking increasingly of the patient in his environment, particularly the ghetto, and the patient in an overseas environment, particularly the underdeveloped nation. One reason why the biological and the social sciences have had difficulty throughout the years in becoming integrated conceptually is that they have used different sorts of dimensions in their measurements. It seems unreasonable that we should employ one set of psychological dimensions within the skin of the organism or one set of social dimensions within the boundary of the society, and another set with no known relationship to them outside in the sciences of the environment. It is essential to produce a conceptual system that will tie the inside and the outside together so that man-environment relations and that particular subset of them, man-machine relationships, can be studied in the same framework. This is becoming more and more important as the artifacts of modern technological society become more sophisticated.

The Critical Subsystems

Table 1 lists the critical subsystems whose processes must be carried out by all living systems. The definitions of each of these critical subsystems, applicable to all levels of living systems are as follows.

SUBSYSTEMS WHICH PROCESS BOTH MATTER-ENERGY AND INFORMATION *Reproducer*, the subsystem which is capable of giving rise to other systems similar to the one it is in.

Boundary, the subsystem at the perimeter of a system that holds together the components which make up the system,

Table 1. The Critical Subsystems

Matter-Energy Processing Subsystems	*Subsystems Which Process Both Matter-Energy and Information*	*Information Processing Subsystems*
	Reproducer	
	Boundary	
Ingestor		Input Transducer
		Internal Transducer
Distributor		Channel and Net
Converter		Decoder
Producer		Associator
Matter-Energy Storage		Memory
		Decider
		Encoder
Extruder	}	
		Output Transducer
Motor		
Supporter		

protects them from environmental stresses, and excludes or permits entry to various sorts of matter-energy and information.

MATTER-ENERGY PROCESSING SUBSYSTEMS *Ingestor*, the subsystem which brings matter-energy across the system boundary from the environment.

Distributor, the subsystem which carries inputs from outside the system or outputs from its subsystems around the system to each component.

Converter, the subsystem which changes certain inputs to the system into forms more useful for the special processes of that particular system.

Producer, the subsystem which forms stable associations that endure for significant periods among matter-energy inputs to the system or outputs from its converter, the materials synthesized being for growth, damage repair, or replacement of components of the system, or for providing energy for moving or constituting the system's outputs of products or information markers to its suprasystem.

Matter-energy storage, the subsystem which retains in the system, for different periods of time, deposits of various sorts of matter-energy.

Extruder, the subsystem which transmits matter-energy out of the system in the forms of products and wastes.

Motor, the subsystem which moves the system or parts of it in relation to part or all of its environment or moves components of its environment in relation to each other.

Supporter, the subsystem which maintains the proper spatial relationships among components of the system, so that they can interact without weighing each other down or crowding each other.

INFORMATION PROCESSING SUBSYSTEMS *Input transducer*, the sensory subsystem which brings markers bearing information into the system, changing them to other matter-energy forms suitable for transmission within it.

Internal transducer, the sensory subsystem which receives, from all subsystems or components within the system, markers bearing information about significant alterations in those subsystems or components, changing them to other matter-energy forms of a sort which can be transmitted within it.

Channel and net, the subsystem composed of a single route

in physical space, or multiple interconnected routes, by which markers bearing information are transmitted to all parts of the system.

Decoder, the subsystem which alters the code of information input to it through the input transducer or the internal transducer into a "private" code that can be used internally by the system.

Associator, the subsystem which carries out the first stage of the learning process, forming enduring associations among items of information in the system.

Memory, the subsystem which carries out the second stage of the learning process, storing various sorts of information in the system for different periods of time.

Decider, the executive subsystem which receives information inputs from all other subsystems and transmits to them information outputs that control the entire system.

Encoder, the subsystem which alters the code of information inputs to it from other information processing subsystems, from a "private" code used internally by the system into a "public" code which can be interpreted by other systems in its environment.

Output transducer, the subsystem which puts out markers bearing information from the system, changing markers within the system into other matter-energy forms which can be transmitted over channels in the system's environment.

Medical Health Care Delivery System

The medical health care delivery system is an abstracted system. It is frequently isolated conceptually for purposes of analysis from the total structure of community as a system (viewed as a subsystem of the American society, which is a subsystem of the international system) and the total process that goes on in the community. We can identify it as being primarily a part of two subsystems of the community, the reproducer and the producer. It is obvious why the reproducer is involved. If a living community is to survive it must be able to create new persons to replace the ones that are becoming incapable of working and are dying in it. Obviously this production is carried on in human beings through the reproductive process, which is a major concern of obstetrics, gynecology, pediatrics, epidemiology, and other specialties in the health sciences.

Why the producer is involved is more complex. It synthesizes matter and energy required for growth of the community; for repair of damage to it, including the persons who make it up; for replacement of its components; for living or nonliving products or for markers, which are matter-energy forms bearing the information which it outputs into its suprasystem; and for movement of its parts. Production of inanimate artifacts, of course, is not a function of the health care delivery system. This is a function of the manufacturing component of the community's or society's producer, which makes buildings, automobiles, airplanes, furniture, clothes, food, and so forth. The functions of the health care delivery system, on the other hand, concern growth, damage repair, replacement of components, and the production of energy for moving and other functions of the human components, the people who make up the essence of the society. It attempts to keep within normal steady-state ranges the processes in all the subsystems of the human organisms in the community, and deals with life from birth to death, from the womb to the tomb, from the sperm to the worm. The health care delivery system attempts also to alter pathological processes, by surgery, by drugs, or by artifacts like glasses or hearing aids for an individual person, fumigants and sanitary facilities for groups, or smoke repressors and sewage systems for communities.

What then are the subsystems of this health care delivery system which we have abstracted out for analysis from the total process of the community? And what are the subsystems and components of the lower-level systems which make up the overall health delivery system? The particular components of these subsystems at various levels in the health delivery system as specialized for this particular health purpose are as follows.

SUBSYSTEMS WHICH PROCESS BOTH MATTER-ENERGY AND INFORMATION *The reproducer.* The reproducer includes, at the group level, the mating dyads who are the sources of new children that add to the population as well as, at lower levels, their reproductive organs and cells. This subsystem is downwardly dispersed to the group level and below by all higher level systems, organization up to supranational system. The people who make up the health care delivery system are no different in this from those in any other organization—they are reproduced by mating dyads.

The boundary. Individual persons and groups carry out

these subsystem processes, sometimes aided by artifacts. In order to get into the health delivery subsystem the patient must somehow cross its boundary. The protective and filtering boundary functions may be carried out by the receptionist in a physician's private office, a hospital admissions officer, a medic on a battlefield, or a visiting nurse from a city health service. The boundaries of the various echelons of governmental jurisdictions ordinarily are "artificial" boundaries. That is, they are determined by information flows—such signals as "You are now entering Cambridge," rather than major changes in matter-energy structure or processes. But they do have an important effect on how health services are delivered. A resident in a large city, for instance, may not have the same access to health services as a citizen in its suburbs. Establishment of a county-wide health department can mean that city boundaries established by law have no effect on where the health services actually are delivered.

Another type of boundary process is carried out by the various professional certifying boards. State certifying bodies and national examining boards provide licenses or diplomas which indicate that certain trained personnel become members of the health delivery system and are qualified to give certain particularly specified types of services.

SUBSYSTEMS WHICH PROCESS MATTER-ENERGY *The ingestor.* The ingestor is made up of the persons who bring the matter-energy into the system to build the clinics and the hospitals and who bring into such buildings the matter-energy needed to operate them, including food, water, drugs, surgical implements, and so forth. It also includes those who recruit trainees, nurses, interns, staff doctors, social workers, and other personnel required for carrying out the system's services.

The distributor. This subsystem is composed of certain specialized personnel: drivers of ambulances, stretcher bearers, pilots of helicopters for evacuation units that bring the patient to a place where care can be provided, and local, national, and International Red Cross transportation personnel and conveyances. Largely this is a function which is upwardly dispersed to the distributors at the level of the entire society or even to supranational distributors. In general, the health delivery system or medicare system makes use of

these just as nonmedical parts of the society do. That is, they use the same roads, public transportation, and transportation personnel.

The converter. When we recognize the wide dispersion of this subsystem throughout the community and at the next higher level of the society, we see how complex the health care delivery system is. It includes the hospital cooks and dietitians, the surgeons who alter the matter-energy in patients from one form to another, other clinic and hospital management personnel who aid in these processes, pharmacists who compound drugs in the hospital and in the community, and at the society level, manufacturers of drugs and medical supplies. All of these take matter-energy raw materials that come into the health care delivery system and put it into a form that can be used specifically within the system.

The producer. This subsystem includes persons all the way from the Boy Scout who gives first aid, to the doctor who sets legs, the surgeon who transplants organs, the physiotherapist who exercises joints, the occupational therapist who oversees handicrafts, and the public health nurse who changes a dressing in a patient's home. It includes also the various members of group medical teams, and in some primitive societies, medicine men. These are the persons and groups that alter the pathological system, reconstruct it after trauma, encourage its growth, and make the changes in human tissue and in the environment which are required to produce health or to maintain it.

Matter-energy storage. This subsystem embraces the home medicine kit and whoever stores it in the bathroom closet, the pharmacy, hospital stores of various sorts—stores of foods, stores of drugs, stores of bedding, the blood bank, the eye bank, the heart bank—and outside the hospital, the firm that stocks surgical instruments, and a series of other such places where specialized sorts of matter-energy used in health care are available on demand.

The extruder. In this subsystem are the doctor who finally approves the discharge from the hospital of a well patient, the nurse who accompanies him to the front door, and unfortunately but unavoidably in some cases, the undertaker who carries a dead patient out the back door.

The motor. Artifacts that move parts of the health care

delivery system, and the people who use them to carry out such movement, are components of this subsystem. Examples are bloodmobiles, mobile chest x-ray units, movable emergency or field hospitals, and hospital ships. Also included are persons who change the environment in order to make it more healthful, such as aviators who spray swamps to kill malarial mosquitoes, engineers who channel the flow of sewage, those who filter and add chemicals to drinking water, and those who inspect meat and other food to be sure it meets health standards.

The supporter. This includes a few human beings, such as an Indian mother who carries her sick papoose on her back or a Boy Scout who helps a cripple across the street. Most of the parts of this subsystem are nonliving artifacts, however, such as a crutch, a cane, a Thomas collar, a back brace, a hip pin, or a cast. Included also are hospital beds, operating tables, and hospital and clinic buildings.

SUBSYSTEMS WHICH PROCESS INFORMATION *The input transducer.* The persons or groups who convey oral or written medical tradition which has come from Aesculapius, from Hippocrates, from five generations of Homanses at Harvard, from Osler, and from Cushing are parts of this subsystem. So are the scientists who convey new research information relevant to medical care which they have discovered, the librarians and readers of professional literature who bring to a particular community health care delivery system health information which was discovered in other places, and those who bring to the community information about where specific services are available throughout the nation or the world.

The internal transducer. Reports are received by this subsystem from components and subsystems of the entire health-care delivery system indicating where actions must be taken in order to maintain it in operation or improve its functions. Components of it include writers and editors of journals who report on the effectiveness of health systems; speakers at conventions and symposia who talk about the system and what could be done to improve it; employees of professional associations who collect health planning data; board members of hospitals and clinics who get reports on operations of their organizations; officers of the Public Health Service; medical administrators who maintain constant surveillance on the status of health facilities in the society; and pathologists who provide data on the health of patients and on the effectiveness of previous treatment by reporting to clinicians pathological findings from tissues obtained in operations or from autopsies.

The channel and net. This subsystem is comprised of those people and artifacts that convey information throughout the system, including professional personnel at hospital ward rounds, teaching conferences, doctors in consultation, persons who prepare hospital records and write articles in medical journals, and broadcasters of radio and educational television programs on health topics. In the future other electronic media will have increasing importance, including community-wide closed circuit television, regional medical program communication networks, the National Library of Medicine, biomedical communication system, and international satellites to convey health information.

As these channels and nets become more complex and more sophisticated, a problem which has been traditional in medicine will become more and more difficult. This is the question of what should be secret or privileged communication. The nature of this privilege in a doctor-patient relationship has been understood for centuries. Generally it has been respected, but now there are more opportunities for getting information. As medical electronic data banks increase in number and electronic networks spread, as they unquestionably will, however, it will be easier for all sorts of people inside and outside the health care delivery system to get access to it. Privacy, secrecy, and privilege about health matters will be threatened. We must develop regulations, ethical rules, and probably laws as to what people with what roles should have access to medical information, when permission must first be received from the patient or from his family, what sort of information should be erased from storage in data banks after what period of time, and so forth.

The decoder. The doctor who listens to the patient's basic English and interprets it into medical terminology, or conversely who changes medical jargon into basic English in telling the patient about his condition or how to take his pills at home, belongs to this subsystem, as does the interpreter who mediates between the patient who speaks only Greek and the doctor who does not. At the supranational level the decoder includes a language translator at the World Health Organization and a multilingual specialist who translates scientific or professional journals from one language to another.

The associator. Dentistry, nursing, and medical students who learn, and also clinicians, professors, scientists, and laboratory technicians, all of whom are constantly learning, make up this subsystem. Most of the learning in the health delivery system is dispersed downward to organisms. Groups and organizations also learn, however. Their learning involves discovery of new procedures, as for handling presurgical patients in a hospital, or filling prescriptions in a clinic, or following up contacts of infectious venereal patients in a community. There is also cultural learning in the community as its members gradually learn to go to an allopathic physician in preference to an osteopath.

The memory. Memories relevant to the health care delivery system are stored primarily in the brains of individual persons and in artifacts in the system. The memories include old wives' tales on how to treat illnesses in primitive societies, and in modern communities, books in a professional library, a local medical library with its librarians and their books and journals, a teletype terminal to the National Library of Medicine in Bethesda or to drug, poison, and other health information centers and data banks. Another form of storage of information is the storage of money—money being after all information concerning credit. This information can be stored in doctors' offices, hospitals, insurance companies, and banks for use by patients to pay for services or by the health delivery system to pay its costs.

The decider. This subsystem includes first of all the patient himself, when he recognizes that he is ill and goes to see a doctor, or when he consents to an operation. It also has as components the families of the patient or the courts when they give their consent to commit him to a mental hospital or give permission for autopsy; doctors' receptionists; x-ray technicians; nurses; interns; residents; internists; pathologists; undertakers; and hospital managers and board members. At higher levels there are the government agencies that approve budgets for medical insurance, the Surgeon General of the United States, the Secretary of Health, Education, and Welfare, and indeed the President himself in their roles as budget makers, policy determiners, and administrators. One of the complexities of a hospital or a community health-care system is the fact that there are so many echelons of deciders. They must be coordinated, prevented from conflicting, and, if possible, made rational.

The encoder. This subsystem is made up of such persons as the doctor or nurse who interprets the knowledge gained by the health care delivery system, explaining what is relevant to the patient, to his family, or to the community at large; hygiene teachers in schools; public health officers who prepare statements in laymen's language to inform the country of an epidemic; or educators of the public. At the highest level, the World Health Organization translator is an encoder as well as a decoder.

The output transducer. The doctor who announces the birth of a baby to the father or issues statements on the illness of the President; teachers of health subjects; professors; and continuing education personnel are output transducers. At the society level there are health attachés, the president of the American Medical Association, the president of the American Hospital Association, the Surgeon General of the United States, and at the highest level, the director of the World Health Organization. All these make announcements or convey information outside the boundaries of the health delivery system. They may do their own encoding, putting their message in a language which can be understood outside. Sometimes, of course, they read speeches that have been prepared or encoded by others.

So much for the subsystems of the health care delivery system. Many of these subsystems are assisted by artifacts like glasses, hearing aids, plastic legs, artificial kidneys, artificial heart pacemakers, hospital furniture, medical buildings in which many of these services are carried out, vehicles, communication equipment, computers, communications media, and so on.

It is incumbent upon modern society to evaluate the matter-energy or information-processing artifacts available to each one of these subsystems in order to determine to what extent these matter-energy or information-processing artifacts can aid health care delivery. If they make services faster, cheaper, or more effective, we should adopt them and incorporate them in the total system.

The systems approach to health care puts emphasis not only on the individual doctor-patient relationship—still central and valid, of course—but also on services to large populations of individual organisms, to groups, organizations, societies, and nations of the world. When you deal with such populations it is appropriate to apply operations research and to ask the sorts of questions that operations researchers do. Such questions have rarely been asked about health care delivery systems. How do we assure flexible use of manpower? Where should we build treatment centers? What kind of treatment centers should they be? For what duration should they be constructed? What various types of institutions for health care delivery should we have—or should there be only a single type? Do we want personal continuity of care or merely continuity of information flow through the whole system? Should all medical information be centrally stored? What sort of educational system should be maintained? How should new recruits be distributed to the system?

In order to answer questions of this sort, I would contend that both applied studies and basic research in systems at all levels should be carried out. This basic research should involve not only study of how variables are controlled and transmissions occur in the critical subsystems of different levels, but also development of mathematical models to answer questions about the fundamental nature of systems process with any given individual, type, or level in mind, and also across levels. Cross-level studies can not only be powerful in basic science but also in improving day-to-day applications.

Hypotheses

In order to begin to carry out such studies of formal identities across levels, it is desirable to state hypotheses. I shall list some of the hypotheses which I have selected at random out of many that I have written about in the past. They are principles about systems behavior which can be evaluated at two or more levels by empirical study. They may give us clues as to how to answer practical and important questions. Each of the hypotheses applies to processes in one of the critical subsystems that I have discussed.

1. The longer a decider exists, the more likely it is to resist change.

2. The larger a system is and the more components it has, the larger is the ratio of the amount of information transmitted between points within a system to the amount of information transmitted across its boundary.
3. The amount of information transmitted between points within a system is significantly larger than the amount transmitted across its boundary.
4. The higher the level of a system, the less are its decider's activities determined by genetic information, and the more are they determined by the information of stored experience.
5. The probability of error in or breakdown of an information channel is a direct function of the number of components in it.
6. There is always a constant systematic distortion—or better, alteration—between input and output of information in a channel or net.
7. Growing systems develop in the direction of (a) more differentiation of subsystems; (b) more decentralization of decision-making; (c) more interdependence of subsystems; (d) more elaborate adjustment processes; (e) sharper subsystems boundaries; (f) increased differential sensitivity to inputs; and (g) more elaborate and patterned outputs.
8. The more decentralized a system's deciding is, the more likely is there to be discordant information in various components of it.
9. Systems do more centralized deciding when under stress than when not under stress.
10. Up to a maximum higher than yet obtained in any living system (but less than 100 percent) the larger the percentage of all matter-energy input that a system consumes in information processing (as opposed to matter-energy processing), the more decentralization and segregation increase conflict among subsystems or components of a system, and a continually higher proportion of adjustment processes must therefore be devoted to resolving conflicts, which means they cannot be devoted to advancing goals of the system as a whole.
11. As a system matures it uses increasingly efficient codes; *e.g.*, codes which require fewer binary digits or equivalent signal per input signal. These codes approach but never actually reach the theoretical minimal number of symbols required to transmit the information. Efficient codes also

have the following characteristics: (a) Simple symbols are used for the most probable messages and more complex ones for the less probable ones. (b) The symbols are selected among them. (c) Encoding involves chunking in units of long rather than short blocks of symbols. (d) Limitations on the transmitter of the signal are taken into account; *e.g.*, if it transmits highly redundant signals, each one is not coded, but some of the redundancy is removed. (e) Limitations on the receiver are taken into account; *e.g.*, distinctions to which the receiver cannot react are neglected.

Conclusion

In the 1930's Chester Barnard and Alfred North Whitehead gave a course at Harvard Medical School. It dealt with a total approach to the study of the patient in his environment, for Whitehead and Barnard were oriented toward systems. Whitehead called them organisms or events. Today he would probably call them systems. Barnard wrote his book, *Functions of the Executive* (Cambridge: Harvard University Press, 1938) based on his experience as president of New Jersey Bell Telephone Company. It was thoughtful applied sociology, expressed in terms of early systems concepts. Barnard referred to the notion of the "unseen hand" that had originated many decades before with Adam Smith. He said something like this:

"My office is up on one of the top floors of the Rockefeller Center in New York City. One day I suddenly decided that I had to hold a business meeting in Chicago. I called the airport ticket counter. A girl was waiting to answer the phone though she had no notice that I was going to call. I made a reservation. I left my office and pushed a button. The elevator came to my floor. An operator was on it, even though he had no previous notion that I was going to signal him. I rode down with him and went out the front door of the building. I arrived there unexpectedly, but a doorman was waiting for me. He hailed a taxicab. The taxi had been waiting in a line nearby although the taxidriver had no idea that I would be coming along. I rode to the airport. There was my plane, manned by a crew that had no previous knowledge that I would be there. They flew me to Chicago, where various people aided me in getting rapidly to the office where my meeting was held."

Barnard made the point that this looks like previous planning, like an "unseen hand" operating the society. To those who are mystical or religious, this "unseen hand" can be interpreted as a divine influence. We can also analyze it objectively in systems concepts. The system components interrelate as they do because they have been so preprogrammed, so organized. Each person in his special job feels free and yet all of them are clearly interrelated in a constantly changing structure of great complexity whose nature is only beginning to become clear to us. As we extend basic research in systems science we may well obtain new understanding which can enable us to improve our health care delivery systems.

Alan Sheldon

5. Toward a General Theory of Disease and Medical Care

Organism and Environment: The Problem of Cause

In his magnificent and sadly unfinished history of medicine, Henry Sigerist (1951, 1961) presents an account of primitive medicine which stimulates important questions about current and widely accepted medical theory. In primitive society, the sick man is believed to have "transgressed a taboo, offended a spirit, or fallen victim to a fellow man's magic. He may have committed a sin quite unintentionally . . . or he may have insulted a ghost or a neighbor in a dream, an offense for which he must accept responsibility. . . . But even the most careful individual will stumble at times or will become the innocent victim of evil powers. As a result, calamities of various kinds will visit him. His cattle may die, his boat may be wrecked, his hut with all his property may burn down, or he himself may have an accident or become sick" (Sigerist 1951,[1] p. 153). For primitive man, disease, like other disasters, is brought about by his transgressions. Rather than dealing with disease in symptomatic terms, primitive medicine deals with it in causal terms. To primitive man, "the cause is the disease, and it is the cause he must diagnose. To that end he may begin, very much as we do, by interrogating the patient and his relatives or—in technical language—by taking a history of the patient. He will ask him whether he remembers having broken any taboo or having committed any other offense by which he might have incurred the wrath of the spirits. He will ask about dreams, because they might very well give a clue about what has happened. Or did the patient recently notice anything suspicious, a strange object at the entrance or in the roof of the hut that might be a fetish? Or has he enemies that could have wished to kill him through witchcraft? Did he quarrel with his son, or his wife, or his neighbor? If so, they would be suspected" (Sigerist 1951, p. 181).

With the dissolution of the extended family, modern man

[1] All citations from H. E. Sigerist, *A History of Medicine* (New York: Oxford University Press, Vol. 1, 1951, Vol. 2, 1961) reprinted with permission from the publisher.

tends to be held less accountable for the actions of his relatives, and sickness as sin is less evident. But just as poverty is often seen as retribution, however obliquely, certain categories of disease, such as alcoholism, are still held to imply a moral deficit. Whether we ignore whole groups, such as Negroes, the old, and the rural, or put them away in mental hospitals and nursing homes, or suppress them in more subtle ways, such as with tranquilizers as Szasz (1963) describes, we are less kind than tidy in our eagerness to dispose rather than to solve.

Cause as disease is very much with us. Organismic theory has provided us with a whole range of causes which we have set about eliminating. Yet the constant diminishing of these causes has left us in a position to question the validity of single-cause theories, as well as to view some of primitive medicine's presuppositions with new interest. In ancient Indian medicine, sin is something to be strived against rather than atoned for, one of the few points of difference from that of primitive societies.

Recent history has been dominated by "scientific" medicine. Observation in nature, and in the ward, has been augmented by experimentation in the laboratory. Rational treatment is now based on a profound understanding of process, in addition to simple cause and effect as in earlier eras. One of the major breakthroughs was the organismic theory of disease, which in its time was a triumph that radically advanced curative and preventative therapeutic approaches. As Dubos (1965, p. 324) points out, "There is no more spectacular phenomenon in the history of medicine than the rapidity with which the germ theory of disease became accepted by the medical profession." This theory, he continues, posits an essentially physiological view of disease "according to which disease is simply an abnormal state experienced by a given individual organism at a given time" (p. 319). But the organismic theory of disease has serious shortcomings. In contrast to "ontological" doctrines, which are concerned with the relationship between organism and environment, it assumes "that disease is a thing in itself, essentially unrelated to the patient's personality, his bodily constitution, or his mode of life" (p. 320).

The concept of disease as isolated from the ongoing activities of the individual and his relationships with his environment is derived from single-cause theories of disease and its management. Criticizing the organismic theory and its implications for medical practice, Engel (1960, p. 461) writes, "Repeatedly we find this preference for the single external cause perverting the new discoveries of medicine and biology. Such distortion indicates the peculiarities of the function of the human mind more than they reflect nature." A more phenomenological view of disease would necessarily be concerned with the relationships among disease, personality, bodily constitution, and environment, for neither organism nor environment is a static structure which can be separated, but both together are opposing directions in the total biological process. Since the distinction between organism and environment is impossible to make on a morphological basis, the determination of the relationship between them may be made by defining the concepts of organism and the environment in dynamic terms. As Angyal (1967) has suggested, this biological total process "results from the interaction of system determined (self-governed, autonomous) factors and factors which are alien to the system (governed from outside the system, heteronomous)."

On the basis of empirical study, Hinkle and Wolff (1958) state that all individuals behave as though there are periods in their lives during which their susceptibility to illness in general is increased. As the numbers of episodes of illness experienced by an individual increase, the number of his organ systems involved in disease increase. As the number of episodes of such experiences increases, he exhibits illnesses of an increasing variety of etiologies. As the number of bodily illnesses increases, the number of his emotional disturbances increases. These relationships have been obtained consistently regardless of sex, race, culture, socioeconomic background, environment, or life experiences.

These periods of illness occur at no special time of adult life and have no specific duration or magnitude. The great majority of these clusters of illness episodes occurred at times when the subjects perceived their life situations to be unsatisfying, threatening, overdemanding, and productive of conflict, and when they could make no satisfactory adaptation to these situations. In general, these situations arose out of disturbed relations with family members and important associates, threats to security and status, and restrictions and limitations which made the satisfaction of important needs and drives impossible.

Hinkle and Wolff conclude that man's perception of his life situation, which appears to be critical in terms of his reaction to his social environment, must be a function of his genetic endowment plus his acquired characteristics—his cultural and social background, the sum total of the effects of all his past life experiences, and the information available to him about the situation in which he is involved. They estimate that at least one-third of the illness episodes among their subjects were influenced in the time of their occurrence or in their course by the attempts of the individuals to adapt to events and situations. They feel that this is probably a wide underestimate and point out that while a pathogen is, by definition, a necessary condition to the appearance of a specific disease, many factors determine the other conditions necessary for the appearance of the disease.

If we accept this phenomenological view of disease, we are forced to consider the elusive line between health and disease, or in other words, the problem of the definition of normality. Normality is generally defined in statistical terms: what is normal is modal; what is abnormal is not. But statistical definitions are not reliable a priori since increasing numbers of studies, which question the time sampling of variables and measure them continuously rather than at intervals as was traditionally the case, have shown wide variations from values previously believed normal (Dubos 1965). In addition, other studies of "normal" populations have demonstrated much greater ill health than hitherto believed (Langner and Michael 1963).

Quite independent of statistical definitions, normality is also defined in social terms. As Dubos (1965,[2] pp. 250–251) states, "Any disease, or any kind of deficiency, that is very widespread in a given social group comes to be considered as the "normal" state and is consequently accepted as a matter of course within the group. . . . Surprising as it may seem to us, there was a tendency in Europe and America not so many decades ago to accept tuberculosis as an inescapable part of human fate . . . [and] witness our lack

[2] All citations from René Dubos, *Man Adapting* (New Haven: Yale University Press, 1965) reprinted with permission from the publisher.

of public concern with the slaughter on the highways." Just as the concept of disease often carries implications of moral deficiency, so do social concepts of normality. Far from being "abnormal," stress is often both normal and appropriate. The avoidance of stress, may even carry great danger:

Since man is able to eliminate or avoid many of the struggles and stresses which used to be his fate, it seems to follow that his biological mechanisms of adaptation have become useless, or at least obsolete. Paradoxically however, the very avoidance of stresses may in itself constitute a new kind of threat to health if it is carried too far, because the body and the mind are geared to responding to challenges; they lose many of their essential qualities in an environment that is so bland as to make life effortless. . . .

Human history shows, furthermore, that the same kind of knowledge that permits man to alter his environment for the purpose of minimizing effort, achieving comfort, and avoiding exposure to stress also gives him the power to change his environment and ways of life in a manner that often entails unpredictable dangers. The ability to adapt to the unforseeable threats of the future therefore remains an indispensable condition of survival and biological success (Dubos 1965, pp. 270–271).

Organismic disease theory has been preoccupied with the role of microorganisms in producing disease. Although they are primarily associated with infectious disease, they may also be implicated in certain forms of cancer. Yet, even their part in producing infectious disease is as necessary rather than sufficient cause, and their mode of action is far from understood, since many normally occurring organisms may under certain conditions become pathogenic. Of course, not all microorganisms are potentially harmful, as their very ubiquity indicates, for they may not only live in harmony with, but indeed benefit, other organisms including man, and many microorganisms classified as pathogens reside in organisms without causing overt disease (Dubos 1965, p. 111).

It is clear, in conclusion, that the type of relationship existing at any given time between hosts and their parasites is the outcome of many different factors, including past racial experience, evolutionary adaptation through genetic changes and immunologic processes, and transient disturbances in the internal and external environments. In the classical infections of exogenous origins, the determining etiological event of the disease is exposure to the infective microorganism. In endogenous microbial disease the immediate cause is the environmental factor that upsets the biological equilibrium normally existing between the host and the microbial agents (persistors).

This profound difference in etiological mechanisms suggests that the methods used in the control of microbial diseases, both prophylactically and therapeutically, must differ from place to place and vary from time to time. The methods of sanitation and vaccination designed to cope with the great epidemics of the past will not prove effective in the control of the disease states caused by microbial agents that are ubiquitous in our communities in the form of dormant infections. It is also very doubtful that the usual antimicrobial drugs can be effective against them (Dubos 1965, pp. 194–195).

But, like all single-cause theories of disease, the organismic theory offers no entirely satisfactory explanation for the persistence of a disease after the alleged causal microorganism has been either eliminated or rendered impotent. The problem then becomes one of taking a more comprehensive view of the total process involved in the relationship between health and disease. This broader view demands that many factors which were irrelevant to single-cause theories of disease become integrated into a conceptual framework that can account for such effects as those of environment, personal and social history, or genetic make-up on individual biological and social relationship to health and disease.

Like primitive medicine, contemporary medical theory is circumscribed by its theoretical precepts and their implications. Much of current medical explanation has perforce remained incomplete and vague because of its reliance on an organismic theory of disease[3] which cannot account for the conditions which are both necessary and sufficient for producing both infectious and noninfectious disease. Nor has it been able to come to a clear and comprehensive definition of disease beyond the development of two quite distinct and potentially contradictory sets of criteria—the statistical and the social—for determining normality.

[3] Some readers will no doubt accuse the author of being a member of Arthur Koestler's Society for the Flogging of Dead Horses. But even if this particular horse is moribund, the simplistic cause-effect approach to medicine is very much alive.

Diagnosis:
Interface between Medical Theory and Medical Practice

Diagnosis is an interface between the medical care system and the phenomena which it is required to correct, where medical theory becomes medical practice. At this point a person who has hitherto sought remedies elsewhere presents himself as a patient. Throughout the history of medicine, diagnosis has been, and is, a sorting-out process to determine treatment.

For primitive man there were two possibilities: in one case he knows what sin he committed and seeks not a diagnosis, but only a remedy. If, on the other hand, he "was stricken out of a blue sky and neither he nor his family have the faintest idea what causes his illness" (Sigerist 1951, p. 181), he seeks from the medical practitioner—the medicine man—a diagnosis which is arrived at by a combination of empirical and supernatural means. In ancient Egypt, the sorting process was similar to our own in form and its reliance on empirical data: "Using all his senses and taking advantage of his own experience and of that of others as related in the literature, the physician examined the patient and on the basis of his examination made a diagnosis. . . . What the physician saw, felt, smelled on the patient were pathological symptoms, changes on the surface of the body, changed secretions and excretions, abnormal functions. But at the dawn of medical history Egyptian physicians had observed that certain symptoms occur in combination as syndromes" (Sigerist 1951, p. 331).

Once freed of metaphysical considerations, diagnosis can be seen as a clearly iterative process. It is an ordering of phenomena based upon observation, with the result that underlying processes become apparent, and subsequent classifications become based upon these. Engle and Davis (1963) define diagnosis as a mental process which recognizes disease from signs, symptoms, or laboratory data. The process is judged to be both "scientific" and "artistic," as it involves intuition. Common to the various definitions they present, Engle and Davis note an increasing recognition of the importance of individual characteristics in the formulation of diagnosis, to the point where no two patients have precisely the same diagnosis.

Despite the importance of individual characteristics in determining the nature of the process of diagnosis, a major purpose of this process is the more general naming and classification of disease and symptoms. Since diagnosis is an interface between medical theory and medical practice, the systems of classification it generates will necessarily be based on the complicated relationships among structural, physiological, and biochemical schemes which are continually being modified and which constitute the science of medicine. But these structural, physiological, and biochemical schemes are not seen in isolation; they are more generally combined under an implicit or explicit theory of disease. Most contemporary medicine, as we have pointed out, can be described in terms of the organismic theory of disease, and the implications of this view for diagnosis and the classification of disease are great.

One major consequence of the accepted view of disease as an isolated phenomenon is the mode of therapy it prescribes. "The traditional attitude toward disease tends in practice to restrict what is categorized as disease to what can be understood or recognized by the physician and/or what he knows to be helped by his intervention. This attitude has plagued medicine throughout its history and still stands in the way of physicians fully appreciating disease as a natural phenomenon (Engel 1960,[4] p. 471). The general failure of the medical system to recognize this basic link between theory and practice is illustrated by recent literature proposing radically new approaches to medical care which does not question accepted categorizations of disease. Yet the basis of the categorization of disease fundamentally determines what gets done about disease, even more than the organizational structures which develop to deal with it. An example of this relationship between definition of disease and diagnosis was offered by a psychiatrist working in a cardiac unit of a large hospital. A patient with chest pains was referred there and when no physical pathology was found, the patient was dismissed. Shortly afterward, he committed suicide.[5] Describing this general problem, Engel notes that "regardless of the nature the severity of the

[4] All citations from G. L. Engel, "A Unified Concept of Health and Disease," *Perspectives in Biological Medicine,* 3 (1960), published by the University of Chicago Press, and reprinted with permission.

[5] Personal communication.

patient's complaint, the failure to discover an abnormality on physical or laboratory examination means to many physicians that there is "nothing wrong." If the patient responds to the simple reassurance, "there is nothing wrong" as some patients do, this may be regarded as demonstration, there really was nothing wrong rather than the patient had been experiencing some kind of disturbance which was alleviated by this type of reassurance" (Engel 1960, p. 471).

Just as there is currently no unified concept of disease and health, there is no logical classification scheme of diseases. Even the latest American Medical Association classification contains some disease categorized by site affected, such as pneumonia; some by the process at work, such as bronchitis; and some by the results of the unknown agent, such as hypertension. A system of classification based upon a series of internally logical sets of characteristics, if no one set suffices, is clearly desirable if not essential.

Engle and Davis (1963) provide an explanation of why such a unified classification has not yet arisen. First, not all diseases have universally accepted definitions. Second, the degree of confidence with which a physician can make a diagnosis varies considerably from disease to disease, since not all diseases are distinguishable from one another. Third, the definitions of some diseases are continually changing, with the result that there are no fixed number of diseases. Finally, the manifestations of some well-delineated diseases are also changing. Engle and Davis's analysis is clarified by their division of diagnosis into five degrees of certainty: (1) those diseases in which etiology in most instances is clear, and the disease picture does not vary much from person to person or from environment to environment; (2) those diagnoses occurring in situations where the etiology is well defined, but in which the clinical picture has greater variability from patient to patient and from environment to environment; when the etiologic agent is found the diagnosis is by definition made; (3) those diagnoses which are almost entirely descriptive since little is known concerning etiology or even the general type of reaction involved (for example, psoriasis, peptic ulcer, essential hypertension, refractory anemia); (4) those diseases where in general the type of reaction is recognized, but the specific cause is not known and individual as well as environmental variation occurs (such as benign and malignant tumors, degenerative disorders); and (5) those diseases based on constellations of signs and symptoms which comprise the disease picture; the etiology is not known, although there is often some general idea as to the type of reaction, and great variability in the clinical picture usually persists (such as in mononucleosis, lupus erythematosus, aplastic anemia).

In another paper dealing with more general issues, Engle (1963a) points out that the characteristics of the individual patient and the abstraction of the diagnosis form two poles of an axis along which the physician's mind shuttles during the process of making a diagnosis. He notes that the classification of disease is a practical aspect of the theory of universals, i.e., (1) natural recurrences, either recurring identities or similarities; and (2) principles of grouping or classifying. One particularly disturbing aspect of the classification of diseases is the bias which results from overlooking or not reporting certain cases which cannot be diagnosed because they seem to lie intermediate between two diseases.

Maruyama (1968) has described a cybernetic mechanism which may provide a further explanation for the lack of a unified concept of classification. In his description of "deviation amplifying mutual causal processes," he shows how an arbitrary or accidental initial kick may become amplified into a major deviation. It is conceivable that a number of diseases are thus caused: an initial or arbitrary event in the environment of the individual becomes amplified within him for some reason, eventually causing a pathological process. After all, much of what we have done in the past, at least in the case of certain diseases, may have been to categorize a series of irrelevancies.

Engle (1963b), in the third of this series of papers, looks to the future. He points out that the biochemical constituents of the cell, DNA and RNA, can be considered as part of the endogenous information system. All of the environmental influences playing upon the person may be considered to contain exogenous information. Interactions occur between exogenous and endogenous information. Exogenous information does not have the degree of stability of endogenous information; it is, in fact, very unstable. Environmental factors have differing abilities to penetrate the various barriers between extracorporeal and intranuclear environments, and most of the diseases recognized are primarily attributable to discrepancies in the environment. However, recent work indicates that some individuals, because of their genetic constitution, are more susceptible to damage by chemicals than are others. When a disturbance occurs in one part of the system, interactions with remote parts of the system frequently occur and often determine the nature of the disease. Which influences are the most important is obviously difficult to determine.

Engle notes that somatic mutation has been implicated in three important groups of diseases: benign and malignant tumors, diseases of the immune mechanism such as the autoimmune group, and the degenerative diseases which are closely related to age. Another author working on this subject, Burch (1963a,b,c, 1964a,b,c) has also implicated some of the psychiatric diseases in a similar process. Intriguing evidence, which suggests that a common mechanism may underly these diseases, is found in some unusual mathematical relationships. If the logarithm of the specific death rate of the disease is plotted against the logarithm of the age of death, there is a straight line relationship starting at age 30. This suggests that there is a common mechanism underlying various groups of diseases. One must assume that there is a train of events such that each insult, possibly trivial in itself, increases the tendency for other insults to develop until death supervenes. A similar process was described in the Mid-Town Manhattan study (Langner and Michael 1963), where it was found that defined stresses acted in an additive fashion to increase the risk of mental illness, this would produce a similar picture. Therefore, one might hypothesize an alternative explanation to somatic mutation: continually added insults may sequentially modify the capacity of feedback mechanisms to maintain a steady state, especially under stress. A similar process has been invoked (Goldman 1968) to account for the characteristics of aging.

Another concept which will probably play an important role in medical diagnosis in the future is that of quantitative disease as contrasted with qualitative disease. Most disease states are considered to be qualitatively different from normal states. However, if one considers just a single constituent or property of an individual man and then quantifies this constituent or property in a population of individuals, a normal distribution curve is obtained. There is therefore not only much undetected disease as defined by customary criteria, but also no clear cutoff point. This has been well described by Israel and Teeling-Smith (1967), who have termed it the iceberg effect; they thus raise an important question for preventive medicine. It may be difficult, if not impossible, to determine what level of an indicator variable (such as blood sugar) is likely to be associated with disease (such as diabetes) at some later date. One approach to this problem might be to use multiple indicators and multivariate analysis based on probability techniques (Schulberg and Sheldon 1968).

The need for a more adequate classificatory system is also highlighted by Payne (1965), who points out that in the United States only 3 percent of those infected with the tuberculosis organism develop the disease, but in underdeveloped areas 30 percent do so. He suggests that adult tuberculosis, schizophrenia, and suicide should be classified together as a category of disease related to identified social factors. "By examining social factors, especially changing factors, quantifying them as best we can, and relating them to the accompanying changes, both favorable and unfavorable, in human well-being, we may be able to classify the latter in terms of the social factors which brought them about, rather than in terms of a so-called specific agent, infectious or otherwise" (Payne 1965, p. 403). The point here is the introduction of the social-psychological element, not simply as an influence, but as an essential part of the classificatory process. We may take this argument one step further. Engel (1968) has cogently defined the "giving-up" syndrome, in which all the patients described felt powerless to influence changes in their environment and died as a result. Dubos (1965, p. 33) states: "Response patterns are so profoundly influenced by the prior conditioning of the body and of the mind that it is often useful to study the phenomena of disease by regarding them as inadequate responses of the organism to a given situation than as direct effects of a noxious agent." This points to the need for a systematic classification based upon a far more complex approach to response than that implied by such processes as "infection," one which intrinsically links the social, psychological, and physiological together. Such a classification might be supplied by a schema categorizing characteristic feedback mechanisms as discussed further below.

Physician and Patient: Changing Roles in Society and the Medical Care System

Not only are social factors important in the classification and definition of disease, but they are central in determining the nature of the care given, whether informally or formally, and the structure of the system which gives that care. In primitive society the role of the medical practitioner was largely undifferentiated. The primitive medical practitioner had a global role which included the roles of priest, lawyer, and teacher in addition to his role as physician. But just as his role was a global one, he was not the only person to perform the function ascribed to that role. Everyone was to some extent involved with treating the sick. As Field notes in Chapter 7 in this volume, "this chapter deals specifically with the problems of differentiation and specialization within the medical care system." Differentiation and specialization within the medical care system is not, however, something peculiar to the development of modern industrial society.

Ancient Egypt knew it, as Herodotus, a contemporary Greek, described: "Medicine with them is distributed in the following way: every physician is for one disease and not for several, and the whole country is full of physicians; for there are physicians of the eyes, others of the head, others of the belly and others of the obscure diseases" (quoted in Sigerist 1951, p. 319). As the Herodotus quotation implies and as Sigerist later points out, the specialization and differentiation of Egyptian medicine was not a reflection of a more sophisticated technology than existed in contemporary Greek or Indian medicine, where such specialization and differentiation were lacking. Field's paper further illustrates this by demonstrating that there are differing degrees of specialization in the medical care systems in the United States, Britain, and the Soviet Union while the level of medical technology in these three countries is relatively similar. Thus, while some specialization and differentiation develops in response to the demands of new technologies, as often it is a reflection of societal structural characteristics and social values, and we can posit that differentiation and specialization do not necessarily reflect a greater capacity to manage disease. The relevance of social values in determining the nature of differentiation is illustrated by the fact that psychiatric care systems in Britain and the United States are structured in very different ways although the same medical knowledge is the basis for both systems (Sheldon and Hooper 1966).

The highly specialized and differentiated system that the patient in the United States today faces when he presents himself for medical care tends to see only a single technological challenge; if the salient features of his disease remain obscure, he is considered a problem and is often shuffled to another part of the system, or expelled from it as though "nothing is wrong." In criticism of this view of the physician-patient relationship as it exists today, Engel presents his view of the importance of the relationship as a psychobiological process:

Is it possible that between physician and patient there transpire certain psychobiological processes (basic to human relations in general) which have significance for the capacity of the individual to maintain health or to develop disease? . . . Now at long last it is becoming clear that a scientific basis exists for what has so far been known mainly through the insights of poets and of the intuitive, sensitive man of all ages. It is the demonstration that certain aspects, processes and characteristics of the external environment are assimilated by the developing organism, internalized, so to speak, and come to constitute conditions for living, if not for life itself. The terms object and object relationship are convenient ones to designate such phenomena . . . object relationship refers to the nature and variety of interactions between a person and his environment which account for someone or something becoming an object . . . in respect to the essentialness of objects, this has long existed as an experiment of nature. I refer here to the phenomenon of grief, the familiar reaction to the loss of an object, be it a loved person, a valued possession, one's job, one's home or one's country elsewhere . . . suffice it to say that grief is a natural response to a loss . . . that it is ubiquitous and in most instances self-limited, not requiring the ministrations of the physician for recovery, can be said as well of a host of other disease states . . . object loss is essentially some change in the fit between this internalized environment and the real external environment . . . the powerful therapeutic influence of the physician . . . is none other than the effect of a substitute object . . . that which is humane is humane because it takes into account the scientific basis underlying human relationship . . . when the humane is based on maudlin sentimentality, . . . on sympathy rather than empathy, then it may as often deviate from as coincide with a sound scientific basis, in which event it may have for certain patients disastrous consequences.[6]

The Need for an Alternative Model

Primitive man looked for cause when he found himself ailing, much as modern man does. He found cause in the association of events, proximal in time. He interpreted these events in the context of his era, and his interpretations were colored by mythical thinking. However, in attempting to unravel the complexity of disease, he often arrived at explanations, such as the Indian and the Greek, which we are only recently beginning to see again as meaningful. The validity of these explanations is affirmed by the success of many of his therapies. Some of these, empirically determined and rationally used, are still found in the modern armamentarium. Some we scoff at or find horrifying. Others, especially those aimed at the tenuous relationship between man and his fellows, are reflected in our current preoccupation with psychosomatic medicine, processes of psychotherapy, and the concept of the "ombudsman" in law, medicine, and other areas.

The inadequacies of our generally held concepts of medical theory, normality, diagnosis, disease classification, and patient-physician relationships[7] illustrate the need for an approach to disease which focuses not upon a classification of the agents appearing to cause disease or of the disease sites, but upon the nature and characteristics of the various factors involved in the total biological and social process of health and disease.

An adequate model for medicine must explain not only rational and scientific fact, but the hitherto inexplicable placebo effect, a patient's unexpected improvement, voodoo, and the giving-up syndrome (Engel 1968). Of particular importance is the relationship of the patient to the medical care system in its nontechnical aspects. The importance of

[6] G. L. Engel, "The Nature of Disease and the Care of the Patient," *Rhode Island Medical Journal, 45* (1962), p. 250, reprinted with permission.

[7] Mechanic (1968) provides an extensive discussion of many of these issues.

such social process in determining the response of patients to the care system and to therapy is described by a number of authors (Egbert, Battit, Welch, and Bartlett, 1964, Menzies 1960, Turner 1963). The participation of the patient (and his family) in the treatment process and even in decision-making is probably also important. It may be that this can best be understood in the light of cross-system feedback linkages at a social-psychological level, rather than at a psychosomatic level. In other words, a general model might best be able to link conceptually the multitude of complex factors involved in the process which we have traditionally dichotomized into health and disease.

The general model outlined in this chapter is based on concepts taken from general systems theory and from cybernetics. The major contribution of cybernetic theory to these formulations is the concept of feedback. The medical care system is regarded as a feedback device which takes certain outputs from society (and from other systems within it) defined by the medical care system as deviating from certain norms, and treats them as inputs into its own system.

The definition of the inputs as deviance is a priori since the medical care system is not called into action unless there is some problem or the likelihood of a problem, as in preventive medicine. The criteria by which these inputs are selected are not clear, however. Some are social, some are purely individual and subjective, and some are empirically objective. The growing awareness of the range of subjective and social criteria which determine who will come in contact with the medical care system has led to the development of such concepts as "illness behavior." Even if no obvious infection or malfunction is apparent, a complaint may be defined as valid and referred to a different part of the system. The concept of the medical care system as a feedback device offers the possibility of better understanding of how the system itself works, and of its weaknesses as well as its relationship to other systems in society. It does all this without altering the basic conceptual scheme or invoking a completely different set of theoretical propositions.

Notes on a Model

THE SYSTEM: ILLNESS AS DEVIANCE As a feedback mechanism developed by society to maintain deviation within certain limits and along specified dimensions, the medical care

(1) Intraindividual	
(a) Intracellular	Physiological
(b) Cellular	
(c) Organ	
(d) Organ system	
(2) Individual (organism)	
(a) Linked organ systems, the body	Physiological
(b) Internal processes	Psychological
(c) Interpersonal processes	Sociological
	and
(3) Group-Family	
(4) Organizations	
(5) Society	
	Psychological
(6) Culture	

system operates to correct deviation at a number of levels. These levels are listed in the above diagram.

Essentially this list is one of increasing size (number) and complexity, based upon intrinsic links among parts. Such concepts as ecosystem and biosphere essentially describe the complex links between different systems, at one or more of the levels proposed here.

The state, or structure and function, of a particular medical care system is therefore determined by the state of each and all of these levels at any point in time: by current theories of disease, by the current state of knowledge of interpersonal transactions in that culture, by the typical structure and function of groups and families in that culture, by the typical structure and function of organizations in that culture, and by the societal and cultural institutions and values prevalent in that culture at that time.

Deviation at any level of the total system will be brought to the attention of the medical care system if it assumes those characteristics regarded as valid input for the medical care system. Other characteristics will be referred as inputs to other social systems, for example, the penal system. Deviation at any level may go through a sequence of uncorrected stages before such characteristics are assumed. These may include sequences within levels and across levels. In general such cross-level sequences will occur, both up and down.

At each level natural and artificial (man-made) feedback loops operate. These are usually multiple and nesting, for this ensures redundancy. In addition, different loops may operate with differing speeds. The loops have general characteristics which resemble each other and unique characteristics appropriate to the level at which they are operating. Thus deviation in the pH of the blood is corrected by overbreathing, in the behavior of an adolescent by parental pressure, in a dissident sect by societal sanctions. But at each level a salient variable at that level is counteracted by negative feedback.

The distinction must also be made between organism and environment. Organism, for the present purposes, may be defined as the system of focus. The environment is then the total milieu in which the system operates, including subsystems and suprasystems, but not restricted to these. At a cellular level, the cell is the organism; and the body and external world, the environment. Feedback loops operate within the system of focus (O-O) within the environment (E-E) and directionally across the O-E boundary (organism influencing environment and vice versa). Normally each level of the total system is maintained in a state of stability by such feedback loops. This state may not be stationary by any means (Wolf 1963), as implied by the general systems concept of homeostasis. It may oscillate (regular periodicity) between various values of the variables relevant to the operation of that level, or it may vacillate (irregular shift) (Thompson 1963). These oscillations may be of shorter or longer periodicity, or the range of oscillation may shift as occurs in growth.

Since each level consists of a complex set of interrelationships of processes, with linked inputs and outputs, usually directional, deviation in an input or output may occur at any point in these processes. Much disease (as usually defined) is attributed to the results of a deviation in input across the O-E boundary which has not been corrected, or where correction is too little or too late. Uncorrected deviation in input at any stage of the processes becomes deviation in output of that stage and hence deviation in input to the next linked stage forming a sequence of events. Since levels are linked, such a sequence occurs not only within levels, but across levels. Disease, in the usual sense, is then defined as progression along a sequence to a point where output (from at least one level) becomes recognized and acceptable (i.e. legitimate) input to the medical care system, even though the link may not be made. It is clear from this definition that it is subjective: the medical care system decides what is disease. An objective definition is logically impossible, since inadequately corrected deviations are always occurring, at least over short time intervals.

INPUTS, LINKAGE, FEEDBACK, AND PROBLEM SOLUTION Essentially disease seems to result either from the action of an input to the organism from the environment (sometimes the input itself, sometimes a change in it, sometimes a reaction to it), or from a failure of an internal process. It is interesting that most inputs considered in disease theory either mediate their effects through end-organs which effectively translate the input into the body's terms (the eye, ear, etc.), or by direct action on body surfaces, whether internal or external. But the possible direct effects upon internal processes of a number of important environmental factors which might have the property of ignoring boundary surfaces have largely been neglected. The effects of magnetic fields and ions, for example (Haley and Snider 1964), are fascinating. It is quite possible that climatic variation is mediated through its effect upon the quantity and quality of ions in the environment, and in this way exerts an influence on physiological, psychological, and social phenomena (Lucero *et al.*, 1965; 1963) (a rationale for astrology). ESP may be an instance of direct transmission to and reception by the central nervous system of inputs (of an undefined nature) not mediated by end-organs.

Inputs may be defined in terms of number, strength, quality, and time relationships. They may be single or multiple; repeated or continuous; clear or ambiguous; simultaneous or sequential. If simultaneous, they may be conflicting, additive, or independent. If sequential, they may be linked (i.e. sensitizing) or not linked. A relevant deviation in input may be not just an increase, but a decrease or cessation. Thus, executives may typically undergo a midlife crisis when relieved of the tensions of their earlier years (Taguiri).

When does a change in input require correction? For not all changes carry negative connotations, and many carry clearly positive ones. This is not simply a function of the characteristics of the input, but of the field. By *field* we mean the total setting or context in which the input is operating (i.e., system plus environment). This includes the environment from which it is coming and the target process to which it is an input. A change in input will be recognized as relevant only if it is distinguishable from its background, and if the state of the organism is such that it can make this distinction. The phase through which the organism is going will determine in part the relevant field against which deviations in input are measured, and also the available responses. It will clearly only be responded to if appropriate feedback mechanisms are linked to it. The sequence of events involved is that the input deviation must be recognized, labeled, and categorized, a choice of feedback loop made, and then action initiated.

Deviations clearly occur in relation to a departure either from an absolute level which may be important to the organism, or from an operationally functional level, desired or expected. Many variables, while continuously varying, do not operate in a similar fashion throughout the range of variation. Therefore an input, while quantitatively different from a previous value, may become significant and relevant only when a certain value is reached, or it may radically change its nature or relationships at this different level. These step functions are important, not only because they imply the need for new methods of measurement, but also for a new conceptual approach. Disease prevention, based on early diagnosis, especially through multiple screening techniques, cannot be successful if the key variable in a sequence has changed in a fashion irreversible by current therapeutic measures. It is quite possible that the detectable presence of a tumor (which is responsive to radiation) may lag behind undetectable and unalterable changes in cell growth control. If this occurs, only a marginal gain in life expectancy due to early diagnosis can be predicted.

Linkage is essentially the connecting of two or more points in a process by a feedback loop, or of two or more feedback loops into a complete circuit. It is therefore a crucial concept, since it is the means by which inputs and outputs are

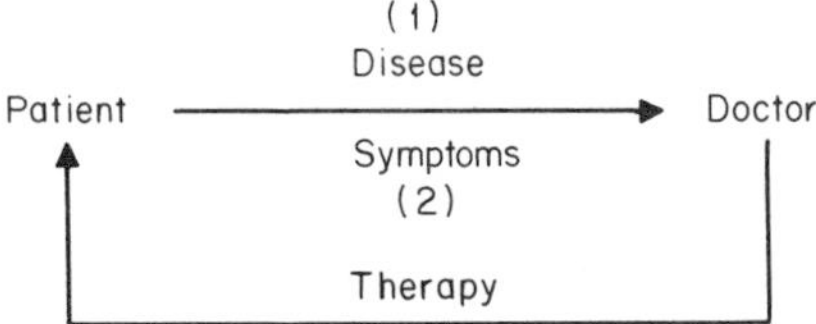

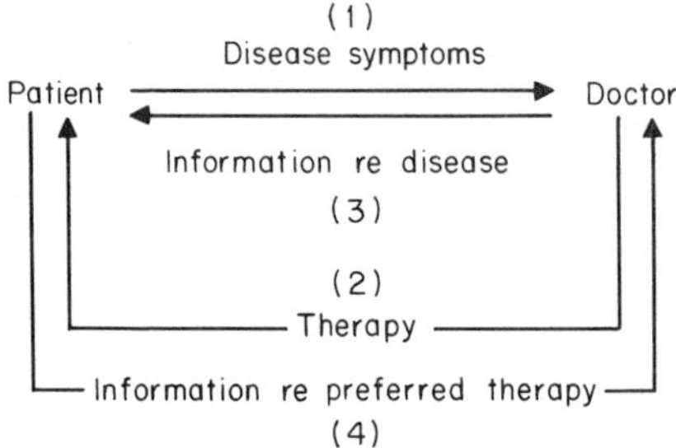

modified. Feedback not linked to an input can obviously not influence it. The number and extent of linkages between points and between feedback loops will determine the availability and rapidity of response. The diagnostic-therapeutic process may be diagrammed as shown in the first diagram. A more effective system, because it has more links, is illustrated by the second diagram. Here the patient is informed in a way he can understand, and is a part of the decision process affecting him.

As has been stated before, feedback loops, whether positive or negative, are linked within (horizontal) and across (vertical) levels. They may be single, or multiple and nesting and thus increasing redundancy and stability of control (Priban 1968). The operation of the loop will be determined by the set of the organism. The state of the feedback loop may be in a normal, hypernormal, hyponormal, or abnormal state. The significance of this is profound. If hypernormal, the feedback response will be overactive; if hyponormal, inadequate. If abnormal, the feedback response may be irrelevant, or it may set off a sequence of responses which become unlinked from the initial input and assume a life of their own.[8]

[8] Richards (1963) has derived Greek terms for somewhat similar states. He defines "homeostasis, a concept which describes admirably the phys-

The importance of positive feedback is highlighted by Phillips (1968). Phillips points out that the excess of poor mental health in lower socioeconomic classes is not necessarily attributable to an excess of stress but is due to a relative lack of positive experiences. Clearly, deviations in input are not all of a kind that require reduction. Many stimulate the organism through positive feedback to develop to new levels of capacity. Maruyama (1968) distinguishes the

---

iological mechanisms that protect and restore the normal, does not encompass the destructive forces of disease." This definition, of course, neglects the potentially maladaptive aspects of homeostasis. He proposes the following additional terms: "the excess response, hyperexis; the deficient response, ellepsis, the inappropriate response, akairia." He adds a further term, "the concept of disorder" and calls it "taraxis." He describes hyperexis as "apparent attempts at homeostasis that either destroy by sheer excess or that, in correcting one defect, involve the organism in other complications caused directly by this same homeostatic effort." The first part of his definition corresponds to the hypernormal state, but in the second, he appears to confuse the nature of the response with its effects. "One of the most striking in the former sub-group is the hyperimmune response, in one or another of its many forms. These range from the abrupt reactions of anaphylaxis—shock, hyperexia, sudden death from these or other fulminating biochemical causes—through the sub-acute, vascular and tissue alterations of the 'arteritis' and 'collagen' diseases to the established chronic conditions associated with fixed fibrosis." In attributing fibrosis to this mechanism, he again seems to confuse consequence with mechanism. Fibrosis is essentially a partial solution to a problem.

Ellepsis "signifies, in general, feebleness, failure and inadequacy." He suggests it as a general term for ineffectual, deficient biological reactions—homeostasis that never arrived or never even began. In his list (nutritional deficiency, starvation, paralysis, atrophy, atresia, ischemia, necrosis, hypofunction, endocrine failure, impotence, senility, idiocy, amentia), he includes for the most part conditions not strictly attributable to this term. Feedback may fail because damped by other forces or because a loop is absent. Perhaps a number of the conditions he describes fall in the latter category. Much of the importance of psychological and sociological inputs may lie in their capacity to depress or enhance normal feedback functions, or to convert deviation reduction into amplification.

Richards defines akairia as: "an ill-timed, inopportune, misguided, inappropriate, blundering reaction of whatever kind." Again he gives examples: "The inappropriately increased reabsorption of sodium and water in heart failure leading to congestion and edema; or salt losses or potassium-losing nephritis. Another is the intimal thickening and the medial hypertrophy of the blood vessels in hypertension, further aggravating the effects of the already existing vaso-constrictor state." These again appear to be the consequences of partial or inadequate problem solution and not defects of the mechanism itself. It is probably more useful to restrict the term "abnormal-feedback state" to the case where feedback mechanisms become themselves destructive to the organism. Examples would include the auto-immune diseases and at least certain forms of cancer. Richards' concept of "taraxis," defined as a stirring up, confounding, throwing into disorder again appears to describe the consequences of inadequate problem solving.

single, simple, positive, or negative feedback loops from those he terms mutual causal deviation-amplifying processes, in which an initial kick, or deviation, possibly accidental and trivial, may become amplified to a significant level.

What determines the choice of alternative feedback loops is not clear. One aspect of growth and development might be defined as an increase in the range, availability, and selectivity of use of feedback loops. It would seem that as the organism develops, in its life, or in evolutionary perspective, it increasingly differentiates feedback devices to deal with specific situations. As complexity increases, different issues are dealt with by specific and differentiated subsystems. This is found to be as true of societal or organizational development as of biology (Lawrence and Lorsch 1967). A recurring problem, however, is the imperative need to provide a reintegration of these differentiated processes, and this is one of the problems facing the medical care system of today, which is so specialized that patients become compartmented.

The fact that there is some discretion in the choice of feedback loops available to deal with a particular situation, whether of a physiological level, has been mentioned. Individuals seem to be characterized by the unique choices they make in this regard, both physiologically and psychologically. Some people find personal problems easy to handle, while others find it difficult even to modify their effects. Some people somatize tension while others release it by engaging in action. This suggests the importance of developing a typology of characteristic styles of feedback handling at the various levels of the total system.

Feedback loops exist within the environment, within the organism, and across the boundary between the two, and feedback devices appear to operate either upon the deviant input or upon its effects. In the instance of a potential infection, organisms existing in the environment are normally kept within certain levels by the pressures of the ecosystem. Thus organisms may be able to exist only within a very limited range of variation in temperature, or may compete with each other for essential nutrients. Linked systems clearly act as feedback devices for each other. Upon the entry of an organism into the body, its potential effects will be determined largely by the state of the body at that point in time. Whether it exists as a harmless intestinal flora, or becomes an arbiter of disease, depends in part upon the characteristics of the organism, and in part upon the state of resistance of the individual. Low resistance implies a low level of operation of the two systems of feedback initially brought into action. One system, including the white blood cells, attacks the input itself—the invading organism; and the second system, including the antigen antibody system, deals with its effects, circulating toxins. Two artificial cross-boundary feedback loops have been developed to deal with the early sequence by man to assist in his capacity to withstand infection. Man may influence the environment by public health measures; the environment may influence him by providing vaccination.

A deviant input essentially presents a problem to be solved. The solution may be total or partial. Total solution would be the eradication of an invading toxic organism, or the repair of a damaged organ. A partial solution is a solution for only a subsystem but not the total system. In coarctation of the aorta, lowered blood pressure in the legs is counteracted by feedback mechanisms which raise the general blood pressure. While solving the problem for the leg region, the rise in systemic blood pressure to "abnormal" levels provides eventual consequences for the total body which can be catastrophic. This is clearly a partial solution. Partial solutions may be optimal or suboptimal.

A problem may be solved, that is, the cause may be eliminated, or if this is not possible, then the results may be counteracted, for example by a reduction in tension or in mediating factors or in effects. At a physiological level, organisms producing toxins may not be eradicated, but the effects of the toxins may be counteracted by antitoxins. At a psychological level, some individuals may not be able to eliminate the origins of stress but may be able to counteract their effects in producing tension by taking, for example, tranquilizers. Or the problem may not be solved at all.

There are in general five ways in which a problem may be handled. There may be a *resolution* of the problem, with its complete eradication. At certain levels *extrusion* is a mechanism used. An individual presenting a problem to a group, if this problem cannot be resolved, may well be excluded.

Extrusion may include altering the frame of reference so that a deviant input is now regarded as valid, that is, rationalization. A third mechanism is *isolation*. The problem may not be able to be resolved, but its effects can be eliminated by isolating it within the system. Fibrosis very often performs this function for chronic infections, isolating an infective focus. A fourth mechanism is *compensation*, where the cause cannot be isolated but the effects can be counterbalanced. Lastly, a problem may be responded to by the organism reequilibrating at a new level of operation, or by developing new devices to counteract it. Essentially, this is *internal change*, which may include growth. Brehm and Cohen (1962, p. 224) note some of the characteristics of problem solution at a psychological level: "When homeostatic drives are aroused, the organism engages in behavior that is directed to reducing drive tension. Cognitive dissonance is included among a psychologist's inventory of drives or motives because its arousal always elicits behavior that is (successfully or unsuccessfully) directed to returning the organism to a state in which the drive is at a lower level of arousal or is entirely quiescent.

Each of these mechanisms has its analogies at all the levels of the total system.

SEQUENCE AND CONSEQUENCE When a deviation in input is uncorrected or inadequately corrected, its effect on the target process will cause consequences which are ramified through linked processes. Clearly this sequence of events is affected by linked systems from other levels, for example psychological processes mediated through the action of the nervous system and of hormones. As a sequence progresses, increasingly higher levels are affected. Thus a pathogenic organism, if not eradicated initially by white cells, starts to cause both structural and functional damage by virtue of its direct action or that of its toxins.

This structural and functional damage then requires correction. At this point either the process itself, or the feedback processes called into play to correct it, may link to a higher level and cause signs or symptoms. A sign is essentially evidence of alteration in function or in structure which is apparent to the observer although not necessarily to the subject. (Of course it is quite possible that the individual may detect signs within himself.) A symptom is the effects of structural or functional damage which become apparent subjectively to the individual, indicating a shift up from the cellular or organ level to the psychological level. The patient may attempt initially to provide his own remedies. These may range from unconscious readjustments, through the taking of various forms of action including going to bed, or talking about the way he feels. Eventually failure to resolve this stage of the sequence results in the development of disease behavior, as the potential patient now presents himself to the medical care system. If the salient characteristics of his deviance mesh with those of that segment of the medical care system to which he first presents himself, he is defined as a patient and appropriate action will be taken to diagnose the cause of his deviance and remedy it. If the salient characteristics do not mesh, he may then either be referred elsewhere or informed that his complaints are not legitimate.

If enough people develop behavioral deviance (an input at the societal level), it then becomes a social problem requiring social definition and response. This accounts for the development of public health measures. An interesting aspect of this stage of the process is that deviance previously defined as falling within the province of one system, may shift to another, if it is large enough and if the first system fails to correct it. Thus until recently drug addiction was defined as being within the province of the medical care system in Great Britain, but as the problem grew sharply and previously successful measures failed, it has increasingly been shifted over to the legal system for solution. At present alcoholism in the United States is a borderline case in which considerable efforts are being made to shift it from the legal system to the medical care system.

The successful reversal of the sequence leads to resolution of deviance and eradication of its effects. However, the sequence may be stopped only part way, or the effects of the feedback processes may be such that, while the initial deviance has been eradicated, the effects remain. Damage may be irreversible, or processes may no longer be able to be stopped. Chronic disease, for example, is essentially one of two types. The first type is where there has been a partial solution of deviation with inevitable consequences and functional adaptation to these has led to some disability. (Disability is defined as the loss of potential capacity to function as a result of uncorrected consequences.) The second form of chronic disease is where the initial deviation is not eliminable, but where there is functional adaptation to it without necessary progression. In addition to the inevitable consequences of progression, where usually the resistance mechanisms have failed and the disease overwhelms the individual, it is also possible for deviations or their effects to be recurrent. Here there is either periodic recurrence of deviation, or the deviation, once adapted to, periodically becomes active by virtue of repeated depressions of the feedback processes.

It is clear that social and psychological factors may influence any part of this chain of events. Their effects on the more molecular processes are mediated through a long set of links. In most work to date such associations have been investigated at a statistical level rather than at a conceptual level. The problem with the statistical approach is that most studies using it focus upon disease defined only if it is seen by a physician, i.e., arriving at a clinic or hospital. However, there have obviously been a number of sequential processes occurring before the patient arrives at a physician, if indeed he ever does. Since psychological and social processes influence these early stages, to look only at their associations with an end stage is highly suspect. It is quite possible that such psychological and social processes influence different steps in the sequence in quite different fashions. Thus their overall effect, when looked at in a later stage in the sequence, may seem to be only negligible. Stressful situations, for example, may depress initial resistance mechanisms so that people are more liable to become ill, but also may make them more sensitive to the signs and symptoms resulting from this process, so that they are more likely to go to a physician at an earlier stage than otherwise. Therefore, stressed people may have more disease than unstressed people, but they may seek medical care at an earlier, and potentially more curable, stage of their illness.

A clearer specification and categorization of the influence of such factors at different stages in the sequence and at the various levels, remains for future work. It should be noted, however, that the presentation of signs and symptoms to the medical care system is by no means simply a function of their intensity or duration. Very often symptoms will be managed by the individual for long periods and presented only when his psychological state for some reason changes and he finds he can no longer tolerate them. Polak (1967) reports that most admissions to mental hospitals, in a series that he followed, were the results of an interpersonal crisis involving the family and not a function of the severity of the clinical state of the patient. Admission to hospital, whether for physical or psychiatric reasons, is not usually sufficiently accounted for by the presence of a physical or psychiatric condition alone. Rejection by the family for a variety of reasons is often the precipitating factor.

Levels within the total system from the point of view of their influence upon one another have been discussed, and the way in which the sequence of events operates through the levels has been described. It is worth noting that disease, again used in its customary sense, is regarded as residing within the individual. While occasionally the term has been applied to higher levels of society, the former has been its general meaning. Within the conceptual framework presented here, any given level in society may suffer the effects of deviations in input which are uncorrected and produce consequences; that is, they may become "diseased." Equally a given level may possess unique strengths or vulnerabilities compared with another level, and so deviations in inputs which have little effect at one level may have a considerable effect at another. In a report in *Science Journal* (1968) it was noted that colonies of bees were far more susceptible to radiation than individual bees. Cages of bees subjected to expectedly lethal neuron radiation showed surprising resistance, while hives of bees subjected to a lower level of radiation were effectively exterminated. This finding was attributed to the initial effect of radiation on the eggs and on the young individuals, and a mechanism was postulated of an irreversible effect upon the adults, possibly mediated through the complex hormonal communication systems known to exist in bee colonies. There is little work of a similar kind within the social organization of humans, although Peachey (1963) has noted that "apparently unrelated episodes of illness in a family will, over a period of time, form repetitive patterns characteristic for a given family." She found four basic patterns: constant illness, regular periodicity, clustering and simultaneity, and certain special types of interaction. This suggests a group level style of handling stress.

Disease at a particular level is a very different phenomenon from that of the influence of one level upon another. Family therapy is an instance of a technology developed for the resolution of group level problems. Hare and Shaw (1965a, b) also note that certain families are particularly susceptible to disease, but it is not clear from their work whether this is an instance of group level disease, or the influence of the group upon the susceptibility of individuals.

A considerable amount of work has been done on this latter problem. Ehrenwald (1963) has identified four major patterns of interaction among members of families which have implications for the climate within the family. Meissner (1966) has suggested that such family interactions influence the emotional adjustment of the individual, the functioning of whom depends upon his degree of involvement and upon the balance of emotional forces within the family system. Disorganization in the family system can precipitate emotional crisis in the deeply involved member who lacks sufficient resources to maintain adequate functioning on all levels. He suggests that the crucial variable may be disruption or disequilibrium within the family rather than stress, and suggests that such disequilibrium may or may not be reflected in individual stress. If so, it is mediated through autonomic and hormonal regulatory systems via the limbic system. Therefore, he is postulating both family level processes of maladjustment as well as ways in which the family can influence the individual through vertical feedback.

Chen and Cobb (1960) have reviewed the literature on the effects of family structure in relation to health and disease. They point out that parental deprivation, whether due to death, separation, sickness, neglect, or rejection, is highly dependent upon the age at which it occurs. Such deprivation has been related to the incidence or prevalence of a variety of physical diseases. Birth order also appears to have some relationship to the incidence of at least some diseases.

Cancer: A Case Example

The purpose of this example is to attempt to outline, with no pretense of expertise, the complexity of possible factors influencing the etiology, course, and therapy of a specific disease. The field of cancer research and therapy, like so many others, is bedeviled by the fact that highly competent experts focus upon a small segment of the problem without necessarily having knowledge or interest in the whole picture.

Cancer is an abnormality of cell growth. Normal growth appears to be a function both of the mass effect of adjacent cells upon each other (horizontal feedback) as well as of central influences (vertical feedback). The cancer process seems to result from an interplay of influences which either cause abnormal growth or depress the normal controlling mechanisms. As Crile (1963) points out, malignant change is most apt to occur in clones of cells removed from all the restraints that the host normally imposes upon cellular growth. Lack of cohesiveness is one of the distinguishing features of cancer cells, perhaps signifying that the growth of the cell is no longer under the control of its neighboring cells.

Lipschutz (1967) provides an excellent account of current concepts of cancer, at least at the time of his essay. He points out that hormones influence the growth of tumors which subsequently may become autonomous and produce metastases. He emphasizes the importance of the naturally occurring rhythmic changes in hormone levels due to natural sexual periodicities (e.g., the menstrual cycle). An alteration of this "law of sexual rhythm" causing tumor responses in the body might be due not only to primary failure of the ovary or pituitary, but also to a failure in the working of the hitherto unknown mechanism responsible for cyclic ovarian function. This mechanism may be related to the hypothalamus.

Tumor production may be a function of both threshold level of estrogen and the timing of estrogen production. Thus, tumor responses in the ovary and elsewhere in the body may occur when steroid homeostasis is shaken by transgression of the law of sexual rhythm. This may be due either to primary failure of the ovary in producing steroids and secondary failure of the hypophysis, or to increased inactivity of steroids in the liver. The maintenance of steroid homeostasis is paramount for the nontumorous condition of the body. Steroid homeostasis is normally subject to transitory changes for the sake of reproduction, but the body succeeds in maintaining and readjusting its levels. For example, normal body defenses against tumor production are relaxed during one part of the menstrual cycle in order to allow the foreign body—the fetus—to grow. Lipschutz is describing the fact that cyclic variations in the levels of important controlling substances within the body may provide periodic opportunities for the failure of feedback mechanisms if an insult should occur. These periodic variations in hormone levels are controlled by the neurohypophysial axis, which in turn is influenced by psychological processes. This gives a pathway by which psychological and social phenomena may be translated into neurohormonal effects which will influence the potential susceptibility of the body to cancer processes.

Maruyama (1968) provides a possible explanation of the effect of such insults as viruses in producing cancer, a possibility Lipschutz by no means dismisses. The concept of deviation amplifying mutual causal processes suggests that a tumor, if it is related to a virus, may not be the direct result of the action of the virus upon cells, but the end result of the initial kick provided by the virus infection which under certain circumstances may become amplified by abnormal positive feedback mechanisms into a disruption of cellular growth control mechanisms. Why then should this disruption of feedback occur? Lipschutz suggests that one possibility is a periodic cyclic depression or alteration of feedback (or linked systems) so that normally deviation-diminishing links become deviation amplifying. Other writers including Potter (1962) have suggested that at least some cancers may be related to the absence of certain negative feedback loops within biochemical processes. This is the so-called feedback deletion hypothesis. The implication of this conceptualization is that the initial apparent cause is seen as irrelevant and therefore therapy should not be directed at the removal of such apparent causes. The problem is then the abnormal process set off by the original cause, and therapy should be aimed at interrupting this process rather than at the cause or at the consequences—abnormal cells. It would seem quite likely that current therapies aimed at destroying abnormal cells will not have any effect on abnormal feedback loops which may cause the abnormal cells.

Earlier it was suggested that an abnormal feedback mechanism may become itself pathogenic for the body, and that this would provide a possible explanation for the development of certain kinds of cancer or autoimmune disease. If a total response mechanism, a set of feedback loops, becomes pathogenic, then various forms of cancer (of the white cells, for example) should be associated with other abnormalities of the particular feedback system affected. Recent work on Hodgkin's disease (Hersh and Oppenheim, 1965) shows that it is accompanied by other types of immune abnormalities and points in this direction.

The possibility that abnormalities of specific feedback systems, such as the hormonal control and feedback system, may be implicated in cancer is confirmed by Marmorston (1966). He shows that hormone-metabolite assays indicate characteristic and statistically significant alterations in hormone excretion patterns which serve to separate cancer groups from well persons and from persons with benign conditions at the same site. Weiner and coauthors (1966) confirm these findings for different types of cancer. The interrelationship of neurohormonal changes with cancer is pointed to by Jonas (1966) who notes that there are a number of abnormalities of the nervous system found in association with various types of tumor, which appear to precede the onset of the tumor and cannot be attributed to wasting. Very often these manifestations are the first evidence of the self-destructive process. Kavetsky (Kavetsky, Turkevich, and Balitsky 1966) presents evidence of the substantial effect of the higher divisions of the central nervous system on the functional state of connective tissue during the development of tumors.

Turning to some of the evidence for the effects of psychological and social factors on cancer, LeShan (1959) reviews the literature on this subject and points out that the psychosomatic concept is a very old one. In medieval times the theory of body tumors was a complex and sophisticated theory of mind-body interaction frequently invoked to account for the development of cancer. The notion that severe emotional trauma contributed markedly to the onset and subsequent course of cancer was not regarded as radical. This approach began to be unfashionable during the early part of this century and reports in the literature were few.

LeShan (1959) himself found that the major factors

seemingly involved included the loss of important social relationships and confirmed this hypothesis with the evidence that age-adjusted cancer mortality rates were highest among the widowed, next among the divorced, and lowest among the single groups. He reports that cancer patients characteristically avoided emotional involvement and tended to withdraw under stress and have difficulty in social relationships. When patients were divided into those with rapidly progressive disease and those with slow progress, the fast-growing cases had more defensiveness, higher anxiety, and less capacity to reduce tension through motor discharge. LeShan has noted marked changes in psychological stress frequently are associated with sudden changes in the growth rate of tumors. He found that such patients typically were incapable of making adjustments or finding solutions to inner problems, and he felt that psychotherapy did seem to slow the process of the neoplasm. Brown (1966), while noting that the evidence for the significance of psychological inputs for cancer was strong, was very critical of most of the studies. His criticisms ranged from poor selection of patients to failure to use control groups to lack of clarity in specifying interviewing techniques. Greene (1966), while agreeing that his patients (leukemia and lymphoma cases) were also dealing with loss or difficult situations, felt that the issue was less that of the situation than of the lack of resources or capacity on the part of the patient. Kissen (1966) also confirms for lung-cancer patients that they had difficulties in emotional expression.

In sum, it seems clear that cancer patients can generally be typified as having some difficulties in the resolution of problems and probably as having life histories which led to their incapacities in this regard. There have been enough control studies to suggest that this finding is not spurious, although since studies inevitably are based on patients who have already developed cancer, it is difficult to tell from literature whether the findings described are a function of reaction to the presence of cancer, or a cause of it.

One provocative study by Schmale and Iker (1966) shows that when women referred for Papanicolaou smears were interviewed psychologically, the authors were able to predict, before the presence of cancer was known, those women who had developed cancer as demonstrated subsequently by the smear. These women were characterized by feelings of despair. However, while the findings of the study are hardly challengeable, various conclusions are possible since the psychological state of these individuals may have been determined by circulating substances deriving either from the cancer or from the disturbed physiological state producing it, rather than being contributory to the disease.

The conclusion would seem to be that cancer is the complex result of a multitude of factors. An abnormal input, in conjunction with cyclic variation in resistance, possibly coinciding with, caused, or exacerbated by psychological stress, may produce unusual adaptive responses which become amplified into disruption of cellular growth and finally tumor production. There is some evidence that reduction of the original cause will no longer have any effect once the process is initiated, and that a different set of factors may well influence the later course of the disease compared with the earlier onset phase. There is also evidence that the psychosocial setting is important in the course of cancer and may well be a determinant of the success of therapy. This influence may be at a physiological level, or may directly affect whether the patient is offered or rejects treatment. It is interesting that there are patients who initially do well on each new therapy they are offered, but who become resistant to it after a time. While this may be explicable on a purely physiological basis, it may also be a reflection of psychological style translated into physiology.

The implications of this general approach for cancer research and therapy are considerable, and not simply for physiological etiology, for there is a great need for learning more about psychosocial influences on the etiology and course of cancer and the effects of treatment.

Conclusions: Implications for the Medical Care System

Describing the problem facing medicine, Dubos (1965, p. 405) writes:

> . . . there is rapidly emerging in the modern world a set of problems that could properly be called social medicine, not to be confused with the very different concept designated as socialized medicine. The health field is no longer the monopoly of the medical profession; it requires the services of all sorts of other skills. This collaboration will become increasingly urgent as the

community demands that steps be taken, not only to treat its diseases, but also to protect its health.

The danger in this inescapable trend is that the medical profession may be progressively edged out of many social aspects of medicine. While persons trained in the physical and social sciences, from engineers to general biologists and lawyers, play an essential role in the total medical picture of our society, it is usually difficult for them to comprehend all the complexities and subtleties of health and disease problems. Limited points of view are likely to generate oversimplified formulae of action, unless technical knowledge is supplemented by broad medical philosophy and guidance. Seen in this light, the care of the social body as a whole presents new and exciting challenges to the medical profession; it constitutes an enlargement of its calling.

The medical care system must develop a new role in society as well as innovate new internal structures and processes which take account of the concepts elaborated in this essay. The pressures upon medicine do not simply come from the need for new conceptualizations, but from society itself. More and more there is dissatisfaction with the quality of medical care, the segments of the population to which it is directed, and its capacity to respond to societal needs. While integrated and comprehensive programs are proposed, they lack as yet any significant degree of comprehensiveness or integration.

Current medical care systems are essentially reactive. When presented with a problem—a sick patient—the system responds and attempts to do something about it. There is very little consistent planning for patients by using past experience to predict likely alternative futures and developing contingent plans against their eventuality. Planning essentially has two functions. The first function is to replace the uncertainty created in the patient and his family by the impact of disease through a delineated plan which gives some structure to the future. Much has been written about the destructive effects of the imposed role of patient when familiar associations and the predictable future are withdrawn. Therefore, anything the medical care system can do to reduce uncertainty is likely to facilitate recovery. Maruyama (1967) has graphically described the impact on him of an unexpected and prolonged minor illness in a setting with which he was unfamiliar.

A second aspect of planning, essential within the framework proposed here, lies in its capacity to integrate action. This integration is essential both in place and time. Thus, rather than responsive to a critical event, action should take into account the total picture in time and space and act accordingly. It may well be that a hospital admission, precipitated by family decompensation, is the worst possible way of handling a patient in the long term, even though it is an answer to his immediate needs. A variety of disciplines come to bear upon the system of the patient and his family, and each may have relevant information and significant parts to play. Rather than priority being given to any one facet, an integrated system must be devised so that all this information is available and used and each member of the team has a valued part to play. As long as the medical care system is at the mercy of a series of hierarchical professional bodies, each of which is seeking only its own professional advancement and power, it is difficult to see how this can come about. Such goals are human and inevitable, but as long as the individual professional finds his loyalties divided between those of his profession and those of the team working around the patient, decisions will not always be optimal.

Current approaches to the problems of disease categorization and differentiation within the medical care system do not take into account similarities across diseases which cannot be recognized when specialists concentrate on one disease alone. An organization which specializes in certain facets of disease management may optimize its capacity to handle the disease but misses the total picture. Differentiation has brought its advantages, but an integrative approach is now also needed. Within the hospital there would seem to be a good rationale for the division of patients into *acute-general* where the issue is the mobilization of maximal care and continuous monitoring, whatever the disease; *subacute-differentiated* where the different technologies available for specific diseases exert their maximum effect; and *chronic-general* where the issues of prevention of disability and rehabilitation, again across diseases, are salient. Much more use could be made of day hospitals, out-patient departments, and domiciliary approaches. Many patients now brought into hospitals for workup and therapy could equally well be treated in local health centers by their own physicians, or in an outpatient department if they were provided with transportation and consultation.

It is clear that the current hierarchical system has many disadvantages. The medical care system of the future will probably be a matrix like other newer organizational systems. Rather than individuals controlling areas and structures, there will be a loose set of relationships among subsystems which will work collaboratively. This implies a team approach to problems so that individuals may belong to sets of different teams working around problems rather than bearing primary allegiance to professions. In order to optimize the collection, analysis and use of the new types of data necessary for such conceptual and organizational developments, traditional medical controls will have to be modified, since the physician is now, for the most part, trained to emphasize only certain aspects of medicine.

A rationalization of the new system would suggest that there be a new group essentially running medical services which might be termed the *human resources group*. This would consist of a series of professionals trained to manage the interpersonal aspects of social situations, and to use data from a variety of sources and transmit it appropriately. The roles of nurse and social worker and allied professions would cease to exist as such and would be differentiated into technical and human resources specialists. Within this latter group there might be a specific role of expediter, as proposed by Hansell, Wodarczyk, and Vistosky (1968), whose job it would be to keep the patient and family informed of the processes affecting them, and to see them through these processes. There would be a series of technical specialists who would range from those performing the functions of technical nursing to the analysis of physiological function (although this latter function would eventually be taken care of by automated processes).

The physician would also cease to exist as such. In a transitional stage, he would serve as consultant to the human resources group on the technical aspects of diagnosis and treatment. Eventually his diagnostic and therapeutic functions would be taken over in part by automated processes and computers, in part by technical specialists of a variety of levels. A new role will emerge in this complex system, that of the supergeneralist. The physician would be a *sys-*

tems manager trained to analyze and integrate information from a wide variety of sources, and to make and implement plans appropriately. His responsibility would be not only to the individual patient, but to the variety of levels of society implicated in disease processes. He would clearly link the care system with systems in the community, so that, as data was collected about disease, *risk* populations or *risk* situations might be identified and modified where necessary.

It is too early to say that, in the present state of ignorance, prevention will become the rule. However, the approach here outlined does emphasize a facet of the interrelationship—the feedback loop—between man and his disease which will increasingly become the focus for therapy. Already therapies based on this kind of conceptualization have begun to be devised in relation to new syndromes identified by the application of feedback concepts to individual function (Whatmore and Kohli 1968). The concept of linking loops also makes clear the impossibility of developing the feedback loops called therapy unless the individual is linked to the system in an integral fashion. Too often those responsible for therapy think that all that is needed after diagnosis is the issuing of orders. It is hardly surprising that so many patients and their families take themselves out of treatment. Thus, it is essential that patients and families become linked to a therapeutic process. One way of encouraging this association is to involve them in the decision-making and planning that affects them. There is no reason whatsoever why patients should not have a much larger say in choosing the alternative courses available to professionals in taking care of them.

In fostering the notion of therapeutic linking, the care system has a new responsibility toward individual personality style. Instead of merely reacting to, or ignoring a style, it behooves the medical care system to change it, if such a change is in the patient's (and not just the medical care system's) interests. How many patients have been rejected because of behavior unacceptable to physician or nurse, with inevitable consequences for the treatment they receive? If such behavior is seen to be a part of a style that is *relevant to the therapeutic process*, it is a necessary part of therapy to alter it. Feedback of the results of such behavior on staff, and sympathetic explanation, as well as demonstrated understanding of its sources, is remarkably effective and requires neither great expertise nor time.

This essay does not pretend to provide a definitive, even indicative statement of a theory; but it is an attempt to lay bare some problems that have concerned many practitioners, and to sketch some possible directions for the future.

References

Angyal, A.
(1967), *Foundations for a Science of Personality.* Cambridge: Commonwealth Fund, Harvard.

Brehm, J. W., and A. R. Cohen
(1962), *Explorations in Cognitive Dissonance.* New York: Wiley.

Brown, F.
(1966), "The Relationship Between Cancer and Personality." *Annals of the New York Academy of Science, 125,* Art. 3 (January 21), 865–873.

Burch, P. R. J.
(1963a), "Autoimmunity: Some Aetilogical Aspects: Inflammatory Polyarthritis and Rheumatoid Arthritis." *Lancet, I* (June 8), 1253–1257.

——— (1963b), "Autoimmunity: Aetiological Aspects of Chronic Discoid and Systemic Iupus Erythematosus, Systemis Sclerosis, and Hashimoto's Thyroiditis." *Lancet, 2* (September 7), 507–513.

——— (1963c), "A Genetic Theory of Inflammatory Polyarthritis." *Lancet,* 2 (September 21), 636–637.

——— (1964a), "Manic Depressive Psychosis: Some New Aetiological Considerations." *British Journal of Psychiatry, 110,* 469 (November), 808–817.

——— (1964b), "Schizophrenia: Some New Aetiological Considerations." *British Journal of Psychiatry, 110,* 469 (November), 818–824.

——— (1964c), "Involutional Psychosis: Some New Aetiological Considerations." *British Journal of Psychiatry, 110,* 469 (November), 825–829.

Chen, E., and S. Cobb
(1960), "Family Structure in Relation to Health and Disease." *Journal of Chronic Disease, 12,* 5 (November), 544–567.

Crile, G., Jr.
(1963), "The Cancer Problem: A Speculative Review of the Etiology, Natural History and Treatment of Cancer." In D. Ingle (ed.), *Life and Disease,* New York: Basic Books. Pp. 267–292.

Dubos, R.
(1965), *Man Adapting.* New Haven: Yale University Press.

Egbert, L. D., G. E. Battit, C. E. Welch, and M. K. Bartlett
(1964), "Reduction of Postoperative Pain by Encouragement and Instruction of Patients, A Study of Doctor-Patient Rapport." *New England Journal of Medicine, 270* (April 16), 825–827.

Ehrenwald, J.
(1963), "Family Diagnosis and Mechanisms of Psychosocial Defense." *Family Process, 2,* 1 (March), 121–131.

Engel, G. L.
(1960), "A Unified Concept of Health and Disease." *Perspectives in Biological Medicine, 3,* 459–485.

——— (1962), "The Nature of Disease and the Care of the Patient. The Challenge of Humanism and Science in Medicine." *The Rhode Island Medical Journal, 45,* 5, 245–257.

——— (1968), "A Life Setting Conducive to Illness, The Giving Up-Given Up Complex." Presented at American College of Physicians, Boston. Mimeographed.

Engle, R. L.
(1963a), "Medical Diagnosis: Present, Past, and Future. II. Philosophical Foundations and Historical Development of Our Concepts Of Health, Disease, and Diagnosis." *Archives of Internal Medicine, 112* (October), 116–125.

——— (1963b), "Medical Diagnosis: Present, Past, and Future. III. Diagnosis in the Future, Including a Critique on the Use of Electronic Computers as Diagnostic Aids to the Physician." *Archives of Internal Medicine, 112* (October), 126–139.

———, and B. J. Davis
(1963), "Medical Diagnosis: Present, Past, and Future. I. Present Concepts of the Meaning and Limitations of Medical Diagnosis." *Archives of Internal Medicine, 112* (October), 108–115.

Goldman, S.
(1968), "Aging, Noise and Choice." *Perspectives in in Biological Medicine, 12,* 1 (Autumn), 12–30.

Greene, W. A.
(1966), "The Psychosocial Setting of the Development of Leukemia and Lymphoma." *Annals of the New York Academy of Science, 125,* Art. 3 (January 21), 794–806.

Haley, T. J., and R. S. Snider (eds.)
(1964), *Response of the Nervous System to Ionising Radiation.* Boston: Little, Brown.

Hansell, N., M. Wodarczyk, and H. M. Vistosky
(1968), "The Mental Health Expediter." *Archives of General Psychiatry, 18* (April), 392–399.

Hare, E. H., and G. K. Shaw
(1965a), "A Study in Family Health: (1) Health in Relation to Family Size." *British Journal of Psychiatry, 3,* 475 (June), 461–466.

——— (1965b), "A Study in Family Health: (2) A Comparison of the Health of Fathers, Mothers and Children." *British Journal of Psychiatry, 3,* 475 (June), 467–471.

Hersh, E. M., and J. J. Oppenheim
(1965), "Impaired *in vitro* Lymphocyte Transformation in Hodgkin's Disease." *New England Journal of Medicine, 273,* 19 (November 4), 1006–1012.

Hinkle, L. E., and H. E. Wolff
(1958), "Ecologic Investigations of the Relationship Between Illness, Life Experiences and the Social Environment." *Annals of Internal Medicine, 49* (December), 1373–1388.

Israel, S., and G. Teeling-Smith
(1967), "The Submerged Iceberg of Sickness in Society." *Social and Economic Administration, 1,* 1 (January), 43–56.

Jonas, A.
(1966), "Theoretical Considerations Concerning the Influence of the Central Nervous System on Cancerous Growth." *Annals of the New York Academy of Science, 125,* Art. 3 (January 21), 946–951.

Kavetsky, R. E., N. M. Turkevich, and K. P. Balitsky
(1966), "On the Psychophysiological Mechanism of the Organism's Resistance to Tumor Growth." *Annals of the New York Academy of Science, 125,* Art. 3 (January 21), 933–945.

Kissen, D. M.
(1966), "The Value of a Psychosomatic Approach to Cancer." *Annals of the New York Academy of Science, 125,* Art. 3 (January 21), 777–779.

Langner, T. S., and S. T. Michael
(1963), *Life Stress and Mental Health.* London: Free Press.
Lawrence, P. R., and J. W. Lorsch
(1967), "Organization and Environment." Boston: Harvard University, Graduate School of Business Administration, Division of Research.
LeShan, L.
(1959), "Psychological States as Factors in the Development of Malignant Disease: A Critical Review." *Journal of the National Cancer Institute, 22,* 1 (January), 1–18.
Lipschutz, A.
(1967), *Steroid Homeostasis Hypophysis and Tumorigenesis.* Cambridge: Heffer.
Lucero, R. J., et al.
(1963), "Seasonal Variation in Aberrant Group Behavior." *Lancet, 83,* 153–156.
——— (1965), "Weather, Crime, and Mental Illness." *Journal of the Minnesota Academy of Science, 32,* 3, 223–226.
Marmorston, J.
(1966), "Urinary Hormone Metabolite Levels in Patients with Cancer of the Breast, Prostate and Lung." *Annals of the New York Academy of Science, 125,* Art. 3 (January 21), 959–973.
Maruyama, M.
(1967), "The Effect of Oscillating Future Perspective." *Journal of Existentialism, 1,* 27 (Spring), 351–357.
——— (1968), "The Second Cybernetics: Deviation Amplifying Mutual Causal Processes." In W. Buckley (ed.), *Modern Systems Research for the Behavioral Scientist.* Chicage: Aldine.
Mechanic, D.
(1968), *Medical Sociology.* New York: Free Press.
Meissner, W. W.
(1966), "Family Dynamics and Psychosomatic Processes." *Family Process, 5,* 2 (September), 141–161.
Menzies, I. E. P.
(1960), "A Case Study in the Functioning of Social Systems as a Defence Against Anxiety: A Report on a Study of the Nursing of a General Hospital." *Human Relations, 13,* 194–200.
Payne, A. M. M.
(1965), "Innovation Out of Unity." *Milbank Memorial Fund Quarterly, 43,* 4 (October), Part I, 397–408.
Peachey, R.
(1963), "Family Patterns of Illiness." *American Academy of General Practice, 27,* 5 (May), 82–89.
Phillips, D. L.
(1968), "Social Class and Psychological Disturbance: The Influence of Positive and Negative Experiences." *Social Psychiatry, 3,* 2 (April), 41.
Polak, O. R.
(1967), "The Crisis of Admission." *Social Psychiatry, 2,* 4 (November), 150.
Potter, V. R.
(1962), "Enzyme Studies on the Deletion Hypothesis of Carcinogenesis." *The Molecular Basis of Neoplasia,* Symposium Papers. Austin: University of Texas.
Priban, I.
(1968), "Models in Medicine." *Science Journal, 4,* 6 (June), 61–67.
Richards, D. W.
(1963), "Homeostasis: Its Dislocations and Perturbations." In D. Ingle (ed.), *Life and Disease,* New York: Basic Books. Pp. 387–400.

Schmale, A., and H. Iker
(1966), "The Psychological Setting of Uterine Cervical Cancer." *Annals of the New York Academy of Science, 125,* Art. 3 (January 21), 807–813.
Schulberg, H. S., and A. Sheldon
(1968), "The Probability of Crisis and Strategies for Preventive Intervention." *Archives of General Psychiatry, 18* (May), 553–558.
Sheldon, A., and D. Hooper
(1966), "Psychiatric Care in Cross-Cultural Perspective." *Human Organization, 25,* 1 (Spring), 3–9.
Sigerist, H. E.
(1951), *A History of Medicine.* New York: Oxford University Press. Vol. I.
——— (1961), *A History of Medicine,* New York: Oxford University Press. Vol. II.
Szasz, T. E.
(1963), *Law, Liberty, and Psychiatry.* New York: Macmillan.
Tagiuri, R.
Personal communication.
Thompson, J. W.
(1963), "Meteorological Models in the Social Sciences." *General Systems Yearbook,* 8, 153–182.
Turner, R. J.
(1963), "Social Structure and Crisis." Syracuse: Mental Health Research Unit. Mimeographed.
Weiner, J. M., J. Marmorston, E. Stern, and C. E. Hopkins
(1966), "Urinary Metabolites in Cancer and Benign Hyperplasia of the Prostrate: A Multivariate Statistical Analysis." *Annals of the New York Academy of Science, 125,* Art. 3 (January 21), 974–983.
Whatmore, G. B., and D. A. Kohli
(1968), "Dysponesis: A Neurophysiological Factor in Functional Disorders." *Behavioral Science, 12,* 2 (March), 102.
Wolf, S.
(1963), "A New View of Disease." *Journal of the American Medical Association, 184,* 2 (April), 143–144.

Sidney S. Lee
and Curtis P.
McLaughlin

6. Changing Views of Public Health Services as a System

All around us we see general dissatisfaction with the health services prevailing in the United States. Some critics prescribe a new "systems" approach to health, implying that no one has been thinking systematically about medical care problems. Yet every well-endowed medical library contains a continuous and extensive literature about medical planning and care that goes back more than half a century. In attempting to put the current issues in a historical context, it will be useful to single out one example, "public health," a gradually modifying systems viewpoint around which scholars and decision-makers have organized systems concepts and structured many useful activities. In fact, the authors think that such a look provides a useful object lesson for all who are interested in health systems.

This chapter will look back on a moving stream of constructs and perhaps leave the reader with an inkling that he has been here before. For example, there was a burgeoning neighborhood health center movement in Boston during and after World War I (Davis 1927). In the late 1930's an intensive effort was begun to rationalize the public health services of the entire nation along the lines of an effective systems analysis. This approach culminated in Haven Emerson's (1945) publication, *Local Health Units for the Nation* a study which developed the basic structure of what we today consider to be the traditional public health department and applied it conceptually and in operational detail to every county in the United States.

Parallel to this majority view, a minority "medical care" construct developed slowly, receiving quiet but significant assists from medical progress and from the political process. Its proponents dealt in key words and phrases now fashionable—comprehensive care, prepaid group practice—and had their own glossary of special terms like availability, accessability, continuity, comprehensiveness, and quality of care. They also gave some deference to the subject of costs.

World War II was a critical period in the development of public health concepts. Out of it came the concept of rehabilitation as a dynamic process. Wartime experiences and conditioning also gave impetus to the emergence of psychiatry as a discipline. As a result, psychiatry could go into the general hospital and subsequently could become the force which is now called community mental health. But, most significantly, it was during World War II that antibiotics were first used on a large scale. Our capacity to deal with infection was increased manyfold, and communicable disease control came of age.

In the wake of these obvious successes came efforts to apply the concepts of this one area of medicine to others. There was a wave of concern over chronic illness detection conceptualized like communicable disease detection (*American Journal of Public Health* 1947). Chronic disease detection on a grand scale became fashionable and multiphasic screening was attempted (Chapman 1949; Taubenhaus 1968). Prevention was redefined into primary, secondary, and tertiary levels. But this activity was followed by a wave of disillusionment. Available technology and medical knowledge really were not up to the task. Organized medicine was opposed to fresh public incursions. In contrast to communicable disease, early detection of chronic disease, virtually by definition, seldom yielded programs effective in either prevention or halting progression.

Today we see a concentration on systems efforts at all levels of health, with the new emphasis being on higher levels of aggregation (Kissick 1967; White 1968). Some analysts attempt to deal with the whole field of health and medical care as a single system (Horvath 1966). Indeed, to some, the term system inherently implies a holistic approach (Rogers and Messinger 1967; Sheldon, chapter 5 in this volume). In part this is the result of a general trend toward more sophisticated analysis. There is intense interest in neighborhood health centers, in regionalization, and in progressive patient care—all older concepts which have achieved renewed relevance in the political and systems-oriented environment of the present. Health has ceased to be merely an area of professional parochialism and has become a focal point of political concern.

Organizational activity in the federal government can serve as an indicator of the flux in system definitions. Because government is expected to maintain a posture of omniscience and leadership, a study of the boxes in the U.S. Public Health Service organization chart, if not of the people in the jobs, should confirm the movements to which we have referred. The administrative structures of the Public Health Service in 1948, 1957, 1965, and 1967 and the HEW reorganization of 1968 do demonstrate this. The key words appear at the times one would expect them. For example, Table 1, which compares the Table of Organization of the Public Health Service for 1948 with that of 1957, shows the addition of a Chronic Disease Branch, a Heart Disease Control Branch, a National Heart Institute, an Air Pollution Medical Program, a Radiological Health Program, and an Accident Prevention Program. By 1967 the charts show an Office of Comprehensive Health Planning and Development, an Office of Program Planning and Evaluation, a Bureau of Disease Prevention and Environmental Control, and an Office of Equal Health Opportunity. In 1968 the announcement was made of a Center for Population Studies and Human Reproduction. Perhaps someone with fewer administrative and teaching duties will apply the techniques developed to study the rates of diffusion of innovation in industry (Mansfield 1968) to health activities. The titles of the professors in schools of public health and the topics of journal articles might provide useful data and intriguing results from such studies.

Now let us turn to a more detailed discussion of one specific systems model that has influenced the structure of public health for years and that illustrates some of our concerns about systems analysis and people and leaders.[1] Few people realize that for the last two decades the traditional public health department, a favorite whipping boy, has been structured to conform to the recommendations of an early, but thorough, systems analysis. There probably has been no more pervasive systems study in the public health field than *Local Health Units for the Nation*, published in 1945 by the Commonwealth Fund and representing the official viewpoint of the American Public Health Association. The report begins with a familiar refrain: "These local health jurisdictions are inherited from the past. They came into being, like many good and bad things in a large and grow-

[1] D. N. Michael (*The Unprepared Society*, Basic Books, 1968) has explored in depth the humanity of scientists, systems analysts, and decision-makers.

Table 1. Comparative Organizational Units, U.S. Public Health Service, 1948 and 1957.

1947 Organizational Units	1958 Organizational Units
Office of the Surgeon General	**Office of the Surgeon General**
Dental Division	(see Bur. of State Services)
Sanitary Engineering Division	(see Bur. of State Services)
Office of International Health Relations	(see Bur. of State Services)
Division of Public Health Methods	Division of Public Health Methods
National Office of Vital Statistics	(see Bur. of State Services)
	Office of Health Emergency Planning
	Office of Civilian Health Requirements
	National Library of Medicine
Bureau of Medical Services	**Bureau of Medical Services**
Hospital Division	Division of Hospitals
Mental Hygiene Division	
Foreign Quarantine Division	Division of Foreign Quarantine
Federal Employees Health Division	
	Division of Dental Resources
	Division of Indian Health
(see Bur. of State Services)	Division of Hospital and Medical Facilities
	Division of Nursing Resources
Bureau of State Services	**Bureau of State Services**
States Relations Division	(see Division of General Health
Communicable Disease Center	Communicable Disease Center
Venereal Disease Division	
Industrial Hygiene Division	(see Div. Special Health Services)
Tuberculosis Control Division	(see Div. Special Health Services)
Division of Hospital Facilities	(see Bur. of Medical Services)
(see OSG)	Division of Dental Public Health
	Division of General Health Services
	Program Development Branch
	State Grants Branch
	Public Health Education Branch
	Public Health Nursing Branch
(see OSG)	National Office of Vital Statistics
	Artic Health Research Center
(see OSG)	Division of International Health
(see OSG)	Division of Sanitary Engineering Services
	Division of Special Health Services
	Chronic Disease Branch
(see Industrial Hygiene Div.)	Occupational Health Branch

1947 Organizational Units	1958 Organizational Units
(see Industrial Hygiene Div.)	Tuberculosis Branch Heart Disease Control Branch Air Pollution Medical Program Radiological Health Program Accident Prevention Program
National Institutes of Health	**National Institutes of Health**
National Cancer Institute	National Cancer Institute
Division of Tropical Diseases	
Division of Infectious Diseases	National Institute of Allergy and Infectious Diseases
Experimental Biology and Medicine Institute	
Laboratory of Physical Biology	
Biologics Control Laboratory	Division of Biologics Standards
Division of Research Grants	Division of Research Grants Research Facilities Branch Research Fellowships Branch Research Grants Branch National Heart Institute National Institute of Arthritis and Metabolic Disease National Institute of Dental Research National Institute of Mental Health National Institute of Neurological Disease and Blindness Clinical Center

Source: *Official Register of the United States,* 1948 and 1957. Washington, D.C.: Government Printing Office.

ing country, without benefit of policy. We know now that we can afford nothing less than coverage of every population and area unit of our nation with a competent local health service. How can we achieve it? Do we continue in an outworn tradition, or shall we boldly redesign our apparatus? The authors of this report propose the latter course."

This report examined the then current expenditures, staffing, and jurisdictions of every state, and concluded that an annual per capita expenditure of $1.00 for health would represent a realistic leap forward. Given the further assumption that every local health district must have a full-time medical officer and a full complement of auxiliaries, then the minimum district would have to have at least 50,000 persons to support an effort of this scale. To service such a district "there would be needed one full-time professionally trained and experienced medical officer of health, a full-time public health or sanitary engineer, and a sanitarian of nonprofessional grade, ten public health nurses, one of whom would be of supervisory grade, and three persons for clerical work." Part-time men and specialists were to be engaged as needed. The study's six-point delineation of the functions of a local health department became the catechism for students in public health for many years.

The six basic functions of local health department include:

1. Vital statistics, or the recording, tabulation, interpretation and publication of the essential facts of births, deaths and reportable disease;
2. Control of communicable diseases, including tuberculosis, the venereal diseases, malaria, and hookworm disease;
3. Environmental sanitation, including supervision of milk and milk products, food prcessing and public eating places, and maintenance of sanitary conditions of employment;
4. Public health laboratory services;
5. Hygiene of maternity, infancy, and childhood, including supervision of health of the school child;
6. Health education of the general public so far as not covered by the functions of departments of education.

Secure in this definition of what public health departments were to do, and buttressed by data on each state, Emerson and his staff prepared maps and manning tables for 1,197 health districts in 48 states and the District of Columbia. These figures were presented to all state health officers, and, while not universally implemented, they have formed the basic construct for the operation of most local departments to the present.

Emerson's study was prepared on the basis of a population distribution and a pattern of transportation and medical technology that existed in the 1930s and before. Although it attempted to provide a forward-looking approach, it clearly has little relevance today. Advancing technology and specialization make 50,000 persons an inappropriate base for the distribution of health and medical services. It probably is too small for specialized purposes and may be too large for other primary and personalized ones.

Emerson's program was never fully implemented, but it went a long way because it fitted our political structure rather well. Historically, the county has been the basic unit for the organization of government services in most regions of the country, especially the rural areas which have had so much political leverage. For example, at one point there were a hundred county health departments in North Carolina, each with a full-time health officer position, regardless of county size, and each of these jobs was filled. The state governments presumably provided leadership, standards were raised, and people were sent off to schools of public health to get master's degrees, which in turn became a requirement for filling such jobs. Even today, the public health journals carry advertisements that read "Local Health Officer wanted for a county of seventy-five thousand in Northwest . . . , requirements: MPH and three years' experience." The Local-Health-Units-for-the-Nation construct is still operative for many people in the field. It was a tight system definition that influenced the activities of a large number of professionals. In fact, that approach and the organizations that sprang from it have been responsible for substantial achievements in public health. But it also can serve as an example of the negative attributes of such analyses. We are now paying a heavy price for accepting such a narrow, albeit quantified, view of the public health system.

More recently, different ideas about the scope of public health have become more popular. They are not new, but they have been eclipsed by the dominant and prevailing Emerson construct. The alternatives were alive in the writings of many scholars, including Herman Biggs, C.E.-A. Winslow, and Joseph W. Mountin. We tend to forget that legislation was introduced in the New York Legislature in 1924 to allow for "comprehensive health centers" (Terris 1963). It was in 1920 that Winslow defined public health as "the art and science of preventing disease, prolonging life, and promoting health and efficiency through organized community efforts . . ." (Winslow 1920). The primary recommendation of the 1932 report of the Committee on the Costs of Medical Care was that "Medical service, both preventive and therapeutic, should be furnished largely by organized groups of physicians, dentists, nurses, pharmacists, and other associated personnel. Such groups should be organized, preferably around a hospital, for rendering complete home, office and hospital care" (*Medical Care for the American People* 1932). Mountin's work and writings (summarized succinctly in Leavell 1953) sound very much like the blueprint for the federal programs of the late 1960's, even though Mountin died in 1952.

Until recently, public health has been a discrete set of organizations specifically enjoined from relating its missions to other health services. Private physicians and hospitals were engaged in what was called "curative medicine" rather than public or preventive medicine. Today, these are not distinguishable functions.[2] A few years ago, the boundary between them, while not entirely static, was at least operationally clear. For example, only very recently has a physician in a "well-baby" clinic in the City of Boston been permitted to treat an illness he detected. The clinic doctor was to refer any abnormality to a family physician or a hospital clinic for treatment. Generally, patients with tuberculosis or venereal disease were treated at public centers, but they were considered public dangers and poor credit risks. Immunizations were provided, but each fresh category of immunizations required an interaction, if not altercation, with private physicians in the community over whether or not that category should be provided and by whom. Wilinsky, who managed the White health centers in Boston, wrote of the need to deal with "sociomedical" problems as early as 1927, but his orientation was toward sanitation, preventive medicine, and social work.

In attempting to overcome the obvious inadequacies of these constructs, the thinking of health planners appears to have shifted more toward the provision of health services for geographic or socioeconomic blocks of people. In dealing with these blocks we use a number of constructs—regionalization, neighborhood health centers, comprehensive health planning, prepaid group practice, etc. Perhaps without thinking about it explicitly, our viewpoint has shifted from a disease-oriented one to a people-oriented one. The older fashions like rehabilitation, chronic disease, psychiatry, and categorical grants, institutes, and centers were attempts to redefine and regroup medical care activities to make rational

[2] While students under Winslow and Emerson, many of us had the opportunity to witness spirited meetings between these tall, imposing, and brilliant men who persistently debated their strongly held, but opposing views. Emerson clearly won the first round, and for about two decades schools of public health concentrated resources on retreading retirees to fill Emerson's slots. There has been a decided change both in the people entering the field and in the field itself in the last several years.

systems for categorical care. Now, partially in response to social and political forces, we are coming to see groups of people as the unifying focus, although we seem to lose sight of that fact in defending our own specific models. If people are provided better health care by the new structures that develop, then the change will have been justified; but we also must recognize that there is nothing intrinsically suitable about categories (or blocks or herds) of people as the building blocks for health systems.

One advantage of the blocks-of-people approach is its consistency with our long history of public care for "disadvantaged" categories of citizens and for people who were deemed to represent a real or potential danger to the community. In more recent years we also have relied heavily on the mechanisms that have developed in our more or less free market of insurance. We did not enact a national sickness insurance program in 1935 as part of Social Security. Only a minute fraction of the population was covered by insurance at the time, and the nation was in the depths of the Depression. One could make a strong case for the government's taking over almost any sector of society under those conditions, yet we did not choose that route. We allowed the private market to build up along with the technology, devised new mechanisms for financing care, and added new public beneficiaries along the way—the disabled, the blind, dependent children, the aged poor, more veterans, etc. Over time, we brought into the public view many new categories of deprived citizens.

By 1965, it became obvious that the aged had low, fixed incomes, needed more medical care, and had less capacity to cope with its rising cost than other groups in our society. They also were an increasing political force. Other beneficiaries were acquired when riders were tacked onto the Medicare legislation originally intended to help the aged. Very few people in this country were cognizant in 1965 that the bill also provided expanded benefits for children and offered the states the opportunity to pay for care for the medically indigent. Only at the end of the 1960's have the realities of the Title XIX become apparent.

By a conjunction of events and causative factors which are virtually impossible to untangle, it now has become politically sound and intellectually acceptable to take the broader systems view of health.[3] Those who have a strong sense of justice, who claim that medical care ought to be a right, have not prevailed on this theme alone. They have prevailed to the stark accompaniment of population shifts and upward spiraling costs of medical care. In fact, it is not too surprising that many of the concepts of neighborhood health care that were advanced as appropriate for the isolated, urban immigrant ghettoes of the early 1900's have taken on renewed vitality in response to the needs of isolated, urban ghettoes of the 1960's.[4] Emerson's model, the paradigm for the intervening period, which appeared in polished form in 1945, can be viewed as a natural response to the perceived health needs of a Depression-ridden, rural America.

Most of the factors of interest to the federal government and to systems analysts are related specifically to pressures from categories of people "needing" care and from the obvious problems of cost. Today there are political pressures which lead fiscally conscious legislators like Wilbur Mills to raise questions like, "Where are the premium savers? How do we control costs?"

To the legislator, the obvious premium savers are outpatient diagnostic services on the front end and the use of less expensive long-term bed facilities on the other (Somers and Somers 1967). In the middle is the hospital, where a cost-pass-through inflation spirals upward (Klarman 1964). Nursing homes have always been a cottage industry, but a high earner on invested capital. Now they are attracting large corporations. Although many will object to the idea of big corporations making profits from nursing home care, this approach, probably unwittingly, has been one of the few that has boosted the supply of medical services as well as the effective demand; and this alone serves to slow the rise in prices, if not costs.

Such premium savers are really macroapplication of the concept of progressive patient care, so strongly advocated for the inside of the hospital by Haldeman (Haldeman and Abdellah 1959). Florence Nightingale enunciated progres-

[3] Don K. Price has suggested that medical decisions now lie in the professional and administrative estates between the poles of science and politics (Price 1965).

[4] A review of the neighborhood health center concept which emphasizes the changes that have evolved over time can be found in Stoeckle and Candib (1969).

sive patient care in the nineteenth century. Her ward design is still the model for military hospitals. Industry has used the same underlying principles for centuries, combining the factors of production to meet the needs of each stage of a process. Unfortunately the gleaming hardware of the intensive care unit is the operational form of the progressive care construct that has really caught on. It takes a lot more space, i.e., capital, as well as trained people and expensive equipment to give intensive care than it takes to give standard inpatient care. One hospital that the authors know of decided to add two intensive care units, and so reduced its bed complement by twenty-five. And we still are far from facing such hard questions as: Who is being saved with intensive care units anyway? Is this good community service?

Regionalization is yet another rationalizing construct which has floated around for some time. Every military medical service is organized on this basis. Among civilian counterparts, the Bingham Associates established a plan to bring services to small hospitals and their doctors in Maine, to improve their skills, and to facilitate the movement of the most complicated cases to Tufts-New England Medical Center. Other applications include the Rochester regional effort and the Puerto Rico and Michigan efforts (Rosenfeld and Makover 1956; McNerny and Reidel 1962). Again, in utilizing the regional construct, the task of the analyst is to hammer out a manageable concept of a system which can be organized so as to respond to the community's need.

At the federal level the response has taken the form of the Regional Medical Program (RMP) (Russell 1966), and the Comprehensive Health Planning legislation (Jacobs and Froh 1968). To Congress, these programs for coordination appeared as mechanisms to rationalize services; they have had the added tactical advantage of being in harmony with the philosophies of those who desired to see decision-making decentralized, emasculated, or both.

To the systems analyst, the two regional programs represent a potentially serious overlap. We recognize that the fifty states are not useful geographical units for the organization of all health services. Health services cannot always be analyzed, planned, or distributed within political jurisdictions. Furthermore, the two programs are competing with each other for scarce dollars and scarcer manpower. Whether either or both will survive in anything like their present form is difficult to predict. For the next few years it looks as if the bulk of the funds for planning will go to the state agencies. Congressmen represent states, and the Regional Medical Program is stuck with the dirty and declining categorical label. As a result, our people currently rely heavily on two bright and shiny new programs which are flawed conceptually: comprehensive state planning is not based on a logical planning unit, and RMP is not comprehensive.

The question of how to provide comprehensive medical care for individuals, however, is about the most difficult the systems analyst faces today. Comprehensive medical care in a clinical sense has not proved to be an operational concept. The number of people in this country who receive comprehensive care is minute. This is not surprising when one looks realistically at the costs, the pathways to treatment, and the manpower required to accomplish the objectives of such programs.

The neighborhood health center is one application of the comprehensive philosophy. It also fits in well with the more pessimistic view that the city as a whole is ungovernable. It is in keeping with both the conservative's desire for premium savers (because it can serve to reduce the demand for hospitalization) and with the liberal's desire for social action. Most observers now recognize that there is little or no primary medical care available in most poor urban neighborhoods, and that an institution is the only alternative. Once the institutional approach is accepted, there are two differing views. One, with Count Gibson as a spokesman, sees the neighborhood center as the primary institution and the hospital as the satellite (Gibson 1968). The more traditional view calls for the clinic to be a satellite of the hospital. The argument goes well beyond the usual questions of geographic or bureaucratic jurisdictions. The question of leadership is critical. Generally, the public health fraternity has come to admit that the hospital, rather than the local public health department, would be the center of the health system.[5] Yet the hospitals, while able to generate

[5] See Baehr (1964). A more middle-of-the-road view is expressed in McKeown (1959).

dollars, generally are devoid of community leadership capability; and the classical public health movement has fallen by the wayside. Some would substitute a town meeting leadership by the community. This is already Office of Economic Opportunity policy. Obviously, only the community or neighborhood can make the decision whether its resources should go for health services or for other purposes. But, when it comes to decisions about the operation of the technical medical system and the provision of health services, it has not been proved that neighborhood or community boards can give leadership.

If we start with the current premise that the health system should be directed at delivering service to blocks of people, the system construct changes substanially. Although we may use the same tools of analysis, we will be much more effective because we have accepted a model for framing relevant questions, even when the answers are not readily available. We must begin by asking what the size and shape of the building blocks should be. Is today's magic number for the delivery of primary medical care a population unit of 30,000 or 75,000 or 100,000 people? Is the building block the same for all regions? Is it the same for all services? If not, then how are the units to be coordinated?

If health care should be provided on a prepaid basis by a group of professionals who are concerned with prevention, including health education; with early detection, prompt treatment, and follow-up; and with the family as the primary unit of care; we must decide now to assemble the package. The unknowns clearly exceed the known factors. What manpower groupings can best provide the desired care? How do we assure flexibility in utilization of manpower? Where should these facilities be located? Should they be physically isolated? In juxtaposition to hospitals? Next to neighborhood schools? How should we view the use of capital for construction in the light of changing urban patterns of land use? Should we build plants for a 50-year expectation or for a 10-year or a 20-year expectation of useful life?

Providing for operating costs raises further questions. How should costs be distributed? Should the care be purchased with general tax revenues, Social Security, direct payment, or should we perhaps imitate the Danes by instituting compulsory membership in voluntary sick funds?

Once we decide what our basic building blocks are to be, we

must determine how best to integrate them. Do we make several levels of institutional care available? Do we want personal continuity of care or merely continuity of information flow through the system? How many building blocks should feed into a hospital? How should determination of need for hospital care be made, and by whom? What of the next level of aggregation of patients with rare conditions? Should we attempt to relate the organization of the care system to a system for environmental health and sanitation. If so, how does a watershed or airshed relate in size and shape to an aggregation of care blocks?

Further, we must ask what sort of information flow system is required. If it is to be longitudinal, with each person having a continuous, life-time medical record, how do we cope with the family as a potential or real unit of care? Should all medical information be centrally stored, or should it be carried by the patient in miniaturized form on his person? How can occupation, place of residence, environmental exposures, etc., be correlated with clinical information? What range of social data is pertinent to health? How are we to feed new knowledge gained from research into the system? What educational system should be used for maintaining and enhancing skills at all levels among the providers of care? How can new recruits into the system be distributed more efficiently in relation to need?

This is but a small sample of the kinds of questions which might be addressed to any system construct in this complex field. What is important to recognize is that the acceptance of a system construct such as blocks or categories of people does enable us to formulate operational questions like these. Surely we are interested in broader issues like decentralization versus centralization, high skill distribution versus low skill distribution, aggregation versus nonaggregation, expenditure of capital versus manpower, etc. What we have to do, however, is to select first consciously, not unconsciously, an organizing definition of a health system which then leads us to ask questions in a less abstract context. Without this context we can make little, if any, headway.

In designing systems one first sets up a set of criteria derived from the context and then performs analyses to see (a) whether he can achieve his criteria at all, and (b) which subset of methods will let him achieve them most efficiently. During this process, he generally examines several alternative systems concepts, continuing until some are proved unsuitable or until one emerges as clearly better (Marples 1961). In using the tools of systems analysis in health, likewise our method may be to think through alternative constructs: disease categories, geographic patient categories, provider categories, socioeconomic patient categories, etc. After seeing what questions each approach can raise, we can select temporarily the best ones. The selection of constructs must be temporary, because as our society changes, the politically relevant factors governing medical care decisions will change with it. The primary lesson to be learned from the Emerson analysis and its impact is that we cannot settle permanently on any one system.

Experts will be needed. Analysis of systems for providing health care will continue to provide an intriguing subject for research. But analysis without syntheses into effective new systems which are socially, economically, and politically viable will only serve to discredit both the analyst and the system.

We have shown our ability to devise new concepts for public health systems and to demonstrate their application, albeit in rather random fashion. It is not enough, however, that a given approach is successful in demonstrations. To be worthwhile, it must lead beyond demonstrations to truly replicable models, to systems which do not necessarily introduce new or renewed concepts, but which do show how to accomplish our goals through widespread programs. We need prototypes that can fly. Concepts which work in the normal environment of the decision-maker will come out on top in the competition among system models. Despite the despair of some over the rate at which changes are made in health, it is important to recognize that medical care is an open system which above all must retain its capacity to adapt. We should not produce another constraining model. The task of systems research may not be so much to find a final solution, as to breed stronger horses for strong men to ride.

References

Baehr, G.
(1964), "The Hospital as the Center of Community Medical Care: Fact and Fiction." *American Journal of Public Health, 54,* 1653–1660.

Chapman, A. L.
(1949), "The Concept of Multiphasic Screening." *Public Health Reports, 64,* 1311.
Davis, M. M., Jr.
(1927), *Clinics, Hospitals and Health Centers.* New York: Harper.
Emerson, Haven
(1945), *Local Health Units for the Nation.* New York: Commonwealth Fund.
Gibson, Count D., Jr.
(1968), "The Neighborhood Health Center: The Primary Unit of Health Care." *American Journal of Public Health, 58,* 1188–1191.
Haldeman, J. C., and F. G. Abdellah
(1959), "Concepts of Progressive Patient Care." *Hospitals, 33* (May 16), 38–42 ff. (June 1), 41–46.
Horvath, W. J.
(1966), "The Systems Approach to the National Health Problem." *Manageagement Science, 12,* B–391–395.
Jacobs, A. R., and R. B. Froh
(1968), "Significance of Public Law 89–749: Comprehensive Health Planning." *New England Journal of Medicine, 279,* 1314–1318.
Kissick, W. L.
(1967), "Planning, Programming, and Budgeting in Health." *Medical Care, 5,* 201–217.
Klarman, H. E.
(1964), *The Economics of Medical Care.* Ann Arbor: University of Michigan Press.
Leavell, H. R.
(1953), "The Role of the Local Health Department." *American Journal of Public Health, 43,* 19–24.
Mansfield, E.
(1968), *Industrial Research and Technological Innovation,* New York: Norton. Chapters 7 and 8 discuss the mathematical approaches applicable to the study of rates of imitation.
Marples, D. L.
(1961), "The Decisions of Engineering Design." *IRE Transactions on Engineering Management, 8,* 55–75.
McKeown, T.
(1959), "A Balanced Hospital Community." *Hospitals, 33* (August 16), 40–44 and 107–108.
McNerny, W. J., and D. C. Reidel
(1962), *Regionalization and Rural Health Care.* Ann Arbor: University of Michigan Press.
Medical Care for the American People: Final Report of the Committee on the Costs of Medical Care (1932), Chicago: University of Chicago Press.
Official Register of the United States, 1948, Washington, D.C.: Government Printing Office.
———, *1957,* Washington, D.C.: Government Printing Office.
"Planning for the Chronically Ill" (1947), *American Journal of Public Health, 37,* 1256–1266.
Price, Don K.
(1965), *The Scientific Estate,* Cambridge: The Belknap Press of Harvard University Press.
Rogers, E. S., and H. B. Messinger
(1967), "Human Ecology: Toward a Holistic Approach." *Milbank Memorial Fund Quarterly, 45,* 25–42.

Rosenfeld, L. S., and H. B. Makover
(1956), *The Rochester Regional Hospital Council.* Cambridge: Harvard University Press.
Russell, J. M.
(1966), "New Federal Regional Medical Programs." *New England Journal of Medicine, 275,* 309–312.
Somers, H. M., and A. R. Somers
(1967), *Medicare and the Hospitals.* Washington, D.C.: The Brookings Institution.
Stoeckle, J. D., and L. M. Candib
(1969), "The Neighborhood Health Center—Reform Ideas of Yesterday and Today." *New England Journal of Medicine, 280,* 1385–1391.
Taubenhaus, M.
(1968), "The Massachusetts Health Protection Clinics: A Case Study." In R. Penchansky (ed.), *Health Services Administration: Policy Cases and the Case Method.* Cambridge: Harvard University Press.
Terris, M.
(1963), "The Comprehensive Health Center." *Public Health Reports, 78,* 861–866.
White, K. L.
(1968), "Research in Medical Care and Health Service Systems." *Medical Care, 6,* 95–100.
Wilinsky, C. F.
(1927), "The Health Center." *American Journal of Public Health, 17,* 6077–6082.
Winslow, C. E.-A.
(1920), "The Untilled Fields of Public Health." *Modern Medicine, 2,* 183.

Mark G. Field

7. The Medical System and Industrial Society

Structural Changes and Internal Differentiation in American Medicine

This chapter sets forth, in a highly tentative fashion, some ideas and hypotheses concerning the medical enterprise of the contemporary, large-scale, industrial, and urban society. Although it is based primarily on the American situation, it has also benefited from a detailed study of the Soviet system of socialized medicine.

The general approach I have taken is macrosociological, with the society as the unit of analysis, and structural-functional in that it seeks to locate the health system as part of the social structure for which it performs functionally significant tasks and services and from which, in turn, it must receive specific "inputs." The medical care system is thus a relatively "open" system with boundaries "at least partially permeable, permitting sizable magnitudes of at least certain sorts of matter-energy or information to cross them" (Miller 1965, p. 203). These inputs or energies are always problematic since they are scarce resources.

In addition to its evolutionary perspective, this chapter also attempts to identify sources of strain in the relationship between society and the health system, particularly insofar

This paper is based on a larger monograph entitled *Technology, Medicine and Society: Effectiveness, Differentiation and Depersonalization* (1968), written while I was a member of the Research Group on Biomedical Sciences, Program on Technology and Society, Harvard University. In its present form it will be part of a volume entitled *Biology, Medicine and Society,* edited by Everett Mendelsohn, Judith Swazey, and Stanley Reiser, to be published by Harvard University Press, whose permission to reprint it here is acknowledged with gratitude. Some minor changes have been made to bring this paper in line with the others in this volume.

I want to express my thanks to the Program on Technology and Society and particularly its Director, Emmanuel G. Mesthene, and to the members of my group and its Chairman, Seymour Kety, and also to the Public Health Service, Bureau of Health Services, for supporting my research on Soviet Medicine and Medical Organization under grant CH–00002. This paper is derived, in large measure, from the insights obtained in the detailed study of Soviet medicine I have been engaged in for several years. I must also acknowledge my intellectual indebtedness to Talcott Parsons, whose views and insights have largely shaped my approach to the sociology of medicine (Parsons, 1951a; 1951b; 1957; 1958; 1960; Parsons and Fox, 1952). Finally, the assistance of Mrs. Judith Koivumaki in editing the text and preparing it for final publication was invaluable and is gratefully acknowledged here.

as the increased use of technology and the effective demand for medical services lead to the inability of medicine to satisfy traditionally expected needs of the population. The chapter therefore also raises the question of the prices that society has had to pay for medical effectiveness and for increased distributive reach, and attempts to project certain already visible trends. It is not meant to be, by any means, a definitive approach to the subject; rather, its purpose is exploratory. I hope that it will stimulate discussion and perhaps controversy, and that it will serve as the starting point for a more detailed, empirical, and comparative study of the subject.

I. The Medical Needs of the Social System

The concept of the social system implies, among other things, a meaningful interrelation among the different and functionally complementary parts of the system, so that change or disturbance in any part of the system is likely to have an effect on the other parts and on the system as a whole. A social system may be defined as a network of patterned and complementary social roles, organized within interdependent and interrelated institutional clusters. As such the institutionalized role (rather than the individual actor or member) is the basic constitutive element of the social system. Any individual actor, in the course of his day or of his lifetime, fulfills a variety of roles, and it is on the performance of these roles that the social system's existence and its adaptation to and mastery of the environment depend, to a very important degree.

Performance by social actors according to society's specifications is a fundamental prerequisite for a certain level of functioning of social systems, and this performance is dependent on a series of mechanisms that are always problematic. One of these is that of *institutionalization,* or the clustering and the ordering of roles around certain central functions. There are family, economic, political, religious, educational, medical, and other institutions, and an institutional structure relating them to each other. Institutions specify prescriptions, proscriptions, and prohibitions upon the actor in his social roles—a situation that permits order in the social system, based to a large extent on the gross predictability or statistical probability of institutionalized role behavior. Closely coupled with institutionalization are the control of deviant behavior, the imposition of sanctions upon society's members who have failed to conform to role expectations, and the provision of positive rewards for appropriate behavior. Deviance stems from the fact that the individual actor is faced in his various roles with a variety of choices of actions, pressures, counterpressures, and conflicts.

Beyond these considerations, the performance of social roles depends on three other sources.

1. First is the process of *socialization,* or "control over the quality of human beings," or the acquisition by the individual from birth of the basic culture, values, and skills that will be significant when he enters adult roles. The process of socialization must go on constantly because of personnel turnover caused by the birth of new members and the death of old ones (and in some cases by immigration and emigration). A shorthand way to express this process might be "the shaping of capacity." Its primary locus is the family, the school, the peer group, and, to some degree, the work group.

2. Once capacity has been shaped, the maintenance of a minimum level of motivational energy is necessary to permit the individual to perform his social roles. Socializing and training an individual for adult roles may not be sufficient if that individual is disinclined to perform these roles for a variety of reasons: low morale, lack of motivation or incentives, discouragement, or lack of reinforcement. A shorthand description of this might be "the maintenance of motivational capacity," and its locus may be the family, the work group, religious counseling, and in some instances psychologic medicine.

3. It is also necessary to protect capacity from the threats of incapacity that result from illness, injury, or premature mortality. Thus the ability to act, and indeed the willingness to act, may be vitiated by physical failure (the ultimate form of which is death), or psychological failure such as mental illness, retardation, or emotional disturbance (the ultimate form of which is withdrawal from society, a kind of social death, which occurs in severely psychotic, retarded, or regressed patients). A shorthand description of this process might be "the conservation, preservation, and, perhaps, enhancement of capacity." By and large, the mechanism that deals with this function is medicine and the

health care system, including psychologic medicine, although some would hold that many forms of so-called mental illness are not illnesses in the medical sense and therefore not the proper responsibility of medicine and psychiatry.

The threat of physical and psychological incapacity touches at least two important resources of society. First, it affects the investment in time, human efforts, education, and economic outlays and supports which the society has placed in the individual from the time of his birth. In other words, how does incapacity or premature mortality affect the return on such investments? For example, of every 100 males who reach the age of 45 in the United States, only 90 will survive to the age of 55, whereas in Sweden the comparable figure is 95. Thus, during the critical period when most men are at the peak of their working and earning capacity, twice as many die in the United States as in Sweden—a mortality rate that is also higher than that of almost every western nation (Fuchs 1968, p. 18). Second, the failure on the part of the individual to perform adequately (or to perform at all) in his social roles because of illness is potentially a threat to the social system (or any of its subsystems) and to its integrity, depending, of course, on such elements as the criticalness of the roles themselves, the availability of replacements, and the proportion of disabled individuals to a given population or subpopulation.

Thus *from the viewpoint of society,* conceived as a system, health maintenance, because it is "capacity maintenance," has a functional significance that transcends personal unhappiness and the anxieties that are related to illness, injury, and death. The linkage between health and society can be demonstrated in many areas, such as the production losses and other costs caused by absenteeism due to illness, traumatism, and epidemics (for example, 540,000 man-years annually in the United States through heart disease alone, worth $2.5 billion); the number of people declared unfit for military or other services (half of those rejected by the military in the United States are rejected for medical reasons); the percentage of the population affected by mental illness or retardation (half of all hospital beds are psychiatric beds); and the inability of underdeveloped countries to modernize because of high birth and death rates, lowered stamina, and low life expectancy, resulting in a large proportion of consumers. In industrialized society, morbidity presents a threat primarily to the complexity and interdependence of that kind of structure. As a recent Canadian Royal Commission Report stated, "A modern industrial and increasingly automated society is highly vulnerable as long as significant segments of the population remain unprotected by a comprehensive system of health services" (Badgley and Wolfe 1967, p. 135).

The significance of the health service or medical system of a society may thus no longer be solely a question of privilege or income, or even a question of "rights." It tends to become, in the modern, industrialized society, an aspect of social policy with important functional implications. If we focus on illness or premature death as a major threat to the functioning and indeed to the very existence of a society, we must also specify the nature of societal responses to that threat in terms of mechanisms and roles addressed to mitigating, neutralizing, and if possible, eliminating the impact of incapacity on the society and its members. By and large, we may distinguish at least four analytically distinct responses to the needs associated with illness, incapacity, and the ever present possibility of death.

The *magical response* is man's attempt to come to grips with, to understand, and to control or affect the course of illness conceived as the result of the action of certain forces, such as deities, which he tries to propitiate through rituals. The magical response must be seen in the light of the uncertainty of outcomes, that is, the aleatory element, and man's attempt to procure favourable outcomes. The magical response thus often embodies a perspective on causality that is anthropomorphic: for example, gods must be placated through offerings and sacrifices. This type of response is action oriented: it answers to the need "to do something" in the face of illness and uncertainty. "If you want the patient to recover, pray for him like you never prayed before" is the kind of familiar verbal formula that epitomizes this response.

The *religious response* stems from man's attempt to get at the "meaning" of illness, disability, and eventual death. It is an attempt to reconcile him to the existence of phenomena that remain mysterious but which he must accept as the work of some higher purpose and providence. The formula "The Lord giveth and the Lord taketh away" reflects this need; otherwise, the death of a loved child, although it can be described in scientific terms, remains essentially meaningless. The religious answer, as defined here, is passive; it is oriented toward acceptance or resignation and it cannot satisfactorily be derived solely from a scientific or rational viewpoint.

The *compassionate* or *pastoral response* stems from the need for comfort, reassurance, love, support, consolation, and "tender loving care" that the suffering, anxiety-ridden, frightened, and often psychologically disturbed or regressed patient, and sometimes those near him, needs in the course of illness, suffering, or disability. The optimistic bias so often displayed by members of the health profession is part of an attempt to provide psychological reassurance that "everything will be all right," although it may be argued that there is also an important magical component, thereby saying that "everything will be all right, one hopes that indeed it will be so." The compassionate response is an intensely human and personal one that only another human being can provide (it cannot be automated); in evolutionary terms, its prototype is probably the mother-child relationship.

The *technological response* is the application of empirical or scientifically grounded knowledge, techniques, and technology in a rational approach to the alleviation or elimination of pathological states. It is, of course, what is often defined as "medical treatment" or "services": that is, primarily an active, interventionist approach such as stopping bleeding, massaging the heart, giving an injection, or reducing a fracture. The usual verbal formula for this kind of activity is that "the doctors are doing everything in their power to save the life (or limb) of the patient."

Illness gives rise to these four needs, and the maximization of one response at the expense of others may create a critical imbalance detrimental to the patient and society. The magical and religious responses are more, though not by any means exclusively, the province of religious specialists and philosophers, and the compassionate-pastoral and technical responses are more the central responsibilities of medical (including nursing) personnel. We might add that not only is there a great deal of "magical" behavior among medical personnel but that in the past, and to an important extent in the present, a great deal of medical care was provided under religious auspices, indicating the closeness of these needs. Comforting, in its etymological meaning of strengthening, is thus one of the essential tasks of medicine and of the physician, as Magraw (1968, p. 290) has pointed out. Comfort is a function that is perhaps even more important than that of curing or providing specific therapy, and yet it is one that has tended to be overshadowed as a result of an overemphasis on technology and the application of science. It is thus with the balance of the compassionate-pastoral and the technical responses that this paper will be centrally concerned, since they constitute, in my opinion, the core of the contemporary medical responsibility.

II. Societal Response to Illness: Structural Differentiation and the Health Care System

A comparative, evolutionary, and historical look at societal and individual response to illness and premature mortality suggests that, in primitive societies, this response was unspecific and undifferentiated, as were the social roles, collectivities, and facilities concerned with morbidity and mortality. There were, in these societies, no health specialists any more than there were full-time teachers and agricultural experts; neither were there clinics and sanatoria any more than schools, factories, temples, or parliaments. To the degree then that what we consider as medical functions were performed, they were performed by practically everybody (especially members of the family or kinship group) or not performed at all. Even today in our highly specialized and complex society, the family still retains some residual medical functions such as the care of sick children by the mother. By and large, however, in our society the provision of medical care has shifted to medical specialists and to settings outside the home. The relatively early emergence of medical specialists indicates the centrality of the human concern with health problems, since these were tied to life itself and the survival of human groups. We have already observed that the religious and the medical concerns were, in the past, often coterminous.

The practice of medicine as a full-time, specialized occupation, whether by itself or in conjunction with priestly functions, and the rise of an individual identified as a physician mark the beginning of the structural differentiation of medicine from other, more diffuse, and differentiated roles and structures (such as kinship) and lead to a series of important changes and necessary arrangements. First, there must obviously be individuals willing to engage in such work, and they must enjoy some degree of trust and confidence on the part of those they are called upon to treat. They must also have some specialized knowledge and techniques which other members of the population generally do not have, and which they acquire through apprenticeship or some other form of training. Finally, certain supports are required for the physician to practice *qua* physician, since he is prevented, by his occupation, from directly providing for his needs (food, clothing, housing, and so on). Thus, some arrangement must be made to *exchange* medical time for the economic support of the physician, as illustrated by Figure 1. Although the size of the income of the physician has often been questioned, particularly by those who consider his occupation a "calling" or "vocation" implying personal sacrifice, one cannot question the necessity for this income or some equivalent, since the physician cannot feed his family or pay his rent solely from the dewy-eyed gratitude of his patients.

Furthermore, in modern, industrial society, the increase in biomedical knowledge and its technological application lead to the emergence of complex tools and facilities with which and in which the physician applies his skill to the management of illness. The modern heavily instrumented hospital is prototypical of such facilities, and indeed is the most dramatic and sophisticated type. The existence of these facilities, and of the instrumentalities used in them, necessitates the rise of a wide array of occupational groups and supporting personnel whose function it is to assist and support the physician in providing medical services.

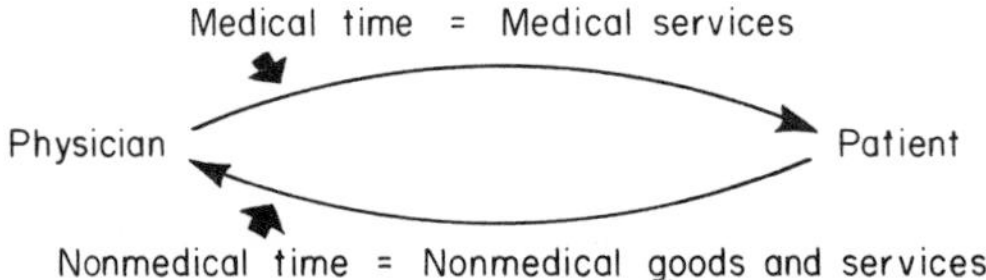

Figure 1. Exchange of medical and nonmedical time.

Modern society thus has a fully differentiated medical care system (or subsystem) that has boundaries (or boundedness); that is, it can be identified in the same way as the educational, economic, political, religious, family, and other systems can be identified and conceptualized. William Kissick (1968, p. 7) has pointed to the amazing diversity of that system:

It is represented by a multitude of resources, both human and material, and a myriad of services derived from these resources. It is composed of programs dealing with people and programs concerned with the facilities, programs related to services, research and educational activities. It requires the labors of physicians, dentists, nurses and other professional and technical health manpower, as well as clerical workers, janitors and so on. It encompasses hospitals, nursing homes, rehabilitation centers and health departments. It includes environmental control and biomedical research programs, the pharmaceutical industry, hospital and medical insurance plans, large national voluntary health agencies, small areawide planning councils. It is an interest of the federal, state and local governments and requires the participation of uncounted individuals from all walks of life. . . . It involves many secular endeavors—education, agriculture, commerce, recreation and conservation. . . . Finally it requires vast and increasing expenditures."

The expression "medical system" or "health care system" is meant as shorthand to designate that totality of efforts and resources, human and material, which a society (taken as the unit of analysis) sets aside for services centered around the health concern. As such, and in the aggregate, the medical system as conceptualized here provides a specialized service or output that is functionally relevant to the members of the society and to the society itself. In turn that system, because of its specialized nature and the narrow scope of its concerns, cannot be self-sufficient any more than can be the physician in full-time practice. Just like the physician, the medical system must receive specific inputs or resources in order to function. Conceptually, the medical system *converts* or *metabolizes* these nonmedical inputs or investments into a medical output or product. There are at least four analytically distinct inputs from society, analogous conceptually to those mentioned earlier with respect to the physician. They will be termed mandate and trust, knowledge, personnel, and instrumentalities.

MANDATE AND TRUST The medical system must receive a mandate from society to care for the health of its population, and it must enjoy the trust of that society. A charter is therefore granted to the medical system specifying its legitimate obligations and privileges. This charter often amounts to a monopolistic license, but it also implies that the medical system will perform its functions to the best of its abilities. This trust is fundamental in light of the life-and-death aspects of illness and the disastrous possibilities due to negligence as well as to the potentialities for the exploitation of the patient. Kerr L. White (1968a, p. 228) has said that society symbolically enters into a contract with medicine. This fiduciary commitment also implies, in many instances, that medicine will police its own house in return for a relatively free hand in most professional matters. Though it may be argued that as medicine, and particularly the work of the physician, becomes more visible (in hospitals, for example, with their tissue-review committees) and can increasingly be monitored in objective terms through computerized medical records, control over the physician's professional actions will increasingly be lodged outside the medical profession as a corporate body. The contract requires, furthermore, mechanisms that articulate the medical system and the rest of society, through spokesmen acceptable to both.

KNOWLEDGE The medical system cannot operate without a body of knowledge and techniques. That is, it requires accumulated cultural resources, the "state of the art," which must be transmitted from one generation of health personnel to another through an educational system which is itself tied to the general education of the society; and it must be added to, revised, and altered through the discovery of new or more advanced knowledge (research). This knowledge may be of a general scientific type, technical, or social-organizational, and it is affected not only by developments and research within the medical field but also to a very significant extent by the state of science, technology, and management in society at large.

PERSONNEL The medical system also requires a contingent of specialized individuals or personnel (physicians, nurses, orderlies, and so on) whose central occupational concern is health. These personnel must be motivated, recruited, taught, trained, socialized, and placed. They apply the results of research as well as the accumulated fund of knowledge, techniques, and technology to the solution of the society's health problems (prevention, diagnosis, clinical care, and rehabilitation); in the aggregate, they must be involved in research and education as well as in services.

INSTRUMENTALITIES In order to perform their mandate, health personnel must be provided with the necessary supports, powers, and instruments. Generally we can distinguish two broad categories of such instrumentalities: political instrumentalities, or the ability to use legitimate power and exercise authority; and economic instrumentalities that may range from an aspirin to a medical center, from the fee paid a physician to the fraction of the Gross National Product devoted to health.

It is thus possible to conceive, at the most general level, of the medical subsystem as providing a certain level of output ("services rendered and services consumed in connection with their work and under their direction" Fuchs 1968, p. 17) provided that it receives certain inputs or investments of the types outlined above. Schematically this might be illustrated as shown by Figure 2.

Of the four major inputs described earlier, two seem to play a major role in the changing nature of the medical system

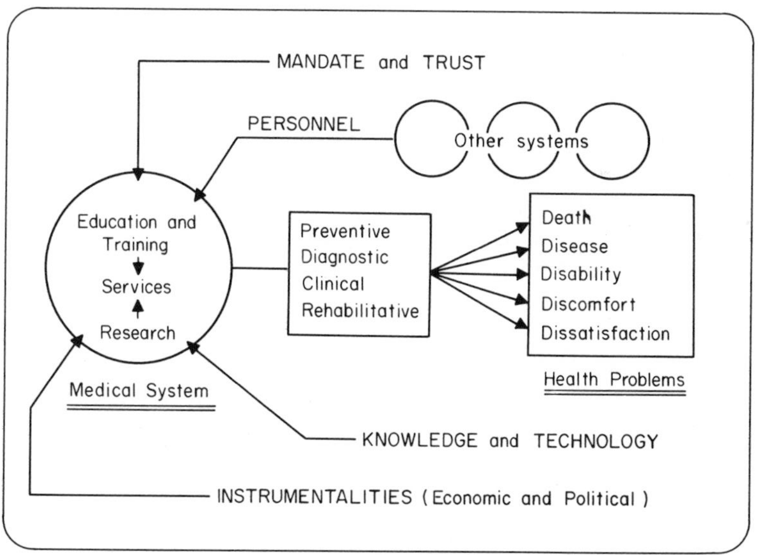

Figure 2. The social system and the medical system.

and medical services. The first is that of science, knowledge, and biomedical technology. This force is truly of revolutionary nature, and it accounts for many features of the contemporary medical system. The other factor, which is of equal significance, is the sheer increase in the effective demand by society for the application, distribution, and delivery of medical knowledge and technology in the form of ever more sophisticated medical services to an ever increasing proportion of the population. This broadened mandate, most often backed by political pressure, not only has ideological components such as equality of access for all citizens to medical care, but also significant functional (particularly economic) correlates.

These two forces account, to a large extent, for increased pressures on the two other inputs mentioned earlier—economic allocations as a percentage of the GNP and the demand for medical personnel as a percentage of the national labor force—particularly since health services, unlike industry, tend to be labor intensive rather than capital intensive. It often happens that the development of knowledge and technology, contrary to the experience of industry, instead of reducing the costs of medical services and the demand for labor, increases them as more personnel are needed to operate, monitor, and service the costly technology. As a result, the role that the society, through the polity, is called upon to play at the national, regional, and local levels gradually and significantly expands. This expansion occurs particularly in the establishment of priorities between competing systems, such as allocations to health as against education, welfare, transportation, housing, defense, and industrial expansion, and in the planning, administration, and collection and redistribution (primarily via taxation) of the necessary monies to finance these services.

Thus in most societies in the world today, and particularly in the industrial and urban ones, the medical care system has, as mentioned earlier, differentiated itself as a subsystem of society, a phenomenon that took place perhaps most dramatically and irrevocably in the nineteenth century with the advent of scientific medicine. Moreover, it presently is itself in a process of accelerated internal differentiation, and is moving from a relatively simple to a highly complex state. This process, as we shall see, has important implications both for the nature of the medical output available to the society and for the members of the population who are the individual recipients of that output, and who pay for it in economic resources, manpower, and political capital.

It may be in order, at this point, to specify what is meant by "differentiation." According to Robert Marsh (1967, pp. 31-32), differentiation is a property of societies and more generally of all social systems.

> It is both a state and a process. As a *state*, differentiation can be defined as the number of structurally distinct and functionally specialized units in a society . . . [such as] roles and collectivities. A society is therefore internally differentiated to the extent that it has numerous specialized roles and collectivities that perform complementary functions in the society. Differentiation . . . must be distinguished from segmentation, in which two or more structurally distinct roles or collectivities perform essentially the same *function*.
>
> As a *process*, differentiation has been defined as the "emergence of more distinct organs to fulfill distinct functions," and as the process of multiplication of one structural unit of a society into two or more structural units that function more effectively in the changed functional exigencies of the situation.
>
> [Furthermore,] differentiation, as state and process is the principal way in which societies (and social systems in general) adapt to their functional exigencies. . . . Changes in the functional exigencies . . . internal or external . . . may require an increase (or decrease) in the number of differentiated roles and collectivities.

Parallel to the qualitative process of differentiation through the specialization of medical and allied roles and of facilities, and partly associated with it, the medical system also experiences a quantitative expansion as the demand for services and hence for personnel increases. More and more personnel are called upon to perform more and more differentiated medical tasks.

The complexity and the size that result from differentiation and expansion may be deemed beneficial only to the degree that they improve the medical system's ability to fulfill the mandate with which it has been entrusted: to deliver an effective product enabling the society and its members better to cope with or master the environment by better dealing with its medical problems. It is difficult, and probably impossible, to make precise and categorical statements on the subject, given the vagueness of the term *mandate* and given the lack of control situations that would permit one to test for two situations, one of a relatively simple medical system, the other of a relatively complex one. This is more, perhaps, a problem for the imagination. The question would become, what would be the state of modern society, all things remaining equal, if, instead of having the kind of medical care system it has today, it had a relatively simple and small one, consisting primarily of physicians trained for general and solo practice as they were, let us say, a hundred years ago?

Note that I am not asking what would happen to contemporary society if, through some kind of strike, disabling illness, or widespread catastrophe that would affect health personnel, the health care system simply ground to a halt and stopped functioning altogether. Such a question might be easier to answer, within gross limits. But the point at issue here is that it is presumed that the differentiation and the increased size of the contemporary medical care system permit it to save more lives, to lengthen life expectancy, to reduce disability and suffering, to eliminate and mitigate many pathological conditions, and to increase the satisfaction of patients. It is my contention that such an assumption cannot, in any way, automatically be made. Differentiation and expansion, in turn, exact prices of their own that make the advantages of such a process problematic, or dependent, in turn, on other arrangements. I will return to these problems and dilemmas in greater detail in Part V. In brief, they are the problem of the assembly of ever increasing narrow outputs into a comprehensive medical product, the increasing chances for technical errors as the system becomes more complicated, and the more depersonalized nature of medical services that go with an advanced division of medical labor and the mounting bureaucratic nature of the medical system. But before these can be examined, it will be necessary to document briefly the evolution of the American medical system toward greater complexity.

IV. The Specialization of Medical Roles and Collectivities

Differentiation, as a phenomenon, is the result of increased specificity of functions and of specialization of roles. Specialization appears to be a hallmark of the contemporary medical system, and it accounts for its phenomenal success in the technical aspects, and for its equally disturbing failures in the area of compassionate care and the therapeutic or psychological support of the patient.

PROFESSIONAL ROLES At an earlier, simpler stage of the medical system, the physician, sometimes assisted by a nurse and a pharmacist, was at the center of the medical stage. Physicians, as such, constituted the vast majority, almost the totality, of the medical contingent. By virtue of his mandate the physician, although a specialist when compared to the other members of the population, was a generalist in medicine and provided almost the entire gamut of medical services. In the last fifty to seventy-five years, the rise of specialty practice within the medical profession has led to a process of differentiation among doctors and to the rise of a large contingent of medical personnel who are not physicians themselves, so that, at present, medical doctors constitute only a small fraction of those working in the medical system.

The first specialty board for physicians was established in 1916, and there were in 1966 over 30 specialties certified by some 20 boards, although legally a physician can simply declare himself a specialist and practice as such if he chooses. Equally significant is the fact that very few medical school graduates go into general practice today. In 1931 four-fifths of all American physicians were in general practice; in 1966 three-fourths of physicians were in specialty practice. According to Magraw (1966, pp. 145–149), the specialization of the entire physician population within another fifteen to twenty years, and perhaps sooner, is likely.

The drawings in Figure 3 are an attempt, not to scale, to represent the past, present, and predicted trends in the balance between general practitioners and specialists in medicine. The starting point, I, is a medical profession consisting almost exclusively of general practitioners, available to all comers and treating all conditions. In stage II, a small core of specialists has differentiated itself from the general practitioners, representing the picture after World War I. The proportion of specialists to all physicians is relatively small, and the number of recognized specialties is quite limited. In stage III, representing the picture toward the end of the 1960's, the specialists represent about three-fourths of all practicing physicians, and the number of specialties has grown from a few to more than 30. In stage IV, a projection of the future if the present trend continues,

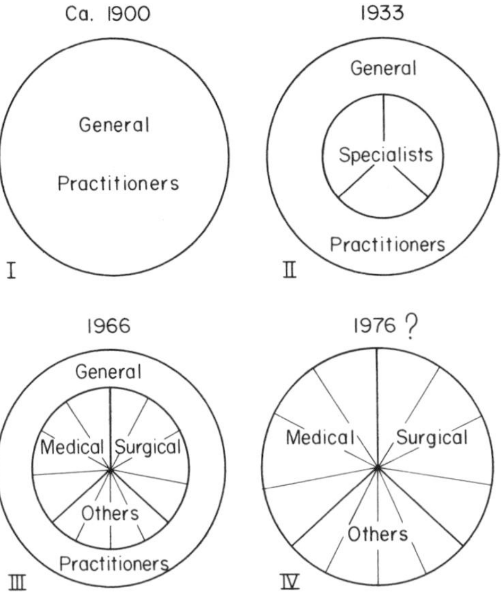

Figure 3. Generalists and specialists in medicine in the United States, 1900–1976.

the medical profession is made up entirely of specialists, the number of specialties and subspecialties is quite large, and the general practitioner is but a fond memory in the medical history books. It might even be tempting to try to predict what will happen after stage IV, let us say by 1984. One possibility is that the process will continue and that "super-specialists," as Kerr L. White calls them, will appear, continuing the trend toward increased differentiation, as illustrated by Figure 4.

ALLIED HEALTH ROLES The traditional characteristic of the physician's role was that he was a *solo* general practitioner. With the changes in the medical system outlined earlier, the physician now works with a team of other physicians and a whole array of allied health personnel. For example, the volume of medical *services* provided under the direction of physicians increased by about 80 percent between 1955 and 1965 in the United States, while the increase in the number of medical doctors has barely kept up, if at all, with population growth. This is due to the existence of an ever increasing number of different allied health personnel, many of whose occupations are due to new biomedical technologies which did not exist before World War II. Similarly, the fact that

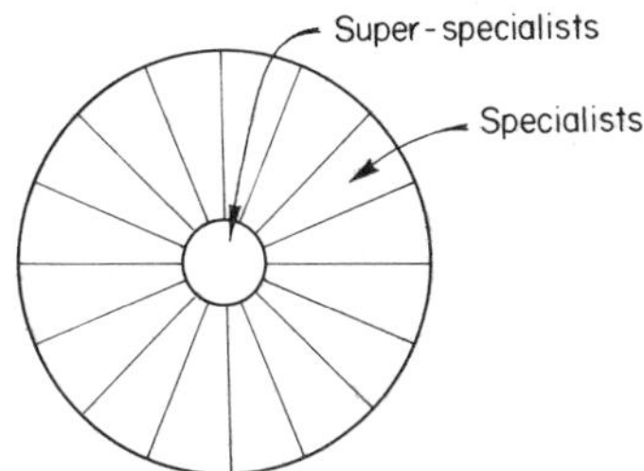

Figure 4. Generalists and specialsts in medicine in the United States, 1984.

the health industry is now the third largest out of 7 industries defined by the Bureau of the Census is due not to a radical expansion of the medical contingent, but to the increased numbers of allied health personnel. Between 1900 and 1960 the total number of such personnel has increased almost sixfold (5.78), while the number of physicians has not quite doubled (1.96). "Other health personnel" (all such personnel except physicians), on the other hand, increased more than 12 times, with the most dramatic rise being that of professional nurses: in 1900 there were 640 professional nurses in the United States and in 1960 there were over half a million professional nurses, an increase of almost 80,000 percent (787.5 times). In these years, as Table 1 shows, the proportion of physicians per 100 persons in all health professions has dropped by two-thirds (from 63 to 21).

In 1960, as seen in Table 2, physicians constituted less than 12 percent of all personnel in health (rather than only those in selected health professions).

NONMEDICAL ROLES IN THE MEDICAL CARE SYSTEM A third category of individuals who play a role of increasing importance in the health system are the nonmedical employees, whose activities are essential to the operations of the health system. The list of these personnel would be extensive. Rutstein (1967, p. 55) mentions the following few: "drug manufacturing employees, pharmacists' clerks, ambulance drivers, the electricians, plumbers, other maintenance workers, the housekeeping staff members in the hospital, and the secretaries of physicians. For obvious reasons, the boundaries of this group are difficult to define." Of the somewhat over 1.6 million people employed in the health service industries in 1950, about 500,000 persons were in

Table 1. Persons Employed in Selected Health Professions in the United States, in Decades, 1900–1960.

Year	All Health Professions	Physicians[1]	Other Health Personnel: Total	Dentists	Professional Nurses	Others[2]
	Number employed					
1900	197,140	123,500	73,640	29,700	640	43,300
1910	307,500	152,400	155,100	40,000	50,500	64,600
1920	408,700	151,300	257,400	56,200	103,900	97,300
1930	600,800	162,700	438,100	71,100	214,300	152,700
1940	692,400	174,500	517,900	71,000	284,200	162,700
1950	871,800	199,900	671,900	75,900	375,000	221,000
1960	1,139,500	242,500	897,000	87,000	504,000	306,000
Increase factor	5.78	1.96	12.18	2.92	787.5	7.11
	Physicians per 100 in all Health Professions		Number per 100 Physicians			
1900	63		60	24	1	35
1910	50		102	26	33	43
1920	37		170	37	69	64
1930	27		269	43	132	94
1940	25		297	41	163	93
1950	23		336	38	188	110
1960	21		370	36	208	126

[1] M.D. and D.O.
[2] Includes persons who are college educated or professionally trained among those employed as biological scientists, biostatisticians, chiropodists, chiropractors, clinical psychologists, dental hygienists, dietitians, health educators, health program specialists, medical laboratory technologists, medical record librarians, optometrists, pharmacists, rehabilitation counselors, sanitary engineers, social workers (medical and psychiatric), veterinarians, and therapists (occupation, physical, speech, and hearing).
Source: U.S. Public Health Service, *Chart Book on Health Status and Health Manpower,* Washington, D.C., 1961, p. 30.

occupations which are nonspecific to the health field. These occupations included about 70,000 stenographers, typists, and secretaries; 75,000 other "clerical and kindred" workers; 12,000 mechanics and repairmen; 18,000 laundry and dry cleaning operatives; 16,000 janitors and sextons; 30,000 cooks; almost 70,000 other service workers; as well as many persons in other occupations (Lerner and Anderson 1963, p. 2).

Problems of definitions make specification of health system

Table 2. Estimated Number of Physicians, Dentists, Professional Nurses, and Other Health Workers in the United States, 1960.

Health Field	Number	Percent	
All health workers	2,179,000	100.0	
Physicians (M.D. and D.O.)	256,000[1]	11.7	39.5
Dentists (D.D.S.)	101,000[1]	4.6	
Professional nurses (R.N.)	504,000	23.1	
Veterinarians (D.V.M.)	20,000[1]	0.9	25.8
Pharmacists (Pharm.D.)	120,000	5.5	
Scientists, therapists, technicians, and other medicial workers	423,000	19.4	
Dental hygienists, technicians, and assistants	115,000	5.3	5.3
Practical nurses	225,000	10.3	28.7
Attendants, orderlies, and aides	400,000	18.4	
Sanitary engineers	5,000	0.2	0.7
Sanitarians employed by health departments	10,000	0.5	

[1] Includes those retired. All other figures are for active workers.
Source: U.S. Public Health Service, *Chart Book on Health Status and Health Manpower,* Washington, D.C., 1961, p. 28.

personnel difficult. According to Lerner and Anderson (1963), of the estimated total of 2.5 million in the health service industries in 1960, 1.75 million belonged to what the census calls health occupations, of which there are 18 distinct types (nurses and student nurses, physicians and surgeons, dentists and medical and dental technicians, as well as others classified as professional, related, or kindred). The balance of about 750,000 would thus be in supportive occupations not specific to health, such as clerical personnel, maintenance workers, laundry employees, janitors and service employees (Lerner and Anderson 1963, p. 221). In 1965, it was estimated that the health manpower of the United States was between 2.87 and 2.90 million, distributed in no less than 35 fields.

As professionals and other health personnel begin to specialize, either because of knowledge and technology or because there is a need to manage an ever increasing number of personnel employed in the health system, many of them cease being generalists and upgraded themselves (or are promoted) to more specialized roles and occupations. As specialists they acquire a scarcity value, and their status and rewards increase accordingly as the scope of their concerns is narrowed and deepened, and as their contribution to the efficiency of the medical dimension, from the topmost super-specialists to the lowliest attendant or orderly, and it widens on the horizontal dimension as more specialties at about the same level of the hierarchy are added to perform new and numerous tasks.

Thus, if we represent *all* personnel involved in any aspect of the medical system graphically in terms of numbers relative to each other and of occupational or professional level or status, we can draw an everchanging pyramid. The top of the pyramid would be occupied by physicians, with professional nurses and other allied personnel below, and the base would be composed of workers in the health field. Over time one would see a vertical, as well as horizontal, proliferation of roles, as shown by Figure 5.

Furthermore, as those who formerly were generalists move into specialties and thereby limit their practices, their previous less specialized functions are vacated, although the need for such functions is in no way eliminated. Indeed, as will be suggested below, the very process of specialization seems to require a parallel process of dedifferentiation that is complementary to specialization. The vacancies created by specialization are filled in a variety of ways: personnel down the line, so to speak, may move up a notch and take

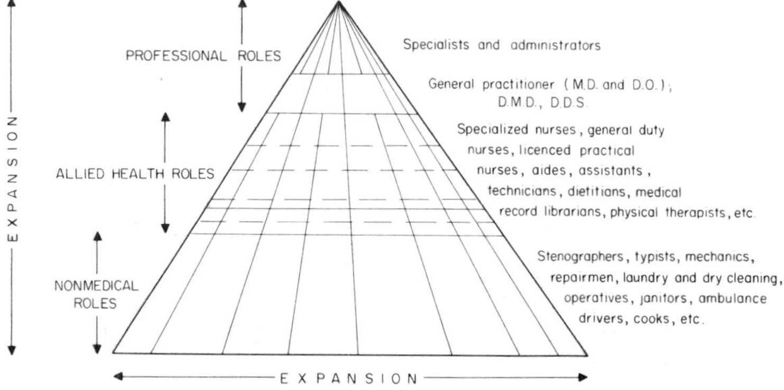

Figure 5. Health personnel.

over some of these functions. This occurs, for example, when nurses are entrusted with tasks that until then only physicians would perform; personnel may be imported from another society, as when physicians and nurses immigrate to the United States; some specialists engage in a kind of general practice, as internists and pediatricians sometimes do, at least in the United States; or the job may go by default, as when the general practitioners disappear from the ghetto areas and are not replaced by any functional equivalent.

The process described here often involves both a downward transfer of responsibilities (physician to nurse, nurse to licensed practical nurse, licensed practical nurse to nurses' aide) and a de-skilling of jobs to permit those with less formal training to perform tasks previously done by more skilled personnel. In New York City, for example, a training program has been instituted to permit nurses' aides to upgrade themselves to the level of licensed practical nurses because of the severe shortage of professional nursing personnel. As it is, in some of the municipal hospitals of that city, "unlicensed and untrained nurses' aides now administer oxygen, perform deliveries, work as obstetrical, radiological and operating room technicians and supervise wards in the city hospitals" (*The New York Times* 1966, p. 31).

The process we have briefly described is not likely to reverse itself in the continued expansion of knowledge, technology, and demand for medical services. For example, while the total civilian labor force increased by about 15 percent in the decade 1950–1960, and while the number in agriculture declined by 38 percent and those in construction by 10 percent, *those in the health service increased by 54 percent.* There is reason to believe that the health services are now the fastest growing segment of the total economy and will continue to be in the future (Magraw 1966, p. 166). The same phenomenon is also visible in Canada, where "the health service industry, one of the biggest in Canada, employs one Canadian in twenty, and ten other persons for each doctor" (Badgley and Wolfe 1967, p. 134). Projections into the future are even more striking, indicating that either health services or education will be the nation's largest consumer of manpower by 1970 (Somers 1968, p. 20). By 1975, according to Dr. Darrel J. Mase of the A.M.A.'s Council of Education, the physician will constitute only 4 percent of those employed in health services, and health may then employ 6,000,000 persons and constitute the nation's biggest industry (*Time Magazine* 1968 p. 36). At the same time as an index of the industrialization, or, as some call it, the institutionalization, of medicine, it should be noted that currently about three-fifths of all persons employed in health occupations are employed by hospitals or related institutions (Lerner and Anderson 1963, p. 219).

Indeed, the strategic role played by the hospital and other medical facilities in the medical system deserves much more attention than can be given in this paper. The modern hospital has become, in the last 50 years, the center of the medical world. Conceptually, furthermore, the process of specialization that has taken place in the medical profession may also be seen if the hospital is visualized as a kind of "collective physician" delivering a medical product. The process of specialization and differentiation between, for example, a community hospital and a research or special-diseases hospital will also require mechanisms such as regionalization and planning to make a more rational use of scarce facilities. The hospital will have, in the words of Cherkasky and Pines (1961, p. 116), "to limit itself to functions that cannot be performed elsewhere. It will concentrate on definitive diagnosis and definitive treatment, delegating all other medical care to closely associated but less expensive satellite facilities."

V. Differentiation and Depersonalization: Technology and the Alienation of the Patient

If the medical care system, under the impact of the twin factors of increased differentiation and quantitative expansion, becomes increasingly large and complex in its internal structure, certain consequences, problems, and dilemmas are produced. These occurrences can be traced in terms of systems theory and, more concretely, in terms of the specific nature of medicine and the kinds of services it gives and the needs it is expected by society and the patient to meet.

One of the prime implications of specialized functions and decreased generalist activities is the necessity for mechanisms that will integrate the increasingly narrow discrete outputs of specialized roles and collectivities into a comprehensive and effective product through planning, organization, integration, management, traffic control, transportation, and communication. The more costly the specialized outputs, the greater the strategic importance of a rational use of these resources to ensure the most equitable functionally adequate deployment of personnel and facilities.

Thus, the first major prerequisite of a differentiated system is the appropriate assembly of the specialized outputs. This entails management, hierarchy, lines of authority, subordination and superordination, and eventually some kind of bureaucratization. The seeds of several important problems are inherent in such needs. One of these, and perhaps from the traditional medical viewpoint (with its Hippocratic legacy of individual responsibility) the most vexing, is that organization and management imply a process in which the physician both becomes part of a larger bureaucratic structure and sees his independence and status threatened by outside forces. At the same time, he himself becomes the manager of a team of professional, semiprofessional, and nonprofessional medical and allied health personnel. The net result, particularly of the second process, is to reduce the time available for direct patient contact. In the aggregate, the proportion of physicians in administration has risen in the last few years. It will presumably continue to rise as the managerial functions of doctors expand at about the same rate as the size and the complexity of the medical system, unless doctors become increasingly willing to delegate these tasks to nonphysicians, which would be a further process of differentiation with its own problems and dangers.

Organization and management have further implications for the two medical needs of the patient outlined earlier, the compassionate and the technical. The technical aspect of medical care, as a result of specialization, differentiation, and allied phenomena, allows an ever greater possibility for error in the chain of activities (the "medical assembly line") as the number of individuals per patient involved in care and treatment increases. Potential conflicts may arise from the need to reach quick decisions (as when a private patient is under the care of the hospital staff and the patient's physician cannot be reached immediately, or when the staff hesitates on whether to bother the physician with what might be considered a trifle), or from the manner in which the instructions of the physician are carried out (for example, in medications), or from errors that are overlooked in the process, and so on. At the same time, the increased number of personnel who handle a patient also has serious implications for the fate of the patient, and particularly for the pastoral element, which I hold is a fundamental component of good medical care.

We can dispose, at the outset, of the argument that in a life-or-death situation the impersonal but effective physician and machine are to be preferred over the tender ministrations of a physician who can only sit through the night at the bedside of a dying patient, and who is powerless to affect the course of illness but who is wise in the ways of comforting the dying. In most instances one can presume that the situation is not that dramatic, and that short shrift often will be given to the patient's emotional needs, though everyone seems to agree that these needs are important. This phenomenon is already highly visible in the heavily instrumented hospital of today. The hospital is, in essence, a kind of medical factory and assembly line in which the patient, because he has the lowest seniority on the hospital totem pole, is sometimes handled as an object to be processed, as a disease inside a human skin, as an interesting diagnostic or scientific problem, or good teaching material, but not necessarily as a flesh-and-bone individual. This malaise is compounded by the fact that the patient is manipulated, percussed, exhibited, trundled, cut into, connected to tubes, swabbed, and wrapped, all the while moving from one person to another.

Thus, as the medical system becomes more technologically advanced, and as more units, personnel, and collectivities become involved in fashioning the ultimate product (the medical service), the more depersonalized or fragmented that product is likely to appear to the recipient and the beneficiary. The understanding of and control of the patient over the process decreases, and the feeling of alienation of the sick man increases. The industrialization or institutionalization of medicine, although increasing the technical efficiency of the service, produces many of the consequences that have been noted for a century or more for industrial workers. It is an alienation, however, of a special medical kind, intensified by the peculiarities of illness and disability and the anxieties related to suffering and possible death. In describing the "maze" through which "consumers wander in search of services to meet their own ideas of need," observers of the contemporary American medical scene have noted that indeed this fragmentation not only detracts from the quality and the continuity of care, but also substantially adds to the overall costs (Stewart 1968, p. 158).

At the same time, to the degree that general practitioners upgrade themselves into specialty practices, and to the degree that no functional equivalents take their place, the loss of the general practitioner is likely to present a serious problem to the patient. It is, of course, the opinion of some that what patients really want is the best technical medical care available and that they will be satisfied when they get it. It is my contention, on the other hand, that the need for the general practitioner (sometimes referred to as the family doctor or primary physician, and defined as the individual responsible for primary care, continuity of care, personal health services, and reassurance to the patient [Rutstein 1967, p. 132]) or some appropriate functional equivalent, has by no means been made obsolete by the increased differentiation, technological orientation, and complexity of the contemporary medical care system. Indeed, the general practitioner may be needed now more than ever.

The process of "upgrading" has been noted for both professionals, as when physicians limit their practice to a specialty, and for semiprofessionals, as when a nurse decides that her role is to see that nursing is done rather than to do it herself. This process depends, naturally, on the availability of less skilled personnel who can with some ease be moved upward into the vacated slots, such as nurses' aide to licensed practical aide, to whom "de-skilled" functions are transferred downward. The process is perhaps not quite the same for physicians as it is for semiprofessional personnel for the reason that *there is no one with medical professional training who stands below the general practitioner.* If one reaches below the GP to scoop someone with medical training who could fit into the physician's shoes, there is, in truth, no one with these qualifications. The upshot is that the functions of the general practitioner are often not being performed by a medical person; or that someone else, without appropriate professional qualifications, steps into that role and performs like a generalist. This is what, to some degree, is taking place in the American medical system. We must, however, attempt to justify why, in an era of specialization and superspecialization, in a system that increasingly relies on automation, computers, and machinery and thus will become technologically increasingly efficient, the generalist role or some adequate functional substitute is important and may not be easily disposed of.

We have already examined, or at least adduced, some reasons for the continuing need for a general practitioner. In the most general terms, illness, by its very nature, gives rise to the need for psychological support and pastoral or compassionate care, and the specialist, by the very nature of his limited mandate, and even though he has had the standard medical training of all physicians, is simply not ready, or perhaps not equipped, to provide that kind of care. And perhaps, in the age of specialization, there is a tendency on the part of physicians faced with an anxious or demanding patient to suggest that he go to another specialist in these matters—the specialist in psychological matters, the psychiatrist—a suggestion the patient may well take as a rejection. Furthermore, it is quite likely that the specialist sees himself as having made large investments in financial resources and time, resulting in a delayed entry into remunerative work, in order to acquire his specialty, and he is thus inclined to get the highest return on his investment by practicing exclusively as a specialist and not engaging in work that does not require his particular expertise. But there are other issues, of a more structural or organizational nature, that come to the fore as a result of the disappearance of general practice. Briefly, they are the following.

ACCESS, DIAGNOSIS, AND PRIMARY CARE: One major characteristic of traditional medical practice in the community was the physician's high visibility and continuous availability. The hanging of the shingle was a symbolic act, signifying to the community that at this identifiable and known geographical location, at almost any time, one could find a doctor, and that medical ethics dictated that claims for primary medical care could not be turned down on any grounds. In this respect, and even though in most instances the physician was in private practice as a member of a liberal ("free") profession, he was a "public servant" in the fullest sense of the words. This meant that in most instances people in the community knew where to find a doctor.

The "open door" also meant, in simplest terms, that the patient could get into the medical system with the least amount of fuss, bother, and barriers, and that he could obtain preliminary diagnosis and care and any further steps which were needed. The patient was thus introduced by his GP to the health care system, however rudimentary that system might have been. With the absolute and proportional decline of general practice in the community, particularly in the underprivileged neighborhoods (the core city and ghettos), and with the exodus of physicians to the suburbs, the potential patient has lost this important portal of entry into the medical system, although substitutes have tended to develop. Moreover, it seems to be a growing phenomenon that even those physicians who remain in general practice in the community often make themselves unavailable during evenings and weekends, a phenomenon described as "5 o'clock medicine" (Helpern 1962).

The importance of the role of the generalist has also been emphasized, as when Badgley and Wolfe (1967, p. 134) commented of the general practitioner in Great Britain, "No health service, private or public, can succeed unless careful attention is paid to the doctor who provides primary care in the community. All other decisions depend on what he decides when the patient is first seen." In the United States, as Jensen and many others observed, despite an annual expense of about 40 billion dollars, the nonavailability of primary care is a common complaint. Although the population has become accustomed to the miracles of modern medical technology, for most people "the greatest medical need is for someone to provide primary medical care for the common maladies" (Jensen 1967, p. 382).

ALLOCATION OR TRIAGE A further, though analytically distinct, aspect of the access and diagnosis problem is particularly important in a highly differentiated and complex medical care system: the question of allocating or directing the patient to the appropriate facilities and specialized personnel who can help him best. This function is seen, perhaps in its sharpest form, during disasters or on the battlefield in the role of the *triage* officer, who in essence makes a summary judgment as to where the patient must be sent next.

The absence of such a role means that patients who need specialized care may not get the right kind of care at the right place at the right time.

At this point, one might also add that the allocative functions usually played by a general practitioner are a necessary complement to specialization. For the GP (or *triage* officer, or whatever one might call this role) has, or should have, a fairly accurate cognitive map of the medical care environment, its resources, strengths, weaknesses, and gaps, and can thus refer patients to the appropriate personnel and facilities. The nonperformance of this role may thus have important negative implications in terms of the nonutilization or misutilization by the patient of available medical resources, a problem that is often compounded by the multiplicity of jurisdictions in the medical system, and by questions of eligibility and selection by hospitals of only certain patients who contribute to their research and teaching functions.

COMPREHENSIVENESS AND CONTINUITY The general practitioner did not only "care for" an individual rather than a condition, organ, or organ system; he often also cared for the patient's entire family by calling at the patient's home and knowing the different members of the family. In addition, through his familiarity with the community in which he lived and worked, the physician could obtain a good picture of the social, economic, and psychological environment in which his patients lived, and the kinds of general pressures and demands they were subject to. The increasingly "scientific" nature of medicine, with its search for the etiological agent in chemical or biological terms, has contributed to deflecting the physician's attention away from the total social and psychological situation of the patient. Further, shifting the locus of medical care to the hospital presents the patient to the physician as an isolated specimen rather than as a person involved in a multiplicity of social relationships, some of which have a bearing on the illness process. Finally, the rapport between the general practitioner and his patient or patient's family permitted, in theory at least, some continuity of care through the different and changing phases of illness, a continuity that often gets lost in the shuffle caused by specialization and by having the same patient treated by various personnel.

INTEGRATION OF CARE AND REASSURANCE OR COMPASSION: Insofar as the general practitioner considered the patient as "his" patient—that is, his *personal* medical responsibility—he could play the role of director or supervisor of the different and specialized medical services his patient was receiving. The physician could call for this or that test or procedure, he could run interference for the patient through the medical maze, and in general he could keep on top of his patient's medical progress while at the same time keep him informed and reassured. In this context, the hospital was the physician's own workshop, replacing either the patient's home (and the somewhat unsatisfactory kitchen table as operating room) or the physician's ill-equipped office or private clinic. What happened to the patient, inside or outside the hospital, was the physician's responsibility, and he had the opportunity to supervise closely what other medical personnel were doing to, or for, his patient. And if he used the services of a consultant, or later on of a specialist, he was still personally organizing the care of his patient. The disappearance of the generalist threatens this function, and failure to replace it by an appropriate functional substitute increases the possibility of error, duplication, lack of proper care, and the isolation of the patient.[1]

I have very briefly examined some of the functions performed in the past by the general practitioner in medicine, and I have raised the question whether failure to replace him would seriously impair the nature and the quality of the medical product delivered to the patient. Indeed, contemporary medicine may, in a symbolic way and seen from the viewpoint of the patient, often be represented as a kind of closed system, a fortress surrounded by walls and barriers. Within the medical compound, the ordinary patient frequently finds a highly confusing and disturbing labyrinth, a Kafka-like medical maze, often what we might call the "medicine of the absurd": technological sophistication and

[1] This is reflected in the following familiar story: A caller phoned the hospital asking the condition of a Mrs. Brown in room 550. After calling the correct hospital floor and getting a report from the nurse, the hospital operator said, "Mrs. Brown is progressing quite well. Her behavior is normal. As a matter of fact, she will be discharged in a few days. May I know who is calling?" The caller answered, "This is Mrs. Brown in room 550 whose doctor never tells her anything." ("Smiling Psychiatry," *American Journal of Psychotherapy,* 22 [October 1968], p. 736.)

the dehumanized handling of the recipients of this sophistication. The patient thus needs both a helping hand in finding the appropriate portal into the medical system (that is, a generalist in the community) as well as a guide within the medical system who will lead him from room to room and procedure to procedure, who will try to make the experience less frightening and more meaningful, and who will speak on behalf of the patient. If a man in court is entitled to counsel, a patient in the hospital is also entitled to an ombudsman. And the more complex and differentiated the medical system, the greater the alienation of the patient, and the greater his need for compassion and understanding.

Space and time do not permit a consideration of the substitutes to the vanishing general practitioner that have tended to arise, or of the controversy surrounding proposals for the training of several types of physicians, including a new type of comprehensive physician who would provide the primary care that is part of general practice. But it may be added that the greater the technological sophistication of medicine, that is, the greater its differentiation, the more important is the process of *dedifferentiation* in the structure of the medical system to permit it to perform satisfactorily its mandate task of "care" in the dual sense of efficiency of treatment and compassion toward the patient. Finally, it was not my intent in any way to idealize or romanticize the general practitioner, especially since his medical competence has often been questioned, and with good reason. Rather, my point was to show that in the light of the fundamental structural changes attendant on specialization, the general practitioner or some equivalent has a critical role to perform in the total picture of a sophisticated medical system.

VI. The Medical System and Society: Some Future Trends

An attempt to project certain future aspects of the medical system by projecting trends of the immediate past suggests, at least, the following developments.

1. There will be continuing increased complexity of the medical care system as a result both of biomedical technology and its application, and of effective political and economic demand for medical services, coupled with the recognition of the functional importance of these services. The changes in the medical system will presumably be similar in intensity and quality to those that have led to the

demise of the corner grocery store and its replacement by the supermarket, or the one-room schoolhouse by the modern high school, or the backyard plant by the automated factory.

2. A greater role will be played by public agencies in the medical care system, and public monies will have increased importance in the support of the many activities of the medical care system, including education and research in addition to the services themselves. The following trends, identified by Falk (1967, p. 6), characterize the prospective role of the polity in the health field: (1) financial underwriting to assure availability of health services to the entire population, either through contributory insurance, taxation, or both; (2) the development of procedures and standards to safeguard the quality of services financed through public funds; (3) the provision of services through nongovernmental practitioners and institutions insofar as they effectively cooperate with public authorities; (4) extension toward comprehensiveness in the publicly financed services; (5) direct financial support for the modernization, construction, and equipment of needed facilities and for the education and training of needed personnel.

3. There will be a growing need for a more rational and economical utilization of increasingly scarce and costly personnel and capital resources—that is, for increasing need for planning at several levels: community, regional, areawide, state, and federal. This will necessitate, first, a better and sharper definition or redefinition of the goals of the health system, in light of the already existing multiplicity of agencies and uncoordinated goals and activities. As Sigmond (1967, p. 118) has stated, "the chief problem in the health-care field centers around lack of systematic attention to goals. Each element appears to have a multiplicity of goals, often poorly conceptualized, with little coordination of interrelationships and priorities. In part this is due to the changing technological and social base in which health care rests. Without explicit formulation and definition of goals, there are inevitable overlapping, duplication, gaps and inefficiencies." This coordinating task, in turn, will require agencies or "bureaucratic" organizations of the medical system for the delivery of services which, in general, "has not kept pace with the advances of science."[2]

[2] It may be noted that the Department of Health, Education, and Welfare

One might expect, in the next decade or two, that the increasing bureaucratization of the medical care system will run against the traditional autonomy of the physician and and voluntary hospital, and will necessitate delicate negotiations and adjustments on both sides.

4. There will be a further evolution of professional roles in the medical care system, marked particularly by the decline and perhaps eventual disappearance of the solo and entrepreneurial practice that was traditional in the nineteenth century. In the words of R. H. Ebert, Dean of the Harvard Medical School, "the omnipotence of the individual physician in providing for all the needs of his patient has been lost" (Ebert 1967). One consequence of this decline will be the decrease of personal contact between physician and patient, a topic to which I shall return.

5. The institutionalization of medical care resulting from the shifting of the locus of medical services to the hospital (the medical supermarket) and the increase in specialty practices will continue.

6. Increased significance will be given to planning, and also to assessing the effectiveness of the health system, in light of the fact that such assessment has been, for a variety of reasons, singularly lacking in the past. As Kerr White (1968b, p. 95) reminds us, there is probably no other enterprise of comparable importance that spends so little in evaluating its operations. It must also be clear that the planning and licensing of facilities and the use of medical personnel will have to proceed, after a most careful analysis, on the basis of the health interests of the population served "rather than institutional autonomy or the convenience and disposition of individual physicians" (*Recommendation of the Committee on Hospital Effectiveness* 1968, p. 16).

7. In line with the increase in planning, there will be a gradual reduction of the importance of market mechanisms in determining investments in health personnel and capital, and increased importance in administrative mechanisms to assure a better and more effective deployment of health resources throughout the nation in accordance with needs.

has completed plans to establish a National Center for Health Services Research and Development in order "to improve the quality, availability, accessibility and effectiveness of health services to make the full potential of medical science available to all citizens" (*Conference on Medical Costs*, 1968, p. xii). This center began operation in 1969.

This will, in turn, affect the nature of the relationship between the society and its health care system in the near future in the following directions.

(a) In light of the increased national significance of health, the formulation of health policies at the federal, state, and community levels will probably become more and more systematic; health policies will thus provide guidelines and frameworks rather than directives.

(b) The problem of priorities, and within that problem, the question of allocations of limited resources, will mean that priorities will have to be established in a competitive situation, and difficult choices will have to be made. It is becoming increasingly clear to Americans that even with their huge national resources there are limitations on what can be done. Such priority establishment will necessitate the cooperation not only of those in the health services, but also of the polity and the recipients of such services.

(c) There will be a problem of the equitable distribution of services in light of a demand greater than a supply, with special reference to claims for high quality services for all that cannot be satisfied in medicine any more than in education. There will be, furthermore, other important issues that will arise in connection with the distribution of health services, particularly when rare supplies such as organs for transplantation and complex and expensive medical equipment are involved, and when the decision of who is and who is not going to be helped must be made. These issues transcend the purely medical area and have moral, legal, and religious implications. Thus, the question of the *locus* of decision in these matters will need resolution: is this to be a strictly professional medical matter, as has been the case with abortion committees, or is the deciding agency to have a broader representation from the legal, religious, and other professions as well as representatives of the polity?

(d) The problem of the invasion of privacy or potential loss of privileged communication resulting from a more extensive use of written records and more personnel, central files, and computers will grow. Thus, one important question is whether there is a sharp conflict between concerns for the health and welfare of the population, and liberty, privacy, and civil rights.

(e) There is a potential problem of behavior control

through biomedical technology. Although at the present time there is some doubt that such control will become feasible in the near future, it is still possible. The question then is one of safeguards; it seems that the professional ethic in medicine, and the trust that society has placed in the profession, provide an appropriate precedent and possible guidelines for control over possible control of behavior. The medical profession, at the present, is already given a mandate that affects the life and the health of patients. Could this mandate be extended to safeguard the manipulation of control devices if these become effective, or should some other mechanisms be contemplated?

(f) The problem, mentioned earlier, of the relationship between the public and the medical system will continue. This will imply, among other things, the recognition that the traditional solo practitioner-patient relationship has been profoundly altered by changes in the technology of medicine, and that these changes have affected communications between the patient and those who take care of him. Furthermore, as more and more of the resources necessary for the performance of the health system will be drawn from tax monies, the public or its representatives will be increasingly concerned with the expenditure of these funds.

Although these issues have been drawn from the American scene, and although the American situation certainly has many unique features, the issues are generally related to forces that are present in most of the medical systems of modern industrial society and are therefore not limited to one social system.

VII. The Present and Continuing Malaise in the Society-Medicine Relationship

If every advance made by man also exacts a price from him, it can then be said that one of the major consequences or "prices" of the introduction of science and its technological applications into medicine has been the depersonalization, alienation, or estrangement of the patient. In one sense, the problem of alienation is endemic in a highly differentiated society of the industrial or postindustrial type, and the individual, in his role as a patient, is confronted with the same general phenomenon as in many of his other roles. Yet it might be proposed that the alienation of the individual *qua* patient is perhaps more difficult to bear than that in most other roles because of the peculiarities of illness and the precariousness of the patient's psyche. The pastoral or compassionate element that had loomed, traditionally, as so important in medicine has diminished under the onslaught of biomedical progress, and tends to be relegated to still another specialty, psychiatry.

It is truly tragic when the patient, in whose interest the medical system has supposedly been established, subjectively feels that he is the low man on the medical totem pole, the forgotten man of medicine, even though one might argue that objectively he receives far better care than he would have fifty or a hundred years ago. The distance between the patient and the doctor, the lack of communication and compassion, cannot but have a negative impact on the medical enterprise. W. McPeak (1959) formerly a vice president of the Ford Foundation, expressed this in the following words: "At the present time, patients feel subordinated by the doctors, not only medically, but also personally. Too often the doctor strikes them as either insensitive or indifferent. Anyone knows of several poignant incidents resulting from such attitudes, and hears of many more. What undoubtedly is involved is a change in demeanour which has come with a change in professional role. As the doctor becomes more the specialized scientist, there necessarily follows a narrowing of the base for human contact. No one doubts that the shift in medicine has brought more gains than losses, but the gains do not permit us to ignore the losses, especially when the latter are so much in the patient's sphere. We must remember what medical care is all about and that the word 'care' has a human, as well as a technical meaning."

The increase in the costs and complexity of health care will force a system of organization that, in many of its aspects, is destructive of the personal doctor-patient relationship while, at the same time, it promises a more rational, more efficacious, more economical, and technologically better medical system. The deemphasis of the personal and sometimes the sociological factors in illness has tended to alter the "mix" in the medical care system in the direction of greater concern about the organic, except in some parts of psychiatry. This alteration may be at the root of a great deal of malaise in the society and in the medical profession at this juncture, and the cause of the near rupture of the dialogue between the two.

And this problem, furthermore, comes precisely at a stage when society is becoming, or has become, increasingly impersonal. The physician traditionally has been the one professional with whom the individual could establish a relationship of intimacy outside his family. The withdrawal of the physician, through specialization, from that role means a further decrease of "lightning rods" for the personal problems and may well affect the emotional balance of society. The ambivalence of the public toward medicine and the medical profession is a revealing aspect of that dislocation. On the one hand, admiration is directed at the scientific and technological achievements of medicine and its "miracles"; on the other hand, there is a fair amount of hostility toward the medical profession in terms of the kinds of incomes and other rewards they are able to garner and display, their apparent decreasing interest in their individual patients, their unwillingness to make house calls, their brusque behavior and crowded waiting rooms. The dean of the Harvard Medical School has stated that a cursory review of what has been written about medicine and the physician in newspapers and in weekly and monthly magazines permits the conclusion that "medical science comes off rather well and the doctor's image not so well. One gains the impression that doctors as a group are motivated by money, are becoming less and less interested in patients as people, and are socially irresponsible" (Ebert 1967).

There is little doubt, as mentioned earlier, that anyone would want to go back to a simpler, more primitive, and less effective medical system for the sake of its "pastoral" component. And yet, there is also little doubt that the loss of that element is at the source of a great deal of discomfort. "Even the best balanced medical care system is unsatisfactory if it does not meet the personal needs of the patient. In my view, the personal evaluation of the patient and his guidance and reassurance by his physician (and by other medical personnel) must continue to be a major attribute of medical care. Indeed, any successful system of medical care interrelating the activities of physicians, other medical personnel, and machines must have as *the* essential ingredient 'tender, loving care'" (Rutstein 1967, p. 96).

One might add that to the degree to which the medical care system fails to provide the supportive element, however well instrumented, automated, and cyberneticized that system may have become, the medical product provided by it will be unsatifactory, or at best incomplete. The fissure that runs between the human and the technological-scientific aspects of medicine may well reflect, in essence, two "cultures," each with its peculiar orientation. One might be called the Hippocratic culture, the other the "scientific" culture. This dichotomy runs like a leitmotif through a great deal of the literature concerned with these matters. Furthermore, it should be emphasized that attention to the pastoral or compassionate aspect of medical care may not be a "luxury" or a "frill" but a basic aspect of adequate medical "care."

The final question that must be tackled in an examination of the impact of biomedical technology and demand on medicine, and thus on society, may be asked as follows. Given the functional need for medical services, how does the contemporary medical care system acquit itself of its mandated task, and more precisely, what is the balance in the final analysis of the following chain of events: need for medical care → demand for medical care and societal response through the medical care system → impact of science and technology on that medical care system → fulfillment both of society's needs and patients' medical (technical) and emotional demands → changes in the society resulting from the intervention of the medical care system (demographic, political, legal, economic). Or, seen from a somewhat different vantage point, have the means of medical production and the exchange of medical products been so affected by science and technology that they have altered the patient-doctor relationship to the dysfunctional point of revolt? In light of past experience, and of the trend toward differentiation noted earlier, it is therefore possible to argue that, in the future, medicine may well be formally split into at least two major streams, with at least two types of physicians, trained under different conditions and performing different and complementary tasks: on the one hand, the specialists and superspecialists who increasingly will tend to speak a *universal* tongue of science and technology that will become increasingly meaningless (in the therapeutic sense) to the patient, and on the other, general practitioners (and psychiatrists) who will speak in the *particular* cultural and social language of the patient, who will address themselves to the individual as a person, and will act as the patient's medical ombudsman.

Although one might deplore a further differentiation within the medical system, the basic structural changes that have accompanied the unfolding of that system in the last hundred years or so seem to suggest that such an informal differentiation has already taken place and that the failure to acknowledge the significance of this differentiation can only increase the chasm between the medical system and the social system. In an evolutionary perspective one can view such a differentiation not so much as a deplorable breaking of the unity of medicine, but rather as increasing society's adaptive response to the physical and the psychological inroads of illness, incapacity, and premature mortality.

References

Badgley, Robin F., and Samuel Wolfe
(1967), *Doctors' Strike.* Toronto: Macmillan.
Cherkasky, M., and M. Pines
(1961), "Tomorrow's Hospitals." In M. K. Sanders (ed.), *The Crisis in American Medicine.* New York: Harper.
Ebert, R. H.
(1967), "Social Responsibility and the Education of the Physician." Eastman Memorial Lecture, University of Rochester, November 10. Mimeograph.
Falk, I. S.
(1967), "Medical Care in a University Teaching Program for Hospital Administration." *Medical Care, 5,* 1, 3–8.
Fuchs, V. R.
(1968), "Basic Factors Influencing the Costs of Medical Care." In *Report of the National Conference on Medical Costs.* Washington, D.C.: U.S. Government Printing Office.
Helpern, M.
(1962), "Inaugural Address to the Medical Society, County of New York." Reported in the *New York Times,* October 6, 1962.
Jensen, R. T.
(1967), "The Primary Medical Care Worker in Developing Countries." *Medical Care, 5,* 6, 382–400.
Kissick, W. L.
(1968), Foreword to "Dimensions and Determinants of Health Policy." *The Milbank Memorial Fund Quarterly, 46,* 1, 7–12.
Lerner, M., and O. Anderson
(1963), *Health Progress in the United States, 1900–1960.* Chicago and London: University of Chicago Press.
McPeak, W.
(1959), "The Small Frantic Voice of the Patient." Paper delivered at

dedicatory exercises, Stanford University Medical Center, September 17. Quoted in Badgley and Wolfe (1967), *Doctors' Strike.* Toronto: Macmillan. P. 158.
Magraw, R. M.
(1966), *Ferment in Medicine.* Philadelphia: Saunders.
——— (1968), "The Purchase of Health Care—Payments, Controls, Quality." In *Report of the National Conference on Medical Costs,* Washington, D.C.: U.S. Government Printing Office.
Marsh, R.
(1967), *Comparative Sociology.* New York: Harcourt, Brace and World.
Miller, J. G.
(1965), "Living Systems: Basic Concepts." *Behavioral Science, 10,* 3 (July), 193–237.
New York Times (1966), "Training Planned for Nurses' Aides." March 30.
Parsons, T.
(1951a), *The Social System.* Glencoe: Free Press. Pp. 428–479.
——— (1951b), "Illness and the Role of the Physician: A Sociological Perspective." *American Journal of Orthopsychiatry, 21,* 452–460.
——— (1957), "The Mental Hospital as a Type of Organization." In M. Greenblatt, D. J. Levinson, and R. H. Williams (eds.), *The Patient and the Mental Hospital.* New York: Free Press. Pp. 108–129.
——— (1958), "Definition of Health and Illness in the Light of American Values and Social Structure." In E. Gartly Jaco (ed.), *Patients, Physicians and Illness.* New York: Free Press.
——— (1960, "Some Trends of Change in American Society: Their Bearing on Medical Education." In *Structure and Process in Modern Societies.* Glencoe: Free Press. Pp. 280–294.
———, and Renée Fox
(1952), "Illness, Therapy and the Modern American Family." *The Journal of Social Issues, 8,* 2–3, 31–44.
Recommendation of the Committee on Hospital Effectiveness to the Secretary of the Dept. of Health, Education, and Welfare (1968). Washington, D.C.: U.S. Government Printing Office.
Report of the National Conference on Medical Costs (1968). Washington, D.C.: U.S. Government Printing Office.
Rutstein, D. D.
(1967), *The Coming Revolution in Medicine.* Cambridge: M.I.T. Press.
Sigmond, R. M.
(1967), "Health Planning." *Medical Care, 5,* 3 (May–June), 117–128.
Somers, A. R.
(1968), "Some Basic Determinants of Medical Care and Health Policy." *Milbank Memorial Fund Quarterly, 46* (January), 13–31.
Stewart, W. H.
(1968), "The Challenge to the Nation." In *Report of the National Conference on Medical Costs.* Washington, D.C.: Government Printing Office.
Time Magazine (1968), "Medicine." March 1, p. 36.
White, K. L.
(1961a), "Organization and Delivery of Personal Health Services: Public Policy Issues." *The Milbank Memorial Fund Quarterly, 46,* 1, 225–258.
——— (1968b), "Research in Medical Care and Health Services Systems." *Medical Care, 6,* 2 (March–April), 95–100.

Frank Baker and Herbert C. Schulberg

8. Community Health Care-Giving Systems

Integration of Interorganizational Networks

Considerable attention has been focused in recent years on federal and state cooperation in planning and organizing comprehensive health services at the community level. Following the report of the Joint Commission on Mental Illness and Health in 1960, Congress made available money for two-year grants to finance comprehensive mental health planning at the state level as the first step toward the development of community-based programs. Since the completion of the state programs for planning comprehensive mental health programs in 1965, considerable effort and funds have been expended in constructing and staffing comprehensive community mental health centers and improving existing mental hospitals.

In 1966 Congress enacted the Comprehensive Health Planning and Public Health Service Amendment which became Public Law 89–749. By this law the federal government authorized each state to establish a single agency which would develop an approach to comprehensive health planning so as to obtain federal support for state and local health activities. This later legislation declared that personal and environmental health were essential to the fulfillment of national purposes. Comprehensive health planning overlaps and perhaps even supercedes comprehensive mental health planning in embracing all of the problem areas of community health, including both mental and physical health, environmental health hazards, and health-related social problems. Although each of these varied developments have been lauded as a major breakthrough, many critical problems still remain to be clarified for the planning and operation of effective community health programs.

A major problem is how to conceptualize, organize, and operate a care-giving system which is capable of effectively operating in such a manner as to provide the full range of services required by a community in a comprehensive program of health services. Although the range of services to be integrated varies from model to model, with each one planning differently for implementation, such a program involves an implicit if not explicit attempt to construct an abstract model characterizing a desired pattern of interdependency and coordination of existing and to-be-developed health and health-related organizations. Since comprehensive health planning is just beginning and its details remain to be spelled out explicitly, the rest of this chapter will discuss the general issues in organizing local community health agencies, with specific examples drawn from the community mental health system model.

It is common place today to speak of medical care "systems," but it is still rare that the user intends to develop the full technical meaning of "system." In conceptualizing an ideal comprehensive coordinated network of medical care facilities, thinking in terms of systems seems the most appropriate conceptual approach available, as it does whenever "the phenomena under study—at any level and in any domain—display the character of being organized, and when understanding the nature of the inter-dependencies constitutes the research task" (Emery and Trist 1965, p. 21). We shall be concerned with two levels of systems in this paper—the medical care agency as an organizational system, and the interorganizational care-giving network as a major community social system.

Health Organizations as Open Systems

Much of the past literature dealing with medical organizations has done so in terms of goal models. The authors have noted in several articles that while goal models are useful, they are limited and do not permit one adequately to conceptualize many of an organization's general properties and processes (Baker 1969).

An organization must fulfill a number of important functions if it is to survive, with achievement of goals being only one of several. In maintaining its autonomy and continued survival, an organization acts (1) to acquire and maintain sufficient levels of necessary resources; (2) to accomplish primary tasks, which involves establishing a hierarchy of tasks and the development of subtasks to be accomplished by its subparts such as departments, roles, and the like; (3) to achieve integration in the face of differentiating environmental influences, in such a way as to facilitate relationships that allow the efforts of individuals and organizational subunits to be effectively coordinated; (4) to adapt to both the environment and its own internal requirements and to some degree to try and control or adapt the environment itself. Only the second of these functions is taken to be of major concern in goal models, while all four functions are of concern in systems models of organizations.

The application of general systems theory to organizational analysis is a fairly recent but rapidly expanding development. As organization analysts have moved from a point of view emphasizing a fragmented and often oversimplified view of organizations to attempt to deal with organizational complexity, there has been increasing agreement that an organization must be studied as a system. General systems theory, with its emphasis on creating a science of organizational universals based on the commonality of elements and procesesses at all levels of systems, offers much to be built upon in the construction of a theory of organizations as systems. As the importance of organizational adaptation to what goes on in the outside world has become the subject of increasing attention by organization theorists and researchers, development in this area has occurred principally through the extension of systems theory. Early systems theory was concerned with the analysis of internal processes in organisms, or organizations, and involved establishing relationships among parts and the whole using a "closed systems" approach. Open systems theory has been employed attempting to relate the whole organization to elements in its environment.

Bertalanffy (1950))first showed the importance through his general transport equation of openness versus closedness to the environment in distinguishing living systems from nonliving systems. An open system is defined as one into which there is a continuous flow of resources from the environment and a continuous outflow of products of the system's action back to the environment. As an open system, an organization depends for its growth and viability upon its exchanges with the environment—that part of the physical and social world outside its boundary. The environment of a health organization includes the community which it serves and the other organizational systems which serve as sources of legal, political, financial, technical, and professional support.

Boundary of a System

Applying the term "system" implies both independence and interdependence. As a distinct systemic entity, an organization must maintain some discontinuity with its environment to continue to exist. This "boundary" of a system may be a line on territory, but in a social system such as a medical care facility, more importantly it exists as a boundary in "social space" representing discontinuity in patterns and clusterings of human interaction.

The boundary of a system functions to separate it from its environment. The system takes in inputs across the boundary, converts these materials within the boundaries of the system, and then exports the products of the system conversion as outputs across the boundary. There is a discontinuity at the boundary of an organization constituted by a differentiation of technology, territory, or time, or some combination of these (Miller 1955).

Organizations differ in the degree to which their boundaries are permeable. Some organization boundaries are easily penetrated while others tend to maintain stricter boundary controls. This applies to people, information, and ideologies; and the relative permeability of an organization's boundaries affects the degree to which the organization can be influenced by various environmental factors. An organization will have different degrees of boundary permeability both of inputs and outputs according to what is being brought in or sent out, and according to variations in the nature of internal and external sources. For example, mental hospitals tend to be more "open" today with regard to both the admission and the release of patients, with a very strong emphasis on outputs of patients to the community. Many mental hospitals in attempting to reduce inpatient census and reduce the iatrogenic effects of hospitalization maintain stronger boundary control on entrance to the hospital and minimal boundary controls on what patients leave the hospital. Many social service organizations, on the other hand, have long waiting lists minimizing input of clients but also have little output in the sense that they maintain the same clients on their rolls for long periods of time. Demographic characteristics of patients or clients have much to do with whether they get in or out of particular organizations. Health organizations also tend to specialize in terms of the problem characteristics of people they admit to their particular services. The trend to multipurpose health and welfare organizations is an example of increasing boundary permeability.

Boundary controls apply not only to patients and other human resources but also to information. Some organizations are more open to informational flows than others. Agencies seem surprisingly unaware and uninterested in the activities of other agencies with which it would appear they should have close functional relationships. Those relationships which do exist often involve strong distrust, prejudice, and a great lack of awareness of the behaviors, goals, and plans of other agencies.

Comprehensive health planning emphasizes the importance of increasing interaction and interdependence among the agency, the community, and other care-giving organizations, with an increasing interpenetration of traditional boundary conditions. For example, since one of the primary aims of a community mental health center is continuity of care, permeability is required not only among the various subparts of the center but also among it and other agencies in the larger care-giving network.

Organizations as systems differ in the degree and type of independence they display to the systems which make up their environment. The particular natures of their boundaries determine how dependent or independent they are to outside influence, as do factors such as physical or social isolation from surrounding systems, and adequacy of communication channels.

Boundary Spanners

Any form of interorganizational relations involves transactions of some kind across organizational boundaries. Organizations develop differentiated subsystems and/or specialized boundary roles to handle the interrelations among organizations. There is a need for the organization to have a representative who interacts with representatives of other organizations. Representatives from several groups, in meeting together to speak for their organizations and establish interorganization relations, tend to encapsulate themselves, and this creates an additional boundary between the representatives as a group and their respective organizations from which they come (Miller and Rice 1967).

Negotiation of interorganizational conflict is frequently done by such representatives. A representative faces the dual problem of: "(1) securing consensus for the negotiated solution among respective group members, and (2) compromising between the demands for flexibility by his opposite number and the demands for rigidity by his own group" (Pondy 1967, p. 313).

Miller and Rice (1967, p. 23) in analyzing such transactions across group boundaries, observe that "it is not uncommon for representatives to be disowned by the groups they represent because they have transferred or are suspected of having transferred their allegiances to the groups they visit or to the 'group' of representatives." Thus individuals who operate at the boundaries become "men in the middle," subject to strains which can be difficult to handle over time. But any organization as an open system must engage in multiple interorganizational transactions. One possibility in meeting the problems of organizational "marginal men" is the rotation of representatives at regular intervals back to more internal organizational position. Another is the use of neutral "go-betweens," such as consulting firms. Some individuals who specialize in such roles and become what Long (1958, p. 258) has called "entrepreneurs of ideas" play a very important role in integrating parts of an interorganizational network.

The attitudes and skills of persons in boundary roles are an important consideration, and organizations would do well to develop adequate training and recruitment programs for boundary-spanners. For example, those staff members of a community mental health center who have frequent commerce with other health and welfare organizations through their selective filtering of information can exercise a great deal of power in affecting whether an organization receives the inputs it needs. Deficiences in communication can lead to needless duplication of services and development of operating subsystems when adequate facilities are available for use in another organization. Schulberg and Baker (1968) have described the importance of boundary spanning personnel in the operation of adequate feedback for evaluation of a health organization's activities.

Nature of the Community Environment

Taking a specific health agency as our focus, the nature of the environment of this organizational system largely determines the nature of its exchange processes of input and output. Emery and Trist (1965) have introduced the concept of "the causal texture of the environment" to refer to the "area of interdependencies that belong within the environment itself" (p. 22). They propose four "ideal types" of environment which vary in the degree to which environmental components are connected as a system. The first type is a "placid, randomized" environment in which there is little or no connection among environmental parts. For a particular system existing within such an environment, environmental systems which offer rewards or adversive effects are relatively unchanging in themselves and are randomly distributed. This corresponds to the economist's "classical market." The second ideal type is a "placid, clustered" environment in which "goods" and "bads" are relatively unchanging in themselves but clustered. This type corresponds to the economist's "imperfect competition." The third type of environment is the disturbed-reactive environment and corresponds to the economist's oligopolic market. This is similar to the type 2 environment except that there is more than one organization of the same kind, and the existence of similar systems in the environmental field constitutes a major qualitative difference. The fourth ideal type of environment is called by Emery and Trist a "turbulent field." In these environments dynamic processes "arise from the field itself" and not simply from the interaction of the component organizational systems. The actions of component organizations and linked sets of them "are both persistent and strong enough to induce autochthonous processes in the environment." Emery and Trist liken the effect produced by organizational actions in the field to that of "a company of soldiers marching in step over a bridge" (p. 26).

Each type of environment calls for different organizational strategies. In a type 1 environment organizational adaptation is easiest, and an organization can proceed by trial and error and survive. In type 2, intelligence about the environment for the development of organizational strategy becomes crucial for survival. Location within the environmental field becomes very important. In a type 3 environment, because of the existence of similar organizations, overlapping effects of the actions of other organizations become important and an organization must calculate the actions and reactions of the other systems. Type 4 is still more complicated, and environmental effects are uncertain. Emery and Trist (1965, p. 26) observe that for this type of organization environment, "The consequences which flow from their actions lead off in ways that become increasingly unpredictable; they do not necessarily fall off with distance, but may at any point be amplified beyond all expectation; similarly, lines of action that are strongly pursued may find themselves attenuated by emergent field forces."

Shirley Terreberry (1968) in reviewing the literature on organizations, concludes that all organizational systems are increasingly finding themselves in environments of the fourth type. Certainly, in the health area there has been a proliferation of local, state, and federal agencies in recent years which seems to be continuing. Although in rural communities the health agency network may still be relatively simple and slow to change, certainly in more urbanized areas any one health organization finds itself increasingly less autonomous and forced to adapt to an environment of great complexity and rapidly changing conditions of interconnectedness.

Understanding the characteristics and needs of the environment in which it is operating is essential for a community health program not simply in theoretical terms but because of very practical implications. A decision by the program to include or exclude discrete segments of the environment from its range of concern of interaction will affect such inputs as people, values, economic resources, physical facilities, and technology. Any alteration of environmental inputs will in turn affect the program's outputs back into the environment. In his analysis of the relationship between large community organizations and their environment, Warren (1967a) found it useful to distinguish between input and output constituencies. In these terms, the input constituency can be conceived of as those other organizations from which a community mental health program receives financing, materials, and support, and to which it acknowledges a responsibility in determining its policy and program. The output constituency is conceived of as those other organizations in the environment acknowledged by the community mental health program as appropriate targets of its activity.

A Community Health Care-Giving System

The set of various community resources, as they are directly or indirectly related in a causal network so that one component of the complex affects the action capabilities of other parts, may be conceptualized as comprising a community system of great importance. The community mental health care-giving system can be distinguished from other community systems such as the educational system, political-legal system, or economic system which comprise its environment by certain boundary conditions which may be more or less well defined, but with which it has commerce in performing the required functions necessary for continued existence. The boundary between a mental health and welfare system and a larger health system are increasingly difficult to define and probably represent a time-bound phenomenon whose disappearance can be predicted. For the present, however, professional distinction and common practice and planning emphasize the boundedness of mental health and welfare as a system with components overlapping other community systems.

A community health care-giving system is a "system of systems" and is comprised of a host of organizational or agency systems at a different level. It should be pointed out that in conceptualizing a community mental health system our focus shifts from the level of the single organizational system to that of a complex network of interrelated organizations, a suprasystem in which agencies constitute components or subsystems. Nevertheless, from the general systems perspective it is still appropriate to apply the neutral terms of open systems theory in making intersystem generalizations so long as we recognize that a molar system may have different characteristics from a molecular one (Miller 1965). Gross (1966) has observed that larger and more differentiated interorganizational systems are likely to be marked by more complicated, divergent, and conflicting roles and relationships than are found within a single organizational system. Thus a community mental health system, comprised of many subsystems with specialized structures and functions, is itself a subpart of other political, social, and professional systems and has many overpapping, complex relationships with them.

The significance of interorganizational relationship and environmental influences in the conceptualization of a care-giving network has become the subject of increasing attention by organizational theorists and researchers. In 1960, Etzioni (1960) observed that comparatively little research on patterns of relationships among agencies had been carried out. However, considerably before that time, Johns (1946) and Johns and DeMarche (1951) had employed mailed questionnaires to study the attitudes toward interagency cooperation. Following the Etzioni article, Levine and his associates (Levine and White, 1961 and 1963; Levine, White, and Paul, 1963) published several articles reporting their studies of interagency patterns within the health agency systems of several communities.

In focusing on a complex interorganizational system cluster such as the "health system" we must view any particular health organization as a component of this larger macrosocial system. *Component interdependence* is a primary attribute of such a system, since any system exists only to the extent that its components or parts are linked in some network of internal relations. Component interdependence is a measure of the interconnectedness of a system, and may be defined as the extent to which a component depends upon other components for resource inputs, decision premises, or as receivers of the component's actions. Each organization comprising an interorganizational system can take various functional roles as parts of whole subsystems in the larger system.

When the activities and decisions of one health organization do not affect what other health organizations do or decide, their component interdependence is low. Component interdependence will be high when two or more organizations in a health system have competing needs for scarce resources, when there is intervention by supraorganizational processes, or when individuals or groups cross organizational boundaries to form intersystems bonds.

Forms of Interdependency

Interdependency of organizations in a particular community environment may be broadly classified as taking the form of cooperation or competition. Thompson and McEwan (1958) have outlined three types of cooperative strategy that organizations may employ in dealing with the other organizations in their environment—bargaining, cooptation, and coalition. Each of these cooperative strategies involve direct interaction among organizations, and this, Thompson and McEwan agree, increases the degree of potential environmental control over any particular organization existing in this interorganizational network.

In bargaining, negotiations are entered into by a formal organization because another organization's support is necessary in developing and maintaining agreement for the exchange of goods or services between the two organizations. To the extent that the second organization's support is necessary to maintain the agreement, that organization is in a position to exercise control over the organizational decision processes of the first organization.

Cooptation makes still further inroads into the goal-setting process, since "not only must the final choice be acceptable to the co-opted party or organization, but to the extent that co-optation is effective it places the representative of an 'outsider' in a position to determine the occasion for a goal decision, to participate in analyzing the existing situation, to suggest alternatives, and to take part in the deliberation of consequences" (Thompson and McEwan 1958, p. 27). From the standpoint of a health system, by providing overlapping memberships, cooptation aids the integration of the diverse parts of such a complex social system.

Coalition refers to a combination of two or more organizations for a common goal. Commitment toward joint action in a coalition may range from a very limited commitment for a short time to complete commitment for an indefinite time, but it is distinguished from a merger in that organizations do not lose their separate boundaries and each member can withdraw from the relationship. Thompson and

McEwan view coalition as the most extreme form of environmental conditioning of organization goals.

Organizations existing within the same social and physical area are also likely to engage in nonfacilitative interaction which may be described as "conflict." They are interdependent in their competition for scarce resources, i.e., situations occur in which the success of one organization in obtaining materials or people is at the cost of another organization in being able to obtain needed resources. Organizations within a health system may compete for either or both inputs and outputs—whether these are legitimation, personnel, finances, physical resources, or clients.

Levine and White (1963) have described the interdependence of health organizations within the health system and their exchange relations, which are determined by three factors: (1) the objective of each organization and the particular functions it carries out, which in turn determine the goods or elements it needs; (2) the access which each organization has to necessary elements from sources outside the system of health and welfare agencies, which may determine an agency's dependence upon other parts of the health system; and (3) the degree to which domain consensus exists within the health system. Organizational domain in the health field refers to the area staked out by individual organizations in terms of the population served, the problems or diseases covered, and the types of services given.

Barriers to Interagency Coordination

COMPLEXITY OF AGENCIES One of the major deterrents to the development of a coordinated system of comprehensive health care is the sheer diversity of agencies providing some kind of specialized health and welfare services. This is not just an urban phenomenon. Roemer and Wilson (1952) found when they attempted to analyze the structure and functioning of all the organized health services (in 1950) having impact on the people in one semirural county of what we now call "Appalachia," that there were more than 600 agencies involved in providing organized health service that had some impact on health care in that county. Of these, 155 were locally based health-relevant organizations (Roemer and Wilson 1952, pp. 77, 78).

Levine and White (1963) identified four main types of

health organizations within the health system, including (1) official or public agencies; (2) voluntary or nonprofit agencies; (3) hospitals and nursing homes; and (4) health-related organizations. By "health-related organizations" Levine and White meant the whole complex constellation of welfare and social agencies. All of these types of health organizations have been increasing in numbers over the years. A report for the Rockefeller Foundation in 1961 observed that an ad hoc citizen's committee had counted, aside from hospitals, over 100,000 national, regional, and local voluntary health and welfare agencies that solicit contributions from the general public (Hamlin, 1961). The increasing complexity of the other types of organization is hardly less striking. Considering the multiplicity of agencies it is not surprising that interagency coordination is often poorly achieved.

MIXED AUTHORITY Most intraorganizational analysis is made under the assumption of the existence of a fairly well-defined authority structure. Litwak and Hylton (1962) point out that, except in societies with a monolithic power structure, interorganizational analysis cannot assume a single well-defined formal authority structure. Agencies comprising the health system have widely deviant sources of authority. The situation operating in the community is one of mixed authority, which means that there is no unitary formal authority which can improve cooperation.

SPECIALIZATION Until recently the trend toward specialization in the health fields has continued unabated. Specialization in medicine, social welfare, and other health-related areas has worked against coordination of both professional persons and organizations. The public has become increasingly disturbed about the number of physicians with whom a family must maintain contact for varying types and degrees of illness. However, although disturbed by cost and loss of time, the public, concerned about getting the "best" in professional skill, has supported specialization.

In planning mental health services for the poor, there has been increasing recognition of the problems of multiple uncoordinated speciality services, and this has resulted in a reemergence of trends toward generalist roles. Both recognition of the problem and emphasis on generalist roles have occured primarily among those professionals working with populations and espousing community mental health ideology (Baker and Schulberg 1967).

STEREOTYPED BELIEFS AND ATTITUDES Beliefs and attitudes of a stereotypic sort can interfere with coordination and development of interdependence of health and welfare agencies. White (1968) investigated local conflicts between two national voluntary health agencies and found that covert beliefs concerning competition for resources, particularly volunteers, funds, and patients, supported the conflicts. Contrary to expectation, research on each of these problems revealed that actual competition in each of these areas did not exist. However, the long history of competition between the agencies coupled with a federated form of organization that allowed national and state levels to put off cooperation for fear that the locals would disaffiliate themselves, indicated that the conflicts would continue.

Baker, Schulberg, and O'Brien (1969) have reported a study of a mental hospital attempting to become more community oriented in which they found that the hospital social workers, perceiving their hospital to have a negative image among local health and welfare agencies, hesitated fully to utilize the services of the local agencies.

As a mental hospital develops into a community mental health center, staff boundary-spanning roles linking the hospital with other community health and welfare agencies become of crucial importance. Without effective human links to form the interorganizational bridges there cannot be the flow of patients, communications, resources, and joint interagency activities necessary for the provision of comprehensive services. In considering the manner in which these bridges are developed and maintained, it is clear that the attitudes and perceptions of individuals linking the hospital system and its community environment are important factors to be studied. The way that an occupant of a boundary-spanning role in the hospital feels about professional and nonprofessional people in the community will affect his interaction with them. Similarities and the differences in perception of the hospital's functioning by hospital staff and agency personnel, furthermore, may be reflected in the way people view the "people-channeling," or referral, patterns among these systems.

Negative attitudes and competition among professional groups also work against the interdisciplinary coordination needed for the effective collaboration of health and social welfare organizations.

DEFICIENT COMMUNICATION We have mentioned earlier the surprising ignorance about services and activities not directly connected with their own activity that exists in many agencies. This applies at both the organizational and individual level. Individuals frequently receive services from several different agencies or several different professional workers within the same organization without the agent or organization being aware or even displaying interest in the involvement of others. Cursory and nonsystematized communication seems to be the norm among professional workers, and this is particularly true of the behavior among health and welfare agencies.

DIFFICULTY IN DEFINING "PRIMARY TASK" In order to comprehend the activities and relationships in a care-giving system it is necessary to consider the network's direct movement toward some goal in relation to its community. Rice (1963) elaborated the concept of "primary task" to distinguish among the varied goals of an organization, and pointed to the difficulty of treating an institution as if it had but a single goal or task. Multiple goals are not necessarily compatible, however, and they may produce competition for scarce resources among those subparts of the organization which are more committed to one goal than to others. Ambiguities usually arise in defining the primary mission or task because certain goals are denied, and the public goals which the organization claims to pursue will fail to be realized because they were never meant to be realized.

Part of the reason for the multiplicity of goals to be found in each component in the health field is to be found in the changing social and technological base on which health care is based in this country. Sigmond (1968, p. 99) has pointed out that "the goals of hospitals in the United States, for example, have been developed in historical sequence with each new goal superimposed upon, rather than superseding, earlier goals."

Like most complex organizations, the care-giving system in a community health program has multiple goals and performs many tasks simultaneously. In addition to providing the patient-oriented essential elements of a comprehensive program, the system engages in such other activities as research, educational programs for various health disciplines, social action programs, the provision of employment for professional and nonprofessional personnel, and self-preservation.

There usually is no clearly established priority of goals within the health care-giving system, and any one of the goals may assume primacy at a given time according to the balance of forces then operating. Priorities are modified as the result of personnel changes, the gain or loss of federal grants, or changing techniques and ideologies, so that any given primary task may have only a limited viability attached to it. A program health administrator is faced with the consequent problem of organizing a stable care-giving system within an ever-changing framework of tasks which clearly affects the composition and motivation of participating staff members.

Although they may share such general goals as promotion of health and prevention of disease, each agency in the community has individual goals and methods of approach. Conflict may occur between the way a particular organizational system defines its primary task and the way in which the larger system defines it. For example, the superordinate health system may define the role of a state mental hospital as primarily custodial, while the hospital itself may define its role as that of an active short-term treatment center with a strong emphasis on primary prevention activities. Environmental definitions of the primary task of the health system may differ from its own definition and may impose constraints upon it. A community may define the primary mental health task for its total health system as that of custodial care, removing the unwanted members of the community, while the health system defines its role as returning the mentally ill to the community as soon as possible to prevent iatrogenic effects.

Based upon his review of interorganizational behavior, Warren (1967b) developed a typology which distinguishes the way in which organizations interact and control the decision-making process, and his patterns are highly relevant to the analysis of community health systems. In the "unitary" pattern a central authority rigidly dominates the subsystem's division of labor and goals, while in the "social choice" pattern, which has no mechanism for division of labor, each unit pursues its personal goals in the manner which it deems most appropriate. Both of these extremes have obvious deficiencies for a community health program, and it is suggested that more effective subsystem interaction will emerge from the "federative" or "coalitional" patterns. These intermediate alternatives are characterized by a willingness of independent facilities to work toward a common goal through formal or informal collaboration. The operations of a coalition are exemplified in Leopold's (1967) description of the West Philadelphia mental health consortium, which has brought together six independent hospitals concerned with the provision of a comprehensive program to a given catchment area.

It is important to recognize that not all participants in a community mental health system openly recognize their interdependence with other facilities. A decade ago Long (1958) described the community as an ecology of games in that much of the local cooperation was unconscious or unnoticed. The resurgent emphasis on coordination among agencies permitting continuity of care once again highlights the importance of conscious awareness by agency personnel of the systemic character of the community health organizational network.

One of the ways to get organizations to relate to each other is through the intervention of supraorganizational regulating bodies (Litwak and Hylton 1962). Health agencies have demonstrated that they will conform to conditions set forth by a wide variety of agencies from which they require some positive act in order to continue to operate. It may be to obtain money, as in the case of Hill-Burton and other types of governmental grant funds. It may be for professional legitimation, as with the Joint Commission on Accreditation of Hospitals and various professional membership organizations such as the Association of American Medical Colleges. Such groups require written plans and statements of goals and control incentives that give them power to affect the development of health agencies. Supraorganizational agencies that control funds and professional status or the licensing of health organizations can affect the operations of these organizations in the direction of providing coordinated community health services to meet the health needs of the local community. A problem in using such supraorganizational agencies is the lack of coordination at this level. For example, Sigmond (1968, pp. 98–99) has said in referring to the discontinuous nature of the federal government:

Probably a half-dozen federal agencies furnish major capital funds for the local health programs, and an equivalent number furnish major operational funds. At least four cabinet-level departments are involved. Instances of noncoordination have arisen in the past; it is likely these will occur more frequently, even within the Department of Health, Education and Welfare. For example, who is attempting to coordinate in the community, the work of Hill-Burton, the Regional Medical Programs, Medicare, the Community Mental Health Program, Social Rehabilitation Services, Medical Assistance and the Veteran's Administration, to name a few.

Pluralism at the governmental level remains a problem in obtaining coordination at community levels, but at these higher governmental levels leverage is offered and increasingly there is sharing of inclusive goals.

Models for Coordinating Agencies in a Community Mental Health System

In spite of the consensus which now exists about the necessity for mental health facilities to collaborate with other community resources, there is still considerable controversy about the optimal nature of such relationships in a comprehensive mental health care-giving system. The contrasting viewpoints, which are complex and varied in their functional and administrative details, can be categorized in an oversimplified manner as the psychiatric medical practice and human services models.

The psychiatric medical practice model of a community mental health system can be described as having a structural arrangement in which the mental health center, under medical leadership, assumes responsibility and perhaps even supervision of all the community's mental health services. The resources of other agencies clearly are seen as being of value but as functioning in a basically supporting role. Foley and Sanders (1966) have schematically represented the comprehensive community mental health program as a circle at the center of which is the community mental health center. Around the periphery are the other community agencies and facilities, each with varying functions and goals. The mental health center's role is described as that of coordinator of existing services, innovator of new services, educator, administrator, and consultant to the community.

Many variations of this model are evident at the present time. Mental health centers, as highly discrete systemic entities, actively interact with their communities by providing specific services to other components of the health and welfare caregiving network. Consultation programs with such agencies as the local school, court, and police department are established, and the mental health professional stands prepared to assist when he is requested to do so. Relationships of both a formal and informal nature can be observed between the mental health facility and other community agencies, but the interaction usually is on an *ad hoc* or special program basis.

Along with the psychiatric medical practice model, increasing attention is being given to the human services model as an alternative administrative arrangement for organizing a community mental health program. Ryan (1963) has characterized as somewhat autistic the tendency to perceive mental health as the hub around which life revolves, and he considered it more realistic to view mental health as a subsidiary area within the broad field of health, education, and social welfare. Many studies have shown that numerous community agencies function as mental health care-givers, and that the mental health of a community is affected by the organization and rules of procedure of these agencies. It is a significant and neglected challenge to consider the potential contribution of these resources within a mental health program, not merely as targets of consultation and education, but as basic components of mental health planning and services. Cumming (1967) has described the arrogance of psychiatric agencies in being willing to tell other care-givers how to do their jobs, but in being unwilling either to learn from them or to collaborate in a genuine partnership.

The structural pattern and network of liaisons in the evolving human services model are such that the mental health center is designated as just one of a variety of community resources which participate in cooperative ways to serve the mental health needs of all citizens. This model is particularly evident in rural areas (Kiesler 1965) and in those instances where mental health programs have assumed a strong social action component (Peck, Roman, and Kaplan 1967). Two-way interaction becomes routinized and the concept of feedback patterns leading to mutual adjustments is institutionalized. The mental health facility and other agencies jointly work with the same troubled family, cooperate in the development of new programs, and try to minimize competition with each other. This pattern could very well become the optimal one for providing comprehensive mental health services to a total population, and it has certain similarities to the comprehensive health programs proliferating throughout the country.

The just developing comprehensive health services model overlaps both the psychiatric medical practice model and the human services model (see Figure 1). It includes part of the emphasis on medical domination and emphasis on physical care and treatment of the psychiatric medical practice model and also part of the emphasis on social welfare and provision of social services of the human services model, but includes elements not common to either of the other two models such as its attention to environmental health.

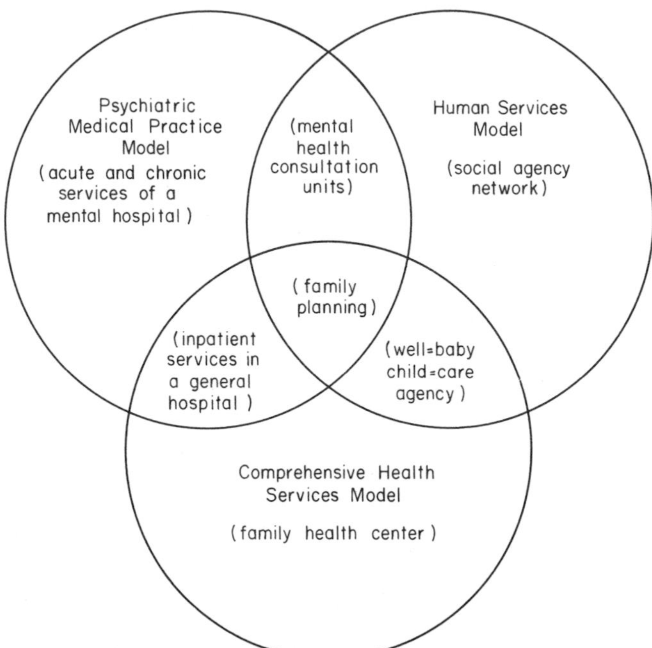

Figure 1. Functional overlap of three models of proving comprehensive health and related community services.

In many ways the distinctions between the medical and human services models are profound and deeply rooted, carrying with them long-standing, emotionally laden stereotypes which are potentially detrimental to effective coordination of psychiatric and nonpsychiatric facilities. Nevertheless, both models feature a mental health program which is broadly based and which incorporates the resources of many facilities rather than being overly centered in any one. This development is most significant since it indicates that programs of primary, secondary, and tertiary prevention cannot be provided without the cooperation of an interacting care-giving network. For the network to be viable it must be sensitive to the aspirations and limitations of its component members, as well as being aware of the varied ways in which environmental forces impinge upon it and change task priorities.

How is the mental health center affected by changing primary tasks under the medical model and the human services model of a care-giving network? Although the center is susceptible to the vagaries of external modifying forces in either model, the medical one provides the center with greater control over its goals and objectives than does the human services model. Positioning itself as the nucleus of a comprehensive program, the mental health center is in a much more potent position to determine its role and tasks vis-à-vis the other members of the network. It can exercise greater influence on the priorities assigned to primary, secondary, and tertiary prevention (usually emphasizing the latter two) and through allocation of its resources it can control working relationships. Although the mental health center gains distinct advantages and stability under the medical model, it also incurs the risk of imposing a task priority upon the care-giving system which does not necessarily meet the wishes of other resources or the community's actual needs. This difficulty is evident, for example, in the strained relationships produced by the primacy of the training task in university-affiliated mental health centers, which contrasts with the emphasis assigned to service by other resources participating in the community network.

The human services model offers the mental health center less absolute control over its task selection. In this model, the center is concerned with and possibly even required to establish task priorities which are compatible with both its internal desires as well as the demands of its environment, i.e., the larger care-giving system of which it is a part and the geographic community in which it is located. The community may see problems of violence control or poor housing as being the issues of immediate concern, and exert pressure on the care-giving system to deal with areas which traditionally have not been of concern to mental health organizations. The internal and external frames of reference for developing task priorities can be in opposition so that the mental health center participating in a human services network must exercise considerable adroitness and flexibility in coping with the potentially contradictory pressures directed at it.

Although the environment is of central importance to both medical-model and human-services model types of community mental health programs, significant distinctions are evident in the manner in which each model designates its specific input and output constituencies. Many exceptions can be noted, but in a general sense the medical-model community mental health program has defined a more limited and familiar constituency as being relevant to itself since its tasks focus more heavily upon secondary and tertiary prevention. More elements of the community are now clearly perceived as significant for the successful completion of these tasks, but expansion of the input and output environment has been relatively limited.

By contrast, the community mental health program employing the human services model has witnessed a major expansion of the environmental constituency to which it is sensitive and with which it interacts. As part of a human services network whose concerns range far beyond the traditional interests of a psychiatric facility, the mental health center in such a program is becoming increasingly involved with problems of primary prevention and thereby is led to accept inputs which go far beyond previous definitions of appropriate endeavor. The outputs of such a center have been similarly affected so that it may be as relevant for the center to help a patient receive a higher welfare check as it is to reduce his paranoid ideation. In general, the consumers of community mental health programs are becoming increasingly restless and we are witnessing a growing concern among them about the formal care-giving network's adequacy and relevance of performance. As a result, pressure is being directed toward the mental health system to reorganize its structure and to realign its priorities. Administrative flexibility and new technical competencies will be required to meet those changing environmental demands.

At the same time, no system can be completely "open" and still survive as an integrated functioning network so that counterpressures will soon develop within the system for boundary control and limitations of service. Effective performance will then be particularly difficult to achieve without a special community subsystem having the responsibility and authority to guide the overall system. The past inability of government to perform this function has resulted in a proliferation of competing and overlapping programs in the same geographic area. We must be hopeful that newly emerging local coordinating and planning mechanisms will permit improved feedback control of the community mental health system.

Conclusion

In conclusion, let us admit frankly that the term "health system" remains operationally a highly abstract concept. Hilleboe (1968, p. 1039) has characterized the present situation in the United States as one in which "Enormous diffusions of sponsorship and organization of health services, maldistribution of resources, and increasing imbalance between expectations predominate." The chief value of the "health system" concept is to highlight the present lack of system in the organization and distribution of health resources. Planning continues with the goal of improving connections among health organizations, and this must involve consideration of ways to integrate interorganizational networks. Application of general systems theory and research, and particularly open systems organizational theory, offer useful tools for furthering this process.

References

Baker, F.
(1969), "An Open Systems Approach to the Study of Mental Hospitals in Transition." *Community Mental Health Journal,* 5, 5, 403–412.

———, and **H. C. Schulberg**
(1967), "Development of a Community Mental Health Ideology Scale." *Community Mental Health Journal, 3,* 216–225.
———, ———, and **G. M. O'Brien**
(1969), "The Changing Mental Hospital: Its Perceived Image and Contact with the Community." *Mental Hygiene, 53,* 237–244.
Bertalanffy, L. von
(1950), "The Theory of Open Systems in Physics and Biology." *Science, 3,* 23–29.
Cumming, E.
(1967), "Community Psychiatry in a Divided Labor." Read at Annual Meeting of American Psychopathological Association, February, 1967, New York.
Emery, S. W., and E. L. Trist
(1965), "The Causal Texture of Organizational Environments." *Human Relations, 18,* 21–32.
Etzioni, A.
(1960), "New Directions in the Study of Organization and Society." *Social Research, 27,* 223–228.
Foley, A. R., and D. S. Sanders
(1966), "Theoretical Considerations for the Development of the Community Mental Health Center Concept." *American Journal of Psychiatry, 122,* 985–990.
Gross, B. M.
(1966), "The State of the Nation: Social Systems Accounting." In R. A. Baver (ed.), *Social Indicators.* Cambridge: M.I.T. Press.
Hamlin, R. H.
(1961), *Voluntary Health and Welfare Agencies in the United States.* New York: Schoolmaster's Press.
Hilleboe, H. E.
(1968), "Administrative Requirements for Comprehensive Health Planning at the State Level." *American Journal of Public Health, 58,* 1039–1046.
Johns, R. E.
(1946), *The Cooperative Process among National Social Agencies.* New York: Association Press.
———, and **D. F. DeMarche**
(1951), *Community Organization and Agency Responsibility.* New York: Association Press.
Kiesler, F.
(1965), "Is This Psychiatry?" In S. Goldston (ed.), *Concepts of Community Psychiatry.* Washington, D.C.: U.S. Government Printing Office. P. 147–157.
Leopold, R. L.
(1967), "The West Philadelphia Mental Health Consortium: Administrative Planning in a Multihospital Catchment Area." *American Journal of Psychiatry* (October Supplement), *124,* 69–76.
Levine, S., and P. E. White
(1961), "Exchange as a Conceptual Framework for the Study of Inter-Organizational Relationships." *Administrative Science Quarterly, 5,* 583–601.
———, ——— (1963), "The Community of Health Agencies." In H. E. Freeman, P. E. Levine, and L. G. Reeder (eds.), *Handbook on Medical Sociology.* Englewood Cliffs: Prentice-Hall. Chapter 12.
———, ———, and **B. Paul**
(1963), "Community Interorganizational Problems in Providing Medical Care and Social Services." *American Journal of Public Health, 53,* 1183–1195.

Litwak, E., and L. F. Hylton
(1962), "Interorganizational Analysis: A Hypothesis on Co-ordinating Agencies." *Administrative Science Quarterly, 6,* 395–426.
Long, N. E.
(1958), "The Local Community as an Ecology of Games." *American Journal of Sociology, 64,* 258.
Miller, E. J.
(1955), "Technology, Territory and Time." *Human Relations, 8,* 292–316.
———, **and A. K. Rice**
(1967), *Systems of Organization.* London: Tavistock.
Miller, J. G.
(1965), "Living Systems: Basic Concepts." *Behavioral Science, 10,* 193–237.
Peck, H. B., M. Roman, and S. R. Kaplan
(1967), "Community Action Programs and the Comprehensive Health Center." In M. Greenblatt, P. Emery, and B. Glueck (eds.), *Poverty and Mental Health.* Washington, D. C.: American Psychiatric Association, pp. 103–121.
Pondy, L. R.
(1967), "Organizational Conflict: Concepts and Models." *Administrative Science Quarterly, 12,* 2, 313.
Rice, A. K.
(1963), *The Enterprise and Its Environment.* London: Tavistock.
Roemer, M. I., and E. A. Wilson
(1952), *Organized Health Services in a County of the United States.* Public Health Service Publication, No. 197. Washington, D.C.: Government Printing Office.
Ryan, W.
(1963), "Urban Mental Health Services and Responsibilities of Mental Health Professionals." *Mental Hygiene, 47,* 365–371.
Schulberg, H. C., and F. Baker
(1968), "Program Evaluation Models and the Implementation of Research Findings." *American Journal of Public Health, 58,* 7, 1248–1255.
Sigmond, R. M.
(1968), "Health Planning." *The Milbank Memorial Fund Quarterly, 46,* 99.
Terreberry, S.
(1968), "The Evolution of Organizational Environments." *Administrative Science Quarterly, 12,* 590–613.
Thompson, J. D., and W. J. McEwan
(1958), "Organizational Goals and Environment: Goal-Setting as an Interaction Process." *American Sociological Review, 23,* 23–31.
Warren, R. L.
(1967a), "The Interaction of Community Decision Organizations: Some Basic Concepts and Needed Research." *The Social Service Review, 41,* 261–270.
——— (1967b), "The Interorganizational Field as a Focus for Investigation." *Administrative Science Quarterly, 12,* 396–419.
White, P. E.
(1968), "Myth and Reality in Interorganizational Behavior: A Study of Competition between Two National Voluntary Health Agencies." *American Journal of Public Health, 58,* 289–304.

Robert Chin and Gregory M. St. L. O'Brien

9. General Intersystem Theory

The Model and a Case of Practitioner Application

I. General Intersystem Models and the Practitioner

In advocating the utility of an intersystem model for purposes of conceptualizing the client system and the practitioner (Chin 1961), we have built upon the models of general systems in relation to developmental models. The practitioner-administrator-advocate-change agent needed special requirements in conceptualizing his job and his function.

This chapter attempts to project beyond concepts of a system into intersystem conditions. It tries to derive the special properties of an intersystem by illustrating these ideas in the specific case of a multipurpose service agency.

Having decided to explore further the proposed intersystem model for practitioners, we are faced with the tasks of spelling out lofty models and deriving prototype tools. Research and development in theory and model building for practitioners should also show the development of concrete action sequences with attendant concepts of "systems analysis." A word about the latter term. As we understand it, systems analysis is partly built directly around "general systems" theories but adds concepts and concrete data gathered empirically, criterion objectives, goals, optimal performance, evaluation of alternatives, and implementation issues. Systems analysis is portrayable in these steps of action: (1) conceptually isolating the system boundaries, equilibrium and subsystems (we would add intersystem dynamics); (2) studying the actual operations and outputs of the existing arrangements; (3) formulating the objectives and defining what is to be achieved in optimal performance; (4) introducing an extrapolation of time into the magnitude and scope of the problem that is being managed by the system; that is, how much variation in the inputs may be expected in the future environments?; (5) examining alternative relationships of input to output in terms of feasibility and acceptability of the contemplated alterations from the existing state of the system (here, cost-effectiveness measures are utilized in assessing the effects of these alterations); and (6) working through the various other issues and problems involved in implementation and decision-making. An intersystem model is based on the concept of two "separate" and open systems in some definable interaction. Doctors and patients, change agents and clients, leaders and groups, health agencies and clients, doctors and nurses, are analyzable in intersystem dynamics. In a sense, intersystem models are analogous to subsystem models.

The purported advantages and the felt necessity for spelling out the intersystem model are summarized briefly in these rather strident overclaims: (1) the linkage functions among parts of systems have tended to be neglected since tight and equally strong connections of parts are assumed in systems and subsystems analysis; (2) the relatively separate autonomy of different components and elements becomes more salient. An intersystem model exaggerates the virtues of autonomy and the limited nature of the interdependence of the interactions between two connected systems; (3) interrelations of two systems are coequal in intersystem models and are not treated as part of a whole, as in subsystems, to subsystems and to the larger systems; (4) the dynamics of change and the source of change, for example discrepancies and tensions arising from within each of the systems, can be seen more sharply as the outcome of intersystem dynamics; (5) The change agent, care-giver, or professional person is seen as an intervention lever who operates both in the context of his own system and in the system of the client-patient. Conceptually treating the patient as a system in intersystem models reconceptualizes disobedience, resistance to change, defense, apathy, and other value-laden terms. The one-sidedness of direction of influence, of cognitions, and assumptions of passivity and inertness, to mention a few, can be alleviated by intersystem models. Collaborative relations require an intersystem model as the conceptual base.

SETS, COLLECTIONS OF SETS, AND DEGREES OF "SYSTEMNESS"

More fundamental than and prior to the discussion of system properties is the question of the conditions under which we can apply the concepts of "system" and "intersystem" to a group of elements. Merely attributing to any collection of elements the properties of systems can lead to false analysis, or at best, nonuseful statements. Vague assumptions of organic unity, interdependency, or organization need to be spelled out.

We shall start with the simple and fundamental term for any grouping, a *set.* A set is a collection of elements which, for some reason, one conceives as belonging together. A set, as the general concept, is known in concrete terms by the following: category, class, attribute, dimension, group. In social terms, sets are stereotypes, status and positional categories, roles, institutions, organizations, and so forth. These elements become classified by names applied by the observer. In approaching and conceptualizing an already existing or a newly planned structure (e.g., a small group, an organization, a health organization, a city) we face alternatives of describing these collections of elements.

The two types of sets to examine before discussing the sets that can become a system are directly concerned with overlap and multiple membership of the elements. The first conception of a collection of sets uses the notion of a tree of sets. A collection of sets forms a tree if and only if for any two sets that belong to a collection, either (a) one set is wholly contained in the other or (b) the two sets are wholly disjointed. In the second type, for structures of complex orderliness, we are reminded of the fact that living structures grow up and take on *overlapping*, though orderly and complex, relationships of elements. These collections, with multimembership of any given sets, are called semilattices.

Indeed, says Christopher Alexander (1965) in his critique of city planning, the heretofore simplistic thinking and conceptual limitations for simultaneously apprehending multivariable sets and collections of sets requires replacement with some conceptions of lattices of sets to hold us to the confronting reality. The youth and old age groups are better conceptualized as semilattices rather than as trees. Hierarchies of organizations may be better conceptualized using lattices. Miller's conceptions (1950) of living systems and their hierarchies of system belongingness is an interesting lead. In acknowledging the nature of sets—the types of collections of sets, trees, and semilattices—we now have open to us for study the nature of the groupings that can form a system. Since multiple and overlapping membership attributes of any set or of an element need to be kept in mind, we need to be careful in treating "systems" not as "trees" but as semilattices.

We call the set of elements a *system* when the elements of a set belong together because they cooperate, interrelate with each other, or work together somehow. In other words, these elements possess a specific characteristic of belongingness. A system, then, is one classification of sets of elements.

There can be graduations of "systemness" in concrete cases. The amount of cooperation, interrelation, and working together is, in fact, the degree of organization of the elements. The notion of degrees of systemness may be helpful in preventing an ordering of interdependency. The degree of systemness can be strung over in some sort of measure; for the present we can typify some stages. Aside from closed systems, sets are related directly to each other, or through some other factors that precipitate a system. For most of us, it is readily visualizable when the elements are somehow in close physical proximity to each other, as the parts of personality or a small group, an organization, a hospital, a health service, a community, or a city.

A fairly low level where things belong together and work together is illustrated by a traffic light on a corner. On the same corner there is a drugstore with a newsrack. During the time of a red light, pedestrians stop and look at the papers in the rack and sometimes buy them. When the light is green, people hurry across and pay little attention to the newsrack. In the simplest sense, the newsrack and the traffic light belong together, cooperate, interrelate, and work together.

It is much harder to see the cooperation, interrelations, and working together when the elements are not in physical proximity. Elements such as individuals forming the sets of youth, old age, mentally ill, or some other such set, *can* take on some properties of a system, and/or at least are analyzable *as if* the elements do form a system. It is important to note that a set of elements can be different in appearance or activity and indeed be a system. In fact, the concept of system allows operation of similar functions or interrelations with different elements, as in systems of body temperature regulation.

A system is conceivable by the observer-practitioner when there is sizable interaction of elements in the presence of each other, or simple interaction in terms of the effect on a third party, namely, the pedestrians-readers-buyers. When no physical continuity is involved, we can at least call the set a conceptual system. But, in addition, we wish to explore the condition where there are third-party elements which are the common elements in the nonoverlapping or noninteractive elements.

For the young, the elderly, the nonhospitalized heart patient, the common elements which make them fit into a set may well be forced upon them by the representatives, legislators, and care-givers of the society as a whole. Age may not be a truly meaningful demarcation for a subset of society until federal regulators make provision for the citizens over the age of 62. Rejection by social groups, laws and regulations defining status, handicaps, limitations, and benefits, and actions of professional care-givers are common elements which bring about coalescence of noncontinuous elements of a set into a system.

The various definitions of system commonly accepted in general systems literature are general indeed. A system, say Hall and Fagen (1956), may be loosely defined as "a set of objects together with relationships between the objects and between their attributes." Or, says Bertalanffy (1956), a system is a set of "elements standing in interaction." Or, a system may be considered to be some form in structure or operation, concept or function, composed of united and integrated parts (Young 1964). In each of these definitions there is some variation of interrelatedness and organization, Hall and Fagen being at the most nonspecific end.

The fourfold classification by O. R. Young (1964), of groups as concepts deemed relevant to describe, explain, and predict the behavior of a general system, provides us with a framework for the examination of the general properties of intersystems: (1) systemic and descriptive factors; (2) regulation and maintenance; (3) dynamics and change; and (4) decline and breakdown. Some of these have been defined and illustrated in a previous publication that attempted to contrast systems and developmental models in relation to change and changing (Chin 1961). Therefore, we shall spend time on those which need special attention.

The systemic factors and concepts that create important distinctions for our purposes are boundaries and environment, interdependence and independence, and integration and differentiation.

Concerning regulation and maintenance, there are concepts of equilibrium and steady state, feedback, and communication. In addition, for this paper we shall add forces creating and pressures reinforcing the boundary.

If one conceptualizes the relations between change agent and client as a relation between two systems in which one system endeavors to facilitate in the other, certain dynamics of the change process are highlighted (Bennis 1961). Concepts of goal, adaptation, learning, growth, and teleology are central issues. Decline and breakdown emphasize problems of disruption and dissolution in systems, involving concepts of stress, disturbance, overload, positive entropy, and decay.

For the purposes of this paper, we shall examine each of the relevant terms in the four areas, suitably modified. For brevity and comprehension, we will focus on a case involving the set of agencies looking after services for the senior citizens and the old age group in the community. Section II will apply these terms and the next stages of systems analysis for action to a specific community agency, a multiservice center for the aged.

First of all, does the collection of old individuals in a community constitute a system? Conceptually, they belong to the social system, the social fabric of the society. They form a subset within this system, conceptually isolatable. They share some properties and to some extent are interrelated in that many people treat them as interrelated. They also share some common problems which force a set of similar behaviors upon them. Part of this commonality comes through third-party interactions rather than through direct actions of the elements or individuals with each other. Other elements of third-party interaction include family members, societal institutions, pressures of governmental Social Security payments, and so forth. All of these factors force interaction among members of this set.

There are also natural circumstances of physical health and stage of life that contribute to commonality of fate and behavior. This set, or quasisystem, then, has many functions filled by other systems in the larger society. The issues and problems it meets are coped with by the societal fabric under normal stress conditions. When there is some stretch imposed on these coping mechanisms, then other forces and institutions (the caretaking institutions and agencies) are set up to take on functions to help the aged.

II. The Senior Citizens Multipurpose Center and Its Place in the Professional Care-Giving System

The Senior Citizens Multipurpose Center (MPC) was inaugurated as a demonstration project for the provision of a variety of services to the senior citizens of a city.

For successful attainment of organizational goals, it is necessary for the multiservice center to act in a number of capacities. It must fulfill different functions as a part of a number of independent, but definitely interdependent, systems. The following portion of this chapter will focus on the future of the multiservice center in its unique role in this intersystem.

DEFINING BOUNDARIES The larger system of which the MPC is organizationally a part was, at the time of this study, undergoing a dynamic change in its operations. All health and social services offered under municipal auspices were being brought under the control of one city department. The other major social service organization in the city is the City Community Services (United Fund) Organization. The MPC office and part of its administrative framework were centered in the Community Services headquarters building to facilitate communication between the MPC and the CCS agencies. This location also provided a critical path (Alexander 1965) between the municipal agencies and the CCS agencies dealing with the set of senior citizens in the city.

In addition to these intersystem connections established by the administrative framework and location of the agency the MPC rapidly developed contact with state, federal, and private agencies and care-givers who also were concerned with services to older people.

In an effort to define the nature and strength of connections between the MPC and various other members of the intersystem, a questionnaire was administered to the professional staff (director, nurse, and social worker) regarding the number and types of contacts they had made in a period of one year. From these data and ongoing interviews with agency personnel, a map of the care-giving and client intersystem for senior citizens was developed from the point of view of the MPC.

There are two types of relations that each agency has vis-à-vis the various systems with which it interrelates. The first type of relationship which must be examined is that which the agencies have with each other. This type of relationship is most clearly determined through observation of the referral patterns which exist among agencies (transducer functions). A second type of relationship which should be examined is that between the agency and its environment. For this particular intersystem relationship, the environment is most clearly represented in the relationships which the agencies have with the client system of the senior citizen set.

While those two types of relationships are quite different from one another, they seem at the same time to be related. If an agency suffers from a chronic overload of its case file, due to its interaction with its environment, then it will be less able to accept referrals from other agencies. It will then begin to limit the types of cases it is willing to accept both from other agencies and from its environment. (This limitation of types of acceptable cases—rigidification of its boundaries—would likewise occur if the pressure to limit numbers of incoming cases came from a large number of cases being referred by other agencies limiting the agency's interaction with the environment.)

In essence, then, the boundaries of the individual agencies may be made more or less rigid depending upon the relative strengths and types of linkages the agency has both with other members of the same suprasystem and with its environment. Because of the nature of its relationships with other agencies and potential clients, the MPC, for example, has found itself defined more as an agency of input into the care-giving system than one of output-maintenance functions.

The health and social care for the senior citizen of the city may then be said to be divided into systems at three major levels, the client system (senior citizens), the societal system of which they are a part, and the professional care-giving system. Within the last level we shall look at the intersystem properties of the element or agencies. The intersystem relationships between the professionals and the aged will not be treated at this time. Another level, the political system, i also represented in the form of city councilmen who de ith members of each of the above systems. Within the cli the societal, and the professional systems exist a numb f largely independent units.

While a crucial question throughout this chapter is the role of the professional care-giving system, we hope that we do not give the impression that all who are senior citizens are removed from the service and function in the societal system through institutions of family, neighborhood, and social-religious institutions. In the professional care-giving system, there are agencies sponsored by, and under the direction of, both governmental and private religious and independent care-givers. While it may be argued that among the professional care-givers there may not exist a unified suprasystem, it is clear that the interdependence among these care-givers provides a basis for analysis of an intersystemic network.

CASES AS INTERSYSTEMIC FUNCTIONING While the existence of a complex intersystem structure has been demonstrated, we have not, thus far, seen how these various systems and subsystems interact within these boundaries. For this purpose we have selected a number of cases from the MPC files and shall review some of the most commonly used paths and critical paths as they exist. It is obvious, of course, that these descriptions and analyses are from the perspective of the MPC. A different portrayal could well emerge functionally if the data were taken from the files of the visiting nurses, the churches, or the other agencies. Hopefully, the principles concerning information flow and properties of intersystem relations among the professional care-giving agencies would be the same. One difference is important; the MPC is formally charged with coordination responsibilities.

A client was referred by a neighbor (transducer within the client system) to the Senior Citizen Club (not a care-giver in the provision of health and social service functions). Client's brother was in a mental hospital on voluntary (temporary) commitment for alcoholism. The Senior Citizen Club contacted the MPC, who, upon visiting the client's home, noted a number of health, financial, and maintenance problems which were simultaneously debilitating the client. As it appeared that the client might be in need of protective (psychiatric) care, the staff psychiatrist of the housing inspector's office, who regularly acts as a psychiatric consultant for the MPC, was called in for an evaluation. While signs of senility were evident, it was felt that, with assistance, the client could maintain herself in the community.

To assist in the client's self-maintenance, the health,

financial, and social problems noted above required professional attention. An independent charitable organization was contacted for financial aid in purchasing clothing and for funds to clean the apartment (both the client and her apartment had been described as "filthy"). Simultaneously, the Visiting Nurses' Association was asked to help the client, an arthritic, in the area of personal cleanliness and to aid her in coping with her arthritic condition.

The Welfare Department was contacted and asked to arrange some supplementary income, as were a sheltered workshop and an alcoholism clinic for the brother, who would be returning from institutionalization within a short time. The housing inspector's office was again contacted; this time it was asked to pressure the client's landlord into making necessary repairs to the apartment.

As is the case with many of the problems of senior citizens, certain of the ties made through the MPC during this period of crisis intervention would be of a continuing nature (welfare, for example). The MPC would cease its active involvement on the case when the crisis had ended.

THE MPC AND INTERSYSTEMIC RELATIONS A number of points are brought into focus by looking at this example. The first point is that the MPC fulfills its role of transducer by utilizing its position to marshal support for the client from a wide variety of sources within the professional caregiving system. The MPC may perform, almost entirely, the transducer function rather than providing direct service through its staff, although this function, too, is often performed by the professional staff.

A second point this example highlights is the relative position that various members of the professional care-giving system hold in the eyes of the community and the societal structure. That is, certain organizations are more visible than others, this visibility being a function of a number of factors relating to avenues of contact between the two systems. While some senior citizens might be aware of the different functions of the various organizations, through their experiences of traveling from agency to agency in order to find the solution to a problem or the answer to a question, those without such active experience with this intersystem would probably not know that such a system existed, much less be aware of the fruitful paths of entry into the system.

A third point, the one perhaps most clearly seen, is that there is a lack of adequate feedback mechanisms among members of different systems whose energies have been brought to bear on this case. While lack of feedback has shown itself to be a problem both within organizations (Miller 1950) and among component organizations of the same system (Young 1964), when intersystemic coordinate efforts are being attempted such a lack is even more threatening to successful handling of the crisis.

Without adequate feedback mechanisms, the possibilities of duplication of effort, or more dangerously, of no one making a particular effort since "another agency is dealing with that aspect of the problem," are greatly increased. Every component of each system in the intersystem is an independent system in and of itself. Each agency makes its own plans and decisions and carries out these decisions in the ways it feels will be most appropriate. While the MPC may request another agency to help in a certain case, it is entirely up to that agency to decide how this help will be forthcoming and with what areas of the problem the agency will deal. The uncertainties placed on the system by a lack of feedback may be predicted to create considerable tensions in the intersystem relations and to decrease the efficient handling of the intersystems operation (Chin 1961, and Bennis 1961).

The MPC is in a particularly difficult position because of its size (there are only three professional workers on the staff) and its defined role in the intersystem. While it has responsibility for marshaling sources of support from a large number of independent systems within the intersystem, it does not have supervisory authority over these independent sources. This lack of control is particularly true for more distant sectors of the intersystem which function on different levels (for example, the political system).

In the structure of the intersystem and its communication network, the lack of adequate feedback mechanisms has further consequences of depriving the MPC staff of adequate information for evaluating the effectiveness of the interventions they suggested and of assessing a client's additional maintenance needs after a particular crisis has been met. Once the members of other systems have taken responsibility for the case, there is no formalized method by which it can follow the case in order to judge if still other members of the intersystem are needed.

While time does not permit us to review a series of cases individually, essentially the same purpose may be served by utilization of some of the techniques of Network Analysis as outlined by Battersby (1964). There are, in this particular situation, a number of questions on which the analysis should focus: (1) What are the intersystem linkages most commonly used at present? (2) Which components of the intersystem serve sensor-receptor functions, and what are the various throughput and output mechanisms by which senior citizens cease contact with the professional care-giving suprasystem? (3) What are the existing mechanisms for feedback and communication? (4) How may intersystem flow be facilitated? From the practitioner's point of view, the first three questions are the important preliminaries to a useful and accurate answer to the fourth question.

The third major stage of network analysis, as is the case with many applied systems analyses, involves the allocation of relevant resources for the purposes of system improvement. It is not solely a time factor we are trying to reduce, and the costs we are attempting to lower are the human costs of suffering, deprivation, and loss of self-esteem. These costs are hard to measure, especially in terms of dollars and cents, and the use of selected aspects of such a network analysis program (particularly those related to critical path analysis) may enable the researcher-practitioner to uncover the critical components of an intersystem which need strengthening for the operation of the intersystem at a superior level.

A sample of cases were selected from MPC files on the basis that the researchers, in consultation with the agency staff, felt that these cases highlighted different aspects of the functioning of the intersystem relations regarding senior citizen care. A further sample of approximately twenty cases was drawn for the purpose of testing the veridicality of the intersystem model as presented below. The only major difference between the intensive study sample and the larger validating sample was that, as would be expected because of the criteria for selection of the intensive study sample, the larger validating sample contained proportionally more cases handled exclusively by the Multipurpose Center without the help of other agencies.

There exist a large number of input and output mechanisms which span the boundaries between the professional care-giving suprasystem and senior citizen (potential and real client) system. These linkages, as pointed out earlier, strengthen the interdependence between the component members of the intersystem. It should be remembered, however, that there are many individuals who are never involved, or are involved only to a peripheral degree, with the professional care-giving suprasystem. For these individuals, the input mechanisms into the set for senior citizens are primarily those determined by age, eligibility for social security, medicare, etc. There are essentially only two ways by which a person can leave the senior citizen set. The first of these is to move to another community, joining the same set in that community; and the second point of departure from the system is death.

In our analysis of the relationships within the care-giving system and between that system and the senior citizen set, we noted that the MPC provides a number of connectors which exert positive forces of attraction between the systems. Mechanisms such as the health education programs, the clublike atmosphere of the drop-in center, the activities of Senior Citizens Day, etc., serve to establish and maintain contact between members of the two systems.

Other characteristics of the MPC operations and those of other care-givers tend to act negatively, that is, to pull the systems apart. The fact that in most instances the client must present himself to the agency with a problem in order to establish the relationship will tend to minimize contact. This pulling apart may be seen as arising from a variety of factors, one such factor being the ideological commitment to independence on the part of the potential client. The individual resists asking for outside help, when all of his life he has been able to manage on his own.

The MPC receives input from a number of senior-receptor mechanisms operating within the confines of the senior citizen community. The receptors, with the addition of cases referred to the MPC by other professional agencies (less than 10 percent of the MPC's total case input), bring clients and potential clients to the boundary of the professional care-giving suprasystem.

Most of these identified sensor-receptor components are organizationally affiliated with the Multipurpose Center but function as foci of activities and interest for the senior citizens of the community, thereby strengthening the interdependence of the intersystems' relationships. At activities such as Senior Citizens Day, and the health education programs, senior citizens become acquainted with the ways in which the MPC can help them, currently or in the future. Also, at these activities agency staff have an opportunity to discuss specific problems of senior citizens. Those who attend center activities regularly are interviewed from time to time in order to uncover problems before they become serious.

DECISION-MAKING AND INTERSYSTEM COMMUNICATION Far more complicated than the input phase of the intersystems operations (particularly from the point of view of the MPC), are the throughput-output aspects. The MPC encounters a situation and contacts a number of independent agencies from both the public and private sectors of the care-giving suprasystem. At this point, certain decisions as to the priorities of needs and some projected plans for the meeting of these needs have been made. Each (treatment) agency contacted must decide what, if any, actions on their part are appropriate. Here is one point of potential conflict within the intersystem which is largely due to the independence of the interacting systems. As the treatment agency to which the MPC recommended the case makes its assessment of the situation, it may decide that it is an inappropriate agency for handling certain aspects of the case. Once the MPC has made its referral, however, it has no control over the other system's output transactions. This is particularly true with nonmunicipal agencies with whom MPC is not organizationally affiliated.

It can be well understood why difficulties in this area should arise. The referral made by the MPC, if accepted, would place an additional strain on what is probably an already overloaded staff. The relationship which exists between the MPC and the other agency may then be seen as placing a strain on the second agency. In order to avoid this strain, the agency may find it necessary only selectively to accept such referrals to avoid an intolerably increased level of tension and strain on the agency's limited resources. The refusal of the referral, however, will probably create an increased level of tension between these interacting systems.

The problem presents itself, here, that the agencies in intersystem relationships must devise mechanisms to control the levels of tensions not only within their own organizational system but also between their own system and other organizational systems. To fail to maintain a tolerable state of tension in either one will force the breakdown of either the systems themselves or the interrelationships among systems. The greater the degree of independence among systems, the more limited is the range of tension increases that intersystem relations can tolerate. The MPC is able to make a wider variety of demands upon the resources of the City hospital, to which it is organizationally tied, than it can upon the independent agencies.

This potential source of breakdown in the efficient operations of the intersystem relations between care-givers and senior citizens can be ameliorated only if there exist adequate communication linkages and feedback mechanisms between the interacting systems. On the basis of tracing the path of communication concerning each of the cases reviewed in the course of this research, and as confirmed in interviews with MPC staff, the paths of communication concerning cases are almost entirely one way. Even if the initiative for gathering feedback were to be taken by the referring agency, it would often be impossible to get information back promptly concerning the progress of the case.

With external pressures facing agencies to attempt integrated operations with minimal "overlap" of services, an increasing need for the development of mechanisms for adequate and rapid communication of relevant information is eminent.

Considering the strain which already exists upon the limited resources of the professional care-giving suprasystem and the ever increasing number of persons in the set of potential clients (now approximately 12,000), a mechanism must be designed which will take a minimum of staff time and yet convey maximal information. The device would serve the multiple purposes of (1) recording the actions taken by the output (treatment) agency for its own records; (2) providing feedback to the transducer or input agency concerning actions which have been taken; and (3) providing background information to any agency to whom the case is further referred for action. While there exist a number of plans for systems of feedback which members of the MPC staff have been investigating, as have other care-givers in the city and state, no such plan has been adopted in the city.

For optimal functioning of the care-giving system for senior citizens in the city, a feedback and communication mechanism must be designed which, in addition to fulfilling the three purposes outlined above, will provide information taken in a uniform manner which covers a large number of potential problem areas in health and social functioning. As the collection of this type of information will be somewhat time consuming, the system should require that the basic information be taken only once (as opposed to the current system whereby each agency takes most of the data at the client's first entry into the agency). The feedback mechanism should also be designed to ensure that information taken once can be passed on from one treatment agency to another without having to be retaken. If the information is to be usable, it must be readily available to a care-giver when it encounters a given client.

As these requirements build upon each other, it becomes clear that one method of meeting the various needs of intersystems communications is by means of a centralized communications resource (information center) which could collect and relay needed information regarding client situations quickly and efficiently. One logical point for the attachment of such a component would be at one of the intersystem's common transducing agents, the MPC. To some extent, this function is carried out when the MPC makes referrals (throughput transactions) of the cases it receives. With the addition of a uniform feedback system to the MPC, such a communication unit could be established.

Because we are dealing with intersystems relations, however, we also are confronted with the task of focusing on the effects of factors such as the location (organizationally and spatially) of such a centralized information center. On the basis of functioning definitions of the various agencies, as noted above, we concluded that an efficient location for the information center would be the MPC. Because of the nature of relationships between the systems involved, there are a number of consequences to this particular location which require further examination. The placing of the information collection and distribution functions within any one agency will greatly increase the power of that agency vis-à-vis those agencies who must both come to it for information and report to it regarding the interventions which it has made in a particular case. In a situation in which there exists less than perfect trust among the interacting agencies, or one in which the agencies see themselves as competitors for a limited quantity of resources (which is almost always the case), it could be expected that agencies would resist full utilization of the information center. The resistance has been shown to be increasing among social service exchanges.

Further, we might expect that an agency would have similar objection to the placement of such a center in any existing or newly formed and independent agency. The existence of any organization to which one must report and from whom one must get information is a threat to the autonomous functioning of an agency. Such an arrangement would be acceptable only if the agencies felt that this information referral system were their property (which brings us to a possible explanation of why there exists such resistance to change regarding referral systems and why there has been such little use of various clearinghouses of information in the past).

We are then posed with a dilemma: to locate an information referral center with any one agency will create intersystems tensions such that communication among the systems may cease; to locate it independently from all other agencies may well result in its ostracism from the rest of the interrelating systems. The possibility of developing a "cooperatively" owned information center depends upon the existence of a rather substantial degree of trust among the agencies as well as a monumental effort at coordination among independent agencies of different systems.

While the above analysis of intersystemic relationships has not pointed the way to an easy solution to a complicated problem, it has given some insight into the complicated nature of the problem and has pointed to potential difficulties. These difficulties might not have been seen had not this examination focused on the unique characteristics of intersystems relations.

III. Some Questions and Issues Arising from an Intersystem Model

By turning back to the first section, where we spelled out

some of the emergent concepts of an intersystem model as based on systems theory, we can raise some questions. It is useful to remind ourselves of why we are pursuing an intersystem model. We do see that intersystem analysis allows for new questions and issues to be raised about boundaries, dynamics and tensions, and feedback and change as a result of the new slant and perspective. The most closely related body of literature relevant in organizational systems literature is that concerned with issues of interface and with the problems of and need for creating linkages and linking mechanisms for parts of a system. In the context of the problems posed, these newly created interfaces and linkages are seen as solutions of and resolutions to the problems between the two systems or components. Here we are equally concerned with the new dynamics, new issues, and new problems which are laid open by an intersystem analysis. In a way, the stance we are taking is that these oft-seen problems ought to be treated as integrally related to the basic notions of the extended system analysis proposed under the rubric of intersystem analysis. We mean that this paper is exploratory in advancing beyond the analysis of system *qua* system into the realm of the unique properties of the intersystem level.

EMERGENT CHARACTERISTICS OF THE INTERSYSTEM MODEL In reviewing the case of the multipurpose center, and in drawing from experiences in other settings where intersystem properties are involved, we might try to abstract some of the specific and newly constructed ideas that are uniquely characteristic of an intersystem model. We have no deep commitment to the particular terms and concepts that follow. What we are trying to do here is locate ideas that seem to represent suitable modifications and/or expansions of systems theory, while staying within the basic terms of general systems theory. Whenever possible, we shall also keep in mind the dynamics of change in the intersystem so as to integrate diagnosis with intervention possibilities.

As an aid in thinking about intersystem conditions, we have found it useful to visualize the intersystem as a dumbbell with large knobs at each end with an interconnecting piece which ties the two ends together. System terms deal with the knobs, the systems, at each end; intersystem terms deal with the connective middle that links both systems and is simultaneously part of both systems.

The presentation will necessarily be brief and somewhat elliptical; the formulations are still tentative. We shall try to refer to the second section to illustrate the emergence and the usefulness of the ideas.

BOUNDARY MODIFICATIONS IN INTERSYSTEM ANALYSIS A boundary of a system is operationally defined as the line where the interchange across the line is less than the interchange within the line. That which is interchanged can be of many kinds: energies, inputs, and outputs. Boundaries are tight or open, require energy to maintain, and have the property of permeability in open systems.

Crossings will be the interchanges between one system and the other system as seen from an intersystem perspective.

Referrals of clients from the MPC to an intake point of another agency will affect the permeability of the boundary of that receiving agency. More generally, under what conditions will an increase or a decrease in crossings affect the boundaries of the system? The boundary of an agency as a system can expand or contract, can become more permeable. As differentiation of functions occur in the care-giving agencies, will permeabilities lessen? Under differentiation and specialization of functions, it seems that boundaries tighten and become more impermeable with attendant increases in crossings.

In a care-giving agency system, there are strong environmental pushes that shape boundaries—funds, social demands, and so forth. Environmental demands, stresses, and turbulences create intersystems. The functional interrelations of an intersystem and its boundaries and other intersystem issues need to be dealt with directly. Such changes as mergers and shifting boxes on organizational charts rarely touch on the functional boundary and the crossings in the intersystem. Collaboration and trust in communication and coordination go beyond boundary concerns, although building these qualities of an intersystem do require, among other things, clarification of boundaries and crossings. In intersystem relationships, energies required for boundary maintenance and for adjustments in the nature of boundary permeabilities are closely tied to the energies required for the maintenance of equilibria and steady states internal to systems.

INTERDEPENDENCE AND INDEPENDENCE MODIFICATION IN THE INTERSYSTEM The essence of the intersystem model is in the nature of and quality of interdependency and independency, simultaneously treated. Treating each of these separately in the first instance leads to more convenient models of one system; the latter leads to separate analyses as two systems.

Interdependency can be conjunctive or disjunctive, that is, pulling closer or pushing away. The degree of interconnectedness is not simply a function of attractiveness of the one for the other. There are many concepts of interdependence and independence that have been developed in personality, small group, and organizational theory, as well as from biological and physical models. Positional concepts such as linkages and linking persons in interfaces, marginality roles, liaison functions, brokers, and gatekeepers, to mention a few, have been extensively developed as systems analysis has come to the foreground of attention. The functional attributes of the dynamics arising from simultaneously and interactively analyzing interdependence and independence have also been deeply explored in these fields. The exaggeration of the autonomy of two systems of two subsystems treated as an intersystem is one of the hoped-for virtues of an intersystem model. At the heart of the intersystem model is the application of concepts and models from numerous areas of inquiry including conflict theory, game theory, exchange theory, and balance theory.

EQUILIBRIUM AND STEADY STATE MODIFICATIONS IN THE INTERSYSTEM By definition, the steady state of relations between two systems is not and cannot be isomorphic with the internal steady state of one of the systems. The simple extension that seems to be required is the concept of equilibrium or steady state of an intersystem. In these terms, following general systems theory, we then look for the mechanisms that maintain, that disturb, that bring perturbations, and that tend to restore the steady state of relations in the intersystem. Most importantly, as a virtue of an intersystem model, we can see the ways in which the steady state and its dynamics of one or both the systems have consequences for the steady state of the intersystem, and how in turn the requirements of the steady state of the intersystem bring about consequences for one or both systems. Perhaps the term *equilibrium of equilibriums* conveys the notions involved in describing the steady state of an intersystem. Whether the properties of the equilibrium of equilibriums are the same as those of any equilibrium requires some further analysis. Given the limited nature of interdependence and the limited interactions—the separateness of boundaries—one would suspect that the assumed dynamics around the steady state of steady states would at least be dampened or even be different. It can be proposed that the issue of change in the structure of a system, the issues of "step-jump" and innovative emergence of new properties of a system, may be relevant to this conception of a steady state of steady states in an intersystem.

FEEDBACK AND STEERING MODIFICATIONS IN THE INTERSYSTEM

Feedback dependence occurs when the sensing, detecting, and processing of the effects of a system are located primarily in the other system, a situation which is the complement of the focal system in intersystem relations. Feedback mechanisms can be located in one system which then must transfer to the originating system the observed data of the effects of action of the acting system. Feedback dependence implicates the nature of the interdependence and connections and the quality of trust within the intersystem.

Feedback and steering of the intersystem can be treated in systems terms. There is one aspect of feedback which is part of the asymmetry of the systems in intersystems relationships, namely, feedback dependence.

CHANGE AND CHANGING MODIFICATIONS IN THE INTERSYSTEM

One of the felt difficulties with systems theory has been the problem of change. While systems theory has been strong on diagnosis and understanding of the interrelations of parts, systems models have been accused of inherent conservatism. Boulding (1966), in discussing "Expecting the Unexpected," reviews the models of mechanical systems, pattern systems, equilibrium systems and evolutionary systems. "In practice, the main cause for failure in prediction is a sudden change in the characteristics of the system itself. Such a change has been called a 'system break' . . . system breaks, unfortunately are very hard to detect. They are virtually impossible to predict in advance; they are even difficult to detect after they have happened for some time, because in the short run it is virtually impossible to distinguish the beginning of a new long term trend from a strictly temporary fluctuation."

In the short run, and for the purposes of intervention and engagement in relationships with a system in order to bring about change, systems models have virtues and limitations. Interest has been shown in applying an intersystems model to this problem. In these formulations, the change agent is one part of the intersystem relationship.

With regard to the processes of facilitating deliberate change from within the system, the intersystems model provides for the assumption of an existential relationship between the "internal" change agent and the system undergoing change. In therapy, training, and organizational development such relationships serve as the basis for the procedures and technologies used.

In more general terms, the intersystems model is better able to focus on deliberately bringing about change, whereas systems models are better equipped for observing and recording change and factoring out the dynamics of change. The intersystems model provides for directionality of planned change, the processes facilitating change, and for alteration of a system, thereby going beyond, in some senses, the systems model. Yet there are conceptual reconciliations possible. Both the "vested interests" source of tension and strain and feedback dependence are installed in a system by the formation of an intersystem relationship. Sometimes these intersystem relationships are in a temporary system.

Concluding Overview

In applying system concepts to the case of a care-delivering arrangement for the aged, we have tried to show an intersystem model has some utility for systematically opening up the issues and problems. We see the system concepts elevated to an intersystems model as a convenient way to conceptualize the arrangements and to lay open the intervention possibilities for bringing about change. A few emergent concepts for intersystems analysis, still in systems terms, are derived for an intersystems model. The ill-formed development of the intersystems approach requires more concentrated effort to delineate more sharply the modified systems concepts for intersystems analysis.

References

Alexander, Christopher
(1965), "A City is Not a Tree." *Architectural Forum, 122,* 2. Abstracted in *Ekistics* (1967), *23,* 139, 344–348.

Battersby, Albert
(1964), *Network Analysis for Planning and Scheduling.* New York: St. Martins.
Bennis, W. G.
(1961), "A Typology of Change Processes." In W. Bennis, K. Benne, and R. Chin (eds.), *The Planning of Change.* New York: Holt, Rinehart and Winston. 154–156.
Bertalanffy, L. von
(1956), "General Systems Theory." *General Systems.* Yearbook of the Society for the Advancement of General System Theory, *1,* 1–10.
Boulding, Kenneth E.
(1966), "Expecting the Unexpected Future of Knowledge and Technologies." In Edgar L. Morphet (ed.), *Prospective Changes in Society by 1980.* Denver: Designing Education for the Future Project. Pp. 199–213.
Chin, Robert
(1961), "The Utility of System Models and Developmental Models for Practitioners." In W. Bennis, K. Benne, and R. Chin (eds.), *The Planning of Change.* New York: Holt, Rinehart and Winston. Pp. 201–214.
Hall, A. D., and R. E. Fagen
(1956), "Definition of System." *General Systems.* Yearbook of the Society for the Advancement of General System Theory, *1,* 18–28.
Miller, J. G.
(1950), "Living Systems." *Behavioral Science, 10,* 193–237.
Young, O. R.
(1964), "A Survey of General Systems Theory." *General Systems, 9,* 61–80.

Curtis P. McLaughlin

10. Systems Analysis for Health

The word "systems" is clearly an all-right word and has therefore had to work very hard. It generally refers to the approach in which an intractably complex problem is divided into a series of more tractable subproblems for the purpose of constructing a model. It also has been used in the sense of "general systems," in which it refers to the search for formal similarities between the attempted solutions of problems in different fields. By a curious but understandable extension it has come to mean approaching an empirical problem with an extensive use of electric data processing and collecting.
L. B. Slobodkin, *Science*, January 26, 1968, p. 415.

This chapter will focus on Slobodkin's first use of the term systems, although it is sandwiched between documents that emphasize the "general systems" approach. These two approaches share strong similarities of point of view, however, despite the unfortunate pressures to professionalize such work under the titles of operations research or systems analysis. Both are philosophically committed to introducing methods derived from any discipline regardless of the field. Both seek the widest possible breadth of view of the system under study. Both view the system as a whole—one as a scientist, the other more as an engineer.

The systems analyst, as systems engineer or operations researcher, or whatever other label he bears, is constrained by circumstances or by choice to a narrower view of most problems than the general systems man, usually by a commitment to produce a recommendation applicable at a specific point in time. To him, "a system is a set of operations organized to satisfy a definable user requirement. You'll find this is more restrictive than the normal ones in the English dictionary. First, it uses the word "operations," rather than "things," therefore, it includes not only structures of tangible black boxes, but manual procedures and computer programs —intangible but very real structures. Note that it implies a way of measuring the effectiveness of a system" (Affel 1964, p. 19).

The systems analyst who takes health as his area of investigation faces real problems in establishing a user requirement and in measuring effectiveness. But only a portion of his problems stem from the unique attributes of the health field. Joseph H. Engel, Vice President of the Operations Research Society of America, defined a generic problem at a recent forum on Systems Analysis and Social Change: "As we move closer and closer to human beings, human life and its goals, we find that we are dealing progressively with more and more difficult problems. . . . We're good at hardware and tactical problems and starting well-defined research and development programs. We're lousy at strategic and philosophical problems." ("Systems Analysts Are Baffled" 1968, p. 28).

Despite this caveat, I am sanguine about the contributions that systems analysis will make to health activities. It is with the hope of encouraging such contributions that this chapter outlines the approaches of people in operations research and systems analysis and relates them to the present realities of health care. Studies are cited and some opinions rendered and rent concerning the exciting road ahead for health professionals and systems analysts. Because of the welter of names, titles, and professional claims, this chapter starts with a historical overview of activities labeled as systems analysis. Then the conceptual process which is its basic method of operation will be described, followed by discussions of the application of specific models to health activities.

The history of systematic management thought traditionally starts with the Scientific Management movement and Frederick Taylor's work at the turn of the century (1911). Taylor acknowledges that the administrator's job involves a social and economic system to be studied scientifically and planned rationally with the aid of any and all available techniques. Although a number of systems analysts preceded Taylor—Charles Babbage, Henry Towne, even Florence Nightingale—Taylor's efforts were the first to lead to an organized movement. The Society To Promote the Science of Management was formed in 1912, and the Society of Industrial Engineers in 1917. While these groups continued to develop their own competences, World War II brought new and more prestigious groups frequently labeled "operations research." Operations research solved problems by grouping together specialists from many disciplines, each of whom brought his own sets of conceptual tools and mathematical models. The wartime successes of these multidisciplinary groups in attacking military problems received much publicity; and that approach was institutionalized in organizations such as The RAND Corporation. When university departments of industrial engineering sensed that they were losing the competition for bright students to departments with a broader mathematics and science base, they began to adopt the quantitative models approach as their substantive base. Like schools of management, they increased their emphasis on operations research.

In the post-World War II defense establishment, the complexity and uncertainty of military decisions increased markedly with new technology, heavy time pressures, and rising costs (Gilmore, Ryan, and Gould, 1967). Many more alternatives had to be considered than possibly could be tested. New methods of a priori technical and economic evaluation were required. At the same time, a number of experiences occurred in which the total system failed to perform acceptably, even though each component seemed to have been developed adequately (Marschak 1964). These failures focused attention on the need to pay attention to the overall architecture of large systems. Defense contractors responded by establishing special systems analysis and systems management groups.

The emerging computer revolution has steadily increased the systems analyst's capabilities for handling large and complex systems. It has continued to ease the constraints on his tools for analysis and control. This is the background of the "curious but understandable extension" to which Slobodkin refers. Indeed, without computers few systems analysts would be willing to tackle problems of the depth and breadth they do today. Life is too short.

Greater capability for solving problems has brought increased prestige and organizational influence to the systems analyst, and this has led to the inevitable tendency to use impressive titles wherever possible. One well-known health systems analyst has the title of Associate Professor of Industrial Engineering, Operations Research, and Systems Analysis. The historical sequence is neatly preserved in that title. Cashing in on the currency of the title, accountants branching out into paperwork control and computer programmers are titled "systems analysts," while computer salesmen and servicers are designated "systems engineers."

Yet beneath this historical and semantic melange there is a relatively consistent approach to problem-solving which is the basis for systems analysis. Although it appears in many shapes and many places, it remains an elemental formula for rational analysis and behavior (see Affel 1964; Ackoff 1956; and Litchfield 1956). What is important is not the label, but what this approach under any label has to offer toward restructuring the health system to meet a real set of user requirements.

Time and time again the systems analyst is called upon to defend the substance of his area. After a full presentation and discussion one legitimate response from the audience is that his approach is essentially the scientific method coupled with a hard-nosed common sense and a bag of mathematical tricks. Essentially the systems analyst is an engineer who deals with large and complex problems which he may choose to treat as systems in the sense described by Affel. As Kershner (1960, p. 141) states, "A system is a collection of entities or things (animate or inanimate) which receives certain imputs and is constrained to act concertedly upon them to produce certain outputs with the objective of maximizing some function of inputs and outputs." This engineering point of view implies a commitment to an explicit objective, to a limited time horizon, to extensive use of the tools of science where applicable, and to "partial control with partial understanding" (Bellman 1964) in the face of complexity and uncertainty.[1]

A conceptual model outlining the systems analysis approach is as likely to halt progress as a definition, but Figure 1 is presented as yet another such model. The first and often the most crucial step in the analytical process is to specify the system in question. The man who calls in the systems analyst usually specifies the system, but the analyst is faced with a dilemma. He must rely on the experience and ex-

[1] Some of us, I think, could get through life gracefully with this definition alone. But the word *systems* may be a depreciating currency following a Gresham's law of semantics. I tend to instruct my students to disregard the word "systems" wherever it appears and to concentrate on the modifying objective in front of it in order to understand what the reader is discussing.

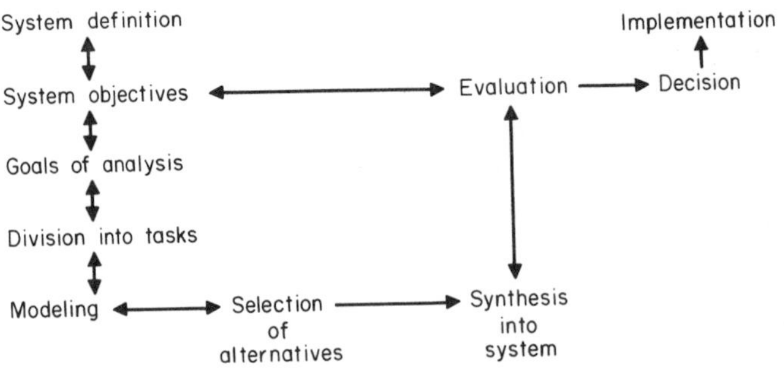

Figure 1. One conceptualization of systems analysis.

pertise of the decision-maker, yet he knows that his informant may not have the most useful definition of the system. If he did, he probably would have solved the problem without a consultation.

On the other hand the analyst must be aware that in substituting his own view he may be imposing a stereotype out of his catalogue of conceptual and mathematical models for the "real" system. Such a superimposition has two dangers. First, it may prevent the analyst from seeking a sufficiently broad (open) view of the system with its myriad interactions with the environment. The second risk is that, having seen a parallel with a known problem or solution technique, the analyst may not take his task seriously, especially the implementation phase. It does neither party much good when an operations researcher hears a description of a nurse staffing problem and snorts, "That is the box-car loading problem and we solved that in 1945." Much of the time the effective health systems analyst must carry at least two models, a closed system for modeling and an open one for evaluating and implementing. The first is necessary for the application of solution techniques available to him. The second is necessary if he is to operate successfully as a change agent in the health environment.

Thus the success of systems projects in health depends as much on diplomacy, if not tact, as on technical competence. Furthermore, the open systems view is as necessary for maintaining relevance as the closed systems view is necessary for mathematical definition. Although the importance of starting with the correct system or problem definitions can hardly be overemphasized,[2] there is a danger that that portion of the process can consume the life of the project. It seems inevitable that redefinitions should come as a by-product of iterations of the cycle. Anyone who has worked on a complex problem usually is impressed by how much his understanding of that problem has improved after he has worked on it for a while. Perhaps there is some merit in studies set up for the sole objective of defining a problem, but my personal evaluation is that real understanding comes only from a commitment to change.

Once an operational definition of the system itself has been formulated, it is important to define carefully the goals of the system. Both the structure of the analysis and the evaluation of the alternatives derive from these goals. Inappropriate goals will be just as harmful as inaccurate application of analytical techniques. Either one will result in the misuse of scarce resources. In open systems like health and medicine, however, setting operational goals is tricky. But that is a hazard of taking on any significant social problem. Biderman (1966) analyzes the problems of setting goals and measuring progress in national social services. Indeed, Boulding (1966, p. B–165) warns us of the dangers of depending on quantitative value functions "simply because the clarity and objectivity of quantitatively measurable subordinate goals can be easily lead to a failure to bear in mind that they are in fact subordinate." In health this problem is just as acute at the community level as it is on the national level (Packer 1968). Although White (1968), Saunders (1964), and others have suggested schemes for comprehensive health measures, none has been accepted, and the outlook for adopting any one objective function in health is poor. At best, goals, like problem definitions, will be transitory; but the best permanent floating set must be kept in the foreground as the analyst proceeds with his work.

The purpose question is a method of starting the analysis as well as a search for an objective. At a conference on

[2] The systems analyst is a mathematically erudite problem solver. A very shaky but occasionally useful analogy compares problems with symptoms and systems analysis with diagnostic and treatment activities involving the disease, host and environment. The systems analyst's armamentarium, has been summarized by Page (1960). It certainly includes a strong background in economics, probability theory, management, and information science, plus some familiarity with the physical and social sciences.

systems analysis, held at Harvard in conjunction with the preparation of this book, Dr. Ed Roberts of M.I.T.'s Sloan School illustrated the effectiveness of this method by asking the physicians in the group to define the objectives of a teaching hospital and the problems of greatest import to them in that setting. Only after these men had framed a series of progressively more refined definitions and broken down the problems into operational questions did answers begin to emerge, but emerge they did.

When the goals of the system have been defined, the next step is to select the strategy for analysis. Failure to accept this as a separate and distinct step is a major pitfall. Horvath (1968, p. B–276) warns that some members of the medical profession

have come to accept change, including that in their own profession, as a sign of progress. They are not only ready but in some respects even eager to seek the help of management scientists in correcting the problems of the organization of health care, especially where they affect matters within their immediate cognizance. In fact, management scientists entering this field should be on guard that the medical profession should not be oversold on the potential benefits from their studies. For, if they are not careful, they may arouse unrealistic expectations of quick solutions to all of the management and organizational problems of the health field. These expectations could quickly turn to disillusionment in the face of the hard realites of dealing with the complexities in the organization of medical care.

In administration many of the diseases are chronic and one seeks temporal mastery over ongoing conditions, not cures. It is important that the patient understands this basic fact.

Obviously, the strategy for analysis must be congruent with the goals of the system. However, the goals of the analysis must be understood as limited ones. The analyst usually intends to contribute to achievement of the goals of the system, but he cannot be all things to all men. He must set forth specifically what he expects to achieve. His expectation will be governed by the methods of analysis available to him and the resources he can command. The goals of analysis will, of course, be constrained by the money, manpower, and capabilities available as well as the tractability of the problem. A responsible study design is built around the capabilities of the men who will do the work. There is nothing quite so discouraging as finding that someone has developed a good study, finally secured a grant or contract to perform it, and then has to scurry around for bodies to do work. Such a project may be a nice educational and financial experience for those who are recruited, but the client probably gets short-changed. Both the client and the analyst must have a full understanding of what is possible with the given resources.

The managers of research and development activities in the aerospace industries have a useful procedure for breaking projects down into "work packages." This involves outlining the job in sufficient detail so that it can be separated into well-defined tasks which can be assigned to individuals or small groups for completion within a specified time period. This procedure also sets the responsibility for completing the work package on the shoulders of one individual. Usually that same individual helps plan the project proposal, contributing his professional assessment as to which parts of the problem are tractable and what personnel will be required. This analysis also indicates where and how men and teams can work independently and where and when they must come together to exchange information. In health, where professionals of many types may become involved in solving a given problem, the work package approach may be especially relevant.

Each team of professionals assigned part of a study will carry out a modeling process. It may range from an implicit problem structure to a large digital computer simulation, but it will be the all-important guide for collecting and interpreting information and it will inevitably be various biases of the investigators. Kuhn (1962) argues effectively that advancement in a science is constrained by the conceptual model that the majority of investigators hold. He points out that experiments are designed with expectations for the behavior of all but one or two variables; and he gives examples of the traumatic impact on cohorts of scientists when their conception of nature underwent a radical change. The investigator's conception of nature determines what data will be collected, what will be observed, and how it will be interpreted. But other factors also affect model building. Each specialist on a project may have his favorite approaches that lead him to follow certain methods of finding the data upon which the final output will depend. He will have fluency with certain types of models and he will adhere to professional standards which may be superfluous or unrelated to system goals, but which may have to be recognized in the project design.

The selection of personnel and allocation of resources by the project director will hinge in part on his judgment about how intensive and extensive the modeling process must be and how he will achieve his goals of analysis. Often, winning acceptance for a project requires kinds of data that are not directly relevant to the final recommendation. Special data may be necessary to impress questioners with the thoroughness of the study or to head off special interest groups or hostile reactions. For example, in a project that involved planning facilities for a small, densely populated state it became evident to the research team that three to five locations would provide reasonable accessability for all residents. Yet we prepared a town-by-town estimate of the case load, so that we could answer questions from legislators and others about the needs in their town or district and then show that the load was below the minimum economical caseload for a service center. Similarily, to safeguard his recommendations, the analyst often may have to devise a program for prevention as well as for treatment, even when the experts cannot agree on any specific mode of prevention. He must anticipate that he will inevitably be asked, What about prevention? Similarily, he also must be prepared to show how his systems analysis fits in with the universal objective of comprehensive care, even though comprehensive care may be out of the question because of its cost.

When the analyst undertakes to implement an efficient system for health care in addition to designing it, he faces some difficult professional and moral choices. He starts with simple conceptual models which he elaborates as he gains knowledge. But he knows that although sophisticated models impress the client and lead to professional stature and advancement, most of their real contribution will be the support and training of graduate students. Does he push on with the most sophisticated model or does he seek only what he needs?

A greater dilemma occurs when some assumptions or results of the analysis will be offensive to the client or to some health constituency. Does the analyst alter his recommendations, does he hide the problem under the rug, or does he boldly charge ahead with what he thinks is right?

A concrete example of this sort of questions is found in recent studies concerning medical facilities to support victims of end-stage renal failure, either by dialysis (artificial kidneys) or by transplantation. Two national systems studies (*Report of the Committee on Chronic Kidney Disease* [1967] and U.S. Public Health Service [1967]) have been completed and studies were conducted in California, Illinois, Massachusetts, New York, and North Carolina. All of these studies are based on epidemiological data projecting the number of persons in the population who will develop end-stage renal failure. Yet for planning purposes the critical variable is the much smaller number of individuals who actually arrive at the door of a renal service before their health has declined below the existing criteria for maintenance dialysis. Does the analyst point out in his report that he is cutting his estimate of the caseload by 20 percent because the physicians in Asparagus and Sassafras Counties probably never will do a good job of diagnosing kidney disease? Probably not. My own inclination would be to compensate by being more conservative in other assumptions and estimates, making sure that the client is informed of this adjustment verbally or in working documents.

Similar problems arise in planning programs for a community or state where racial barriers or rural poverty preclude health care for much of the population. Again the analyst's decision is a matter of conscience, although my personal choice would be to face the fact in the public report.

An even trickier situation occurs where the analyst finds himself in the midst of an arms race among local medical institutions and the hidden agenda for his project includes heading off the proliferation of uneconomically sized special facilities. Does he come out and say that Hospital X and Y should not build a burn center or purchase cobalt bombs? I doubt that that is the most effective approach. Perhaps the best solution is to hide behind the professional cloak and merely specify the assumptions, facts, and results which outline the best system, ignoring for the moment the planned location and number. If the community agrees with the assumptions and analysis, then they are boxed in by the results. The analyst may not stop the power struggle among major institutions or medical schools, but he has given some authoritative leverage to those with stature to apply pressure without arousing direct attack. Chances are that those who would not respond to facts and community pressure, would not have gone along with a direct recommendation either.

Another major reality of the health field, which complicates the moral dilemmas, is the dilemma of incompatible goals. An example of this is the desire for comprehensive care for all at reasonable cost. Norman R. Baker (1967) has pointed out that this is a natural hazard of service organizations in general. He observes and supports with a quasiquantitative model the fact that the user, the funder, and the provider all develop perceived goals, constraints, and policies which may be mutually irreconcilable. For example, when discussing the kidney dialysis problem with a relatively sophisticated group of laymen, one frequently encounters the response that we should mass produce artificial kidney machines and supply them to those who need them. Such a suggestion, however, assumes that the supply of doctors, nurses, and technicians is relatively flexible, and that thousands of these people would choose to concentrate their efforts and institutional resources on this disease entity instead of others. Making dialysis machines in the same manner that we make automobiles would be simple, but operating an adequate care system is quite another thing.

The typical operations researcher is ill equipped to deal with such dilemmas. Universities teach the operations researcher the models, but not the art of modeling. Morris (1967, p. B–709) makes a distinction between the "teaching of models" and the "teaching of modeling." He suggests that the modeling process has three basic phases in that it begins with a real problem, adopts a much simplified analogy or association as a model "quite distinct from reality, and attempts to move in an evolutionary fashion toward more elaborate models which more nearly reflect the complexity of the actual management situation." If the systems analyst operates in this manner, he forces himself to judge at each step whether enrichment will be worth the extra effort and investment. In addition he is in the position of producing an interim analysis which can be fed into the cycle shown in

Figure 1 until that uncertain day when the newly enriched model works.

Morris illustrates the process by describing a systems study of a transportation network. Here the Massachusetts Kidney Disease Planning Project, in which the writer participated, serves as a health-oriented example. The discussion of the project scope centered on the task called for by a contract with the Kidney Disease Control Branch of the Public Health Service, on what realistically might be accomplished, on operational definition of kidney disease, on what personnel were available, on how they might be best utilized, etc. Out of those initial discussions the model shown in Figure 2 emerged. That diagram also served as a precedence network of the type used by specialists in PERT (Program Evaluation and Review Technique) (Levin and Kirkpatrick, 1966). As soon as a rough project scope was devised, we could begin to put people to work on tasks.

The first iteration of the entire cycle really occurred within the first meeting or two, because certain implementation requirements were readily evident, for example, effective

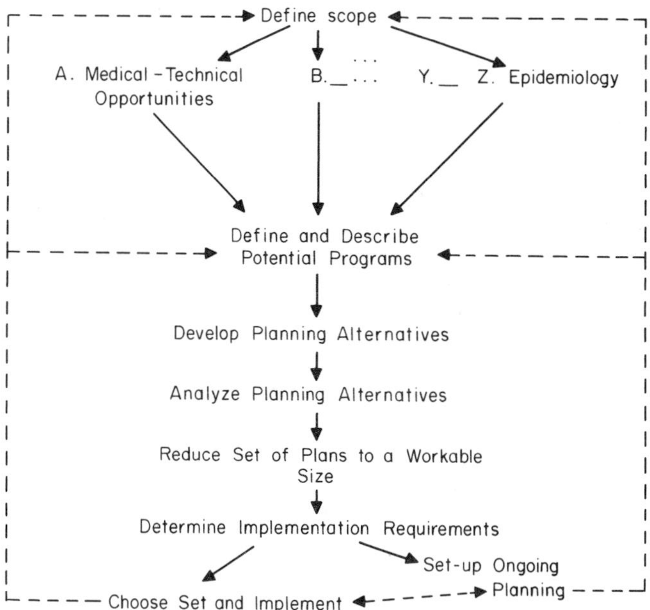

Figure 2. Preliminary model of a state kidney disease control program.

implementation by the powerless project group depended on the active participation of the physicians providing services. They would have to be involved in the earliest phases, the study of medical-technical opportunities. Therefore, one of the earliest steps was to call these physicians together as a technical advisory committee to educate the project staff (which included two physicians) on the operational implications of medical science information about kidney disease. Substantive areas of disagreement among these specialists were uncovered and narrowed down considerably. Information was presented about current programs and future plans.

During this period other work packages were defined and assigned. A trained physician epidemiologist gathered the fragmentary data available on kidney disease in Massachusetts, reviewed the literature, and prepared a background paper, giving his estimates of the occurrence of end-stage renal failure in the state and other data pertaining to the design of a prevention program. The writer and the staff gathered data on the distribution of hospital service areas in the state, their population densities, travel times for patients, and hospital plans for expansion into dialysis and transplantation. A welfare consultant canvassed the hospitals, insurance carriers, voluntary agencies, and state bureaus for information about the amounts and conditions of aid for patients.

The writer prepared a computer model to determine the year-by-year facilities needs under various assumptions about caseload, facilities available for dialysis and transplantation, survival rates, and transplant success rates. Although he considered using Markov chain analysis (Howard 1960) or a stochastic digital simulation (Naylor, Balintfy, *et al.* 1966), these were rejected as gildings of the lily. A deterministic computer model was prepared and used to calculate monthly the expected value of the outcomes of the care system.[3] The degree of control that the project might have excercised certainly did not warrant more refined analysis. In fact, the tables in the final report were based on hand calculations using successive year-end figures.[4]

3 All the variables were uncertain and could have been represented by probability distributions, but single point estimates were used for simplicity. A further simplification was the use of the monthly calculations to represent what was a continuous process.

4 Although the problem may not change, a change in context may call for a change in strategy of analysis. In a comparable study for North Carolina,

As the preliminary studies fed out conclusions, the project staff could begin to see the size of the problem to be faced, the resources available, the possible avenues for prevention and treatment, and the possibilities for financing. They discovered that no significant programs for prevention could be implemented, except as federally funded research projects. Transplantation activities would be expanded in due course by the teaching hospitals, and this would rapidly reduce the rate of expansion required for dialysis facilities. In fact, it appeared that expansion could cease after about seven years. This, however, was based on an assumption that the present rigid medical standards for dialysis candidates would continue in effect. The actual result is more likely to be a relaxation of these standards if facilities become available. Since it appeared unlikely that the project would have much influence on the amount of transplantation done by the wealthy and relatively independent medical schools, the planning for this service was only rudimentary. More emphasis was given to dialysis facilities.

The project staff discussed policies and procedures for state agencies and sought such changes as might improve patient care. Plans were made to channel more patients to agencies or bureaus with aid money available and to assure fuller use of insurance benefits. A recommendation was made for the minimum size, number, and general location of dialysis centers. Authorizations and appropriations were sought and received from the legislature to allow the state Department of Health to assist in establishing such centers. Other potential activities, such as case finding, medical education, and research were evaluated and temporarily set aside because of limited personnel and time and the lack of a clear mandate or a high payoff.

The project conducted studies or drew upon prior studies that applied a number of concepts and modeling tools from operations research, including network planning, decision

geographic variables obviously were extremely important. Travel times and distances had to be considered much more carefully than in Massachusetts. Therefore, patient loads were estimated for each population center, and patient travel costs were compared for alternative locations in an attempt to identify the configurations that would hold down the patient travel costs. In Massachusetts these costs were virtually negligible. Similar analyses were made of the socioeconomic factors affecting the adaptability of the patient and his family to home dialysis, since this factor was considered a potential cause of nonuniform variations in the demand at the regional dialysis centers.

theory, cost-benefit analysis, returns to scale, present value, and computer programming. A more extensive study could have applied information theory, linear programming (which was in fact applied in North Carolina), simulation, and Markov chains.

During the project the staff also was heavily concerned with the activities shown on the right of Figure 1. Many community groups and skilled professionals were drawn together in various meetings to discuss and set the stage for implementing the medical, economic, and social conclusions of the study. The structure of the whole study was predicated on the objective of getting recommendations implemented. Alternatives were weighted heavily on their ease of implementation and their likelihood of contributing to ongoing cooperation and communication among the individual decision-makers in the community. Certainly the project was not as polished or as mathematical as a transportation and logistics study for a military command, but it represented an attempt to deal with the difficult system attributes of the health field and the serious challenges faced by one who attempts to bring about coordination or change in an open health system.

The world of medicine may seem like a fairyland to the systems analyst. He will be awed by the technology, the contributions to the quality of life, and the association with incisive, wealthy minds. At the same time it will no doubt seem unreal and nonrational to him. As Flagle (1967, p. 40) puts it, "The way of life in the health services has been reminiscent of medieval guilds and religious orders." The loose organization, the training and attitudes of people, the lack of data, the social nature of the goals, and the fragmented pressures on the system all pose difficulties for the systems analyst. He is likely to reach the same conclusion as G. C. Szego of the Institute for Defense Analysis, who is reported to have said at the symposium on Systems Analysis and Social Change. "We have been ducking the issue. We are not dealing with a system" ("Systems Analysts are Baffled" 1968).

Gilmore, Ryan and Gould (1967) cite "market fragmentation" as a barrier to applying defense systems resources to health and medicine. Aside from drugs and insurance, health services are highly decentralized, both institutionally and geographically. The druggist, the physician, the nursing home, the ambulance service—each is usually an independent business operating within a complex framework. Hospitals and social agencies proliferate and within each specialization, the decision-maker's authority is diluted and the range of his decisions is narrowed.

This decentralization not only blocks coordination; it promotes competition for status and resources and reduces the scale of capital available. What often is not recognized is that the reduced capital and expense base of individual local organizations cannot support systems studies effectively. Such studies are a capital investment and have to compete for scarce resources with cobalt bombs and open-heart surgery teams. A $50,000 study can be a major outlay to a hospital, but hardly enough to pay for preparing a proposal and administering a contract at a systems analysis firm. Cooperative efforts such as CASH (Edgecumbe 1965) may be a partial answer, but I suspect that Flagle (1967) is quite correct in his assessment that diffusion and the education of "a new breed of managers" will be the vehicle for meaningful change.

Winning respect for the analyst is not an easy task. At first the medical professionals treat the analyst or the administrator with aloofness and a patronizing positiveness. This aloofness is a vestige of the professional role and a result of past unhappy experiences with administrators. Any professional is conditioned to view the administrator as his natural enemy, as the nay-sayer. The physician, unlike the analyst, does not hesitate to reach a decision and convince himself that he is right. He has to do so for his own sanity. The medical professional also is minted by a process which emphasizes technical competence, memorization, repetition, and quick response. He comes from an academic elite and will study and master technical concepts in a short time. He expects authoritative and authoritarian instruction, and he has had little or no formal exposure to complex, solutionless problems. Unfortunately, only the younger men seem at ease with quantitative approaches. One strategy which may work for the analyst is first to illustrate that he does have a special area of competence, before he turns to administrative reality.

The analyst also has to overcome the bad taste often left

by administrators and businessmen-trustees who continually argue for more effective or "businesslike" decision-making. This counsel ends up being interpreted as tighter budgetary control, a firmer hand with the help, and a tougher collection policy. Once these measures are taken and reach a point of diminishing returns, further counsels are dismissed as classical Babbittry. Platitudes have so often served as a substitute for leadership that the administrative skills in the community often are totally devalued. But few successful organizations endure on the basis of successive belt tightenings only. A growing organization emphasizes policy formulation, personnel development, assessment of needs, adaptation to changing technologies, continuous information gathering and evaluation, and a host of other constructive activities.

These constructive activities require a staff and an effective information system. Anyone experienced in health systems analysis recognizes the paucity of information at both organizational and social levels. Much has been written about the information-handling problems of the hospital, particularly patient records, but that is only one of the information requirements for dealing with health systems. There is a need for information systems that collect, process, and report the data necessary for control, evaluation, and planning. Without good data, a systematic analysis or a program plan produces more GIGO (Garbage In-Garbage Out) material.

This problem of lack of management information has been brought home to me numerous times when, as a consultant or a would-be preparer of case studies, I have been stymied by lack of data in a health organization. Such data would have been readily available in most business firms, and the analysis could be done properly. In the health organization, data collection literally is a "federal case" because no one gets the information unless he secures a grant to collect it. Examples of important missing data that the writer has encountered include the capacity of a renal dialysis unit, the waiting times of patients in an orthopedic clinic, the impact of geographic service area on the costs of a prepaid medical group practice, the costs of laboratory procedures, the capacity of a transplant team, and the comparative costs of antihemorrhagic blood fractions.

The medical system is characterized by independent units making choices on limited grounds. Many critical management decisions literally are no one's responsibility. One can verify these phenomena by comparing the number of fact finders, analysts, decision-makers, and evaluators in the hierarchy of any medical organization with a comparably sized unit in other fields. Minimizing the staff may keep down the overhead; but the use of overhead staff has developed in our society as a mechanism for ongoing organizational improvement, and it has survived the test of time.

A similar information problem occurs at the national level, and has evoked a response in the form of the "social indicators" movement. The state of the art is evaluated carefully in the book, *Social Indicators* (Bauer 1966) and outlined succinctly in Bauer's article on "Societal Feedback" (Bauer 1967). We have many fact-finders at this level, but there is no clear attempt to make their activities fully relevant. We have to develop a way of knowing what is going on in order to apply our techniques and human effort to planning, controlling, and improving the health system both at the local operating level and as a national system.

Part of the lack of staff and the resulting scarcity of information and social change derives from the charitable origin of many health services. Since these constituted undesirable drains to the Puritan society, they were pared to the bone. Pett (1965) points out that we need to adopt a broader view of the medical system to get both efficiency and effectiveness, to strike a balance between scientific breakthroughs and minimal progress in patient care. The problem is not that we have four hundred people employed in a two-hundred-bed hospital, but rather that twenty of them are not actively engaged in finding ways to reduce that number.

Flagle (1967, p. 40) points out that historically health organizations have been "bypassed by the stream of events, the constructive conflicts of other industries." But he notes that legislation has brought work practices in health services in line with other industries. Payment schemes also have failed to develop any real incentive for cost reduction. But the rise in costs and the political visibility of health are rapidly changing some attitudes toward efficiency (Horvath 1968).

Horvath (1966, 1968) has observed that the social system

of medicine has evolved as the result of a number of expedient responses to individual problems. Initially it centered on a patient-healer relationship, but new technical knowledge has led to specialization, and larger and more complex organizations have developed. Further fragmentation has occurred in spite of the growth of large organizations which, under most circumstances, would have lead to the division of labor and the development of extensive control systems. Thus, a strangely organized system has developed in medicine. The systems analyst needs to understand this history, lest he become overly cynical about the past activities of the medical profession.

One way of explaining how the system has evolved draws on the sociological theories of organizational slack. Cyert and March (1963) discuss organizational slack extensively. They describe the focusing behavior observed by Horvath and point out that all organizations, even those driving hard for profit, are run with some slack. All organizations are coalitions that proceed toward highly ambiguous goals which constitute a facade over disagreement and uncertainty about goals. As they note, "payments and demands are met in the form of a variety of money payments, perequisites, policies, personal treatments, and private commitments . . . Subunits are permitted to grow without real concern for the relation between additional payments and additional revenue; public services are provided in excess of those required" (pp. 36–37). An alternative view based on exchange is offered by Levine and White (1961). Lortie's (1958) analysis of the movement of responsibility for anesthesia from the nurse to a physician specialist fits their model very well. Scott (1966) goes further than Lortie and develops an analysis of the whole health system based on current concepts of organizational theory.

In medicine, this willingness to avoid the discipline and organization necessary to have an efficient system is enhanced by the dual line of authority—medical vs. administrative (Smith 1958)—and by the presence of many professional groups. In their book of readings Vollmer and Mills (1966) have collected the attributes of professional groups. Physicians epitomize the professional role, since they (1) require specialized training, (2) have a professional organization, (3) have a code of ethics, (4) set their own schedule of fees, (5) establish minimum qualifications for entrance, and (6) attempt to enhance their status in society as a whole. Medicine has remained relatively unaccountable for its actions and costs because the profession has a viable underlying base in a systematic theory, a professional culture sustained by formal sanctions, authority recognized by the client, and support for this authority by the broader community.

In short, the health professional has autonomy because he performs a necessary function which only he can evaluate. This gives him a tremendous advantage for gathering in the payments of organizational slack as the system evolves. He defines the client's needs. It would be surprising then if the definition of the patient's needs were not biased by the physician's desires. Dean Ebert (1966) of Harvard has pointed out this tendency with respect to the organization and financing of the medical schools. If the systems analyst is to gain leverage on the health system, he must understand the system of side payments. He must realize that the goal structure of the professional is not oriented to the institution but includes a strong component aimed at peer-group status. A model for control (in the weakest sense) in a professional environment has been suggested by Saxberg and Slocum (1968).

The movement to define the quality of medical care may also contain seeds for destroying the professional's stranglehold on the system. If a viable professional position rests on being the acknowledged definer of need and evaluator of quality, then systems analysis presents a threat to the professional's autonomy, as do the efforts of Peterson *et al.* (1956), Donabedian (1968), and a host of others.

The analyst, too, has his Achilles heel. Boguslaw (1965) emphasizes the biases of the system analyst in his role as a formulator of social policy. Tagiuri (1964) outlines the similarities and differences of the orientations of administrators and professionals. Certainly, the analyst has a strong bias in favor of numerical argument and a closed system analysis. McDonough (1968) argues that this is a major weakness of the Program-Planning-Budgeting System (PPBS) when it is applied to health activities. McDonough studied the history of PPBS at the Office of the Surgeon General and observed that the two competing systems analysis groups, one attached to the Surgeon General's office and the other reporting to the Secretary of HEW, held much different views of the tasks at hand and how to handle them. McDonough notes that these differences related in part to the differing roles of the two offices and that they ultimately weakened the relations between them. He quotes one man as saying, "They get points for cutting our throats," a syndrome that is common, I'm afraid, to government auditors and analysts, and one which undermines the analyst's function as a weaver of political, social, economic, and technical forces inside and outside the host organization.

A bias for numbers and against people is not the only way a systems analysis can go wrong. We already have mentioned several problems: the tendency to oversell, the power of the approach in the face of inadequate data, and lack of understanding of the medical system. Others stem from the professional structure of systems work.

Most often the analyst has a consulting role. This means that he serves a client who desires results, and he must be impressive every time out. Certainly few men can achieve this constantly, and each unsuccessful venture confirm's people's suspicions that the old ways are better. Good systems analysis comes from a thorough understanding of the environment and mutual respect between the analyst and the administrator. It generally benefits from a continuing relationship. This would seem to indicate that in-house services would be the most effective, but the small size of most health institutions rules this out.

A second problem of the consulting *modus operandi* is the tendency to equate written reports with results. This problem is especially acute where the defense firm turns to health as a civilian application of its skills. Although reports are the lifeblood of aerospace teams, alone they do little to improve health services. The study, as well as the report, may go off in one of two unfortunate directions: it may try to justify an expanded or continued effort, or it may try to achieve professional recognition at the expense of the goals of the analysis. As a professional consultant, the analyst has multiple goals directed at the client's needs, his organization's needs, and his own needs. The client is interested in answers, the organization is interested in survival and growth, and the man is interested in his own survival and development.

Thus the analyst will certainly try to keep the client contented, but he also will desire to enhance the professional competence and stature of both his organization and himself. This generally will lead him to bias his approach strongly in favor of greater sophistication.

In the literature of operations research, one frequently is confronted with the word "optimal." Implicit in most models providing optimal answers is the assumption that the client is going to invest in the full analysis. Yet the decision-maker has no assurance that the cost of the study will not outweigh the improvement in results. It is necessary for the decision-maker to calculate or obtain from the proposing source, not only an estimate of cost, but also an expected value of the improvement to be achieved. Rosenbloom (1965) offers a useful discussion of the expected value of information as a guide to decision-making. Too often it is overlooked in the search for work and for professional status.

If the analyst lacks sufficient depth of experience, his model building is likely to be unrealistic or downright unappropriate. He may omit variables or make recommendations that are so absurd that the opportunity to stimulate change is lost. One of the primary laws of self-preservation in any professional field is to avoid looking stupid. Personally, however, I believe that taking for granted what the experienced physician says is an even greater danger of naiveté. At least the analyst should take the precaution of asking the exact same question of a number of people in a health institution or field, before accepting any information. This will illuminate the facts, as well as the points of view of all parties.

The problem of finding out what is really going on is illustrated by a recurring event in my experience. It goes something like this: An outpatient clinic is believed to require improved scheduling. There have been a number of apparently valid complaints about waits in the clinic of four hours or more. Everyone is concerned, and everyone is puzzled as to why the present methods of spacing appointments have not eliminated this problem. Each patient receives his appointment at the time of a previous visit, and spaces are left in the schedule to accommodate emergencies and walk-ins.

A check with the scheduling clerks indicates that the schedule is kept in a relatively accurate fashion and that overbookings are held down to the extent possible. Thus far everyone tells the same story and the system looks like it should work. Then one checks on the procedure followed in the clinic. The patient announces himself to the receptionist. She pulls his chart, if he has an appointment and it is not lost, puts it in a rack behind those of the other waiting patients, and asks him to take a seat. The attending physicians or nurses take the files from the front of the pile as examining rooms become available. At this point, of course, it becomes evident that one no longer has a functioning clinic schedule, and that patients are being taken on a first-come, first-served basis. Regular patients have observed and learned from this behavior, and they have begun to come earlier and earlier in order to get out early. The poor patient who follows instructions and arrives on time for his 9:30 a.m. appointment ends up waiting four hours. Of course, his wait also may be compounded by clinic overload, late physician arrival, calls to the house floors, etc. But the primary step in avoiding these delays involves retraining the clerks, staff, and patients to honor the existing appointment system.

The inexperienced analyst who believes what he hears about the system would begin by gathering data for a standard waiting line analysis[5] of the clinic, assuming that the scheduling system should be designed to operate with much greater precision. Actually that analysis may be a second step to be taken after he observes the existing system. The arrival times of patients and physicians could be recorded, together with the distribution of the length of time spent with the physicians and the number of late or no-show patients. Then a schedule could be devised allowing for the small (Fetter and Thompson 1966; Fry 1964; Jackson 1964) amount of overbooking necessary to assure full physician utilization and allowing for emergencies and walk-ins. In

[5] The literature of management and operations research is full of articles on waiting lines and queues, most of which are not applicable to field situations. Waiting lines, exemplified by turnpike toll booths, checkout lanes at the supermarket, and barbershops on Saturday, is a characteristic of most service organizations. The important thing to remember is that one's linear intuition about waiting lines rarely is appropriate. Thus one must study their behavior explicitly or seek expert guidance. Very simple situations can be analyzed mathematically, while the realistic or more complex ones can be evaluated by simulating hundreds or thousands of patient arrival and doctor service times in a few minutes on a large computer.

the process, however, the analyst may encounter yet another set of myths about medical care.

Health services, like other service industries, operate in an environment of uncertain needs and demands. In a limited number of situations time is of the essence, but most services can be prescheduled and the scheduling improved by a statistical approach. The analyst will encounter a built-in professional abhorrence of the statistical approach even though it is the basis for research and treatment evaluation. Physicians will tell him that all cases are different and that efficiency criteria are unprofessional. The fact remains, however, that medical services must be planned on the basis of statistical distributions of events, accompanied by a full understanding that there must be provision for wide day-to-day fluctuations in actual events. Unfortunately, since one cannot tell a priori whether the chaos that one witnesses is the result of these fluctuations or of poor planning, the planning is not attempted. Yet effective planning could bring organized confusion out of chaos.

What the analyst really may be bucking is an underlying suspicion of efforts to increase efficiency that derives from three causes. Two of these have been cited above. Better systems limit the individual's ability to extract side payments from the organization; pious pleas or demands for efficiency without methods and personnel to implement them have poisoned the well; and few medical people understand the differences between efficacy and efficiency.

Most of us have been raised on the homily that "you get what you pay for," and observe that the more one puts into a system, the more one gets out of it. Thus the usual reaction to any efficiency-oriented program is to assume that it will end up producing a net reduction in inputs and in outputs. But efficiency, in its pure engineering sense, is a dimensionless number. It is the ratio of output to input; it does not determine the volume of either input or output until one or the other is specified. The analyst in health is more likely to seek more output per unit input than to reduce output, provided that he has access to the total system. It is true that some subunits may lose inputs to others, or even be required to reduce outputs, because other subunits have greater need. The "cost-effectiveness" label which today is often the analyst's basic approach implies that policy-makers set the availability of inputs from which the analyst is to devise a system that gives the greatest output, or that he is given a set of results to achieve and asked to design the most efficient system using the potentially available inputs. His activities do not necessarily lead to a reduction in efficacy in any system.

The companion to cost-effectiveness is benefit-cost analysis. It implies an attempt to gain an absolute value of the outputs per unit input in a form that allows later comparisons of the total value of one system with the values of quite different systems. In practical terms this means that a benefit-cost study in health must end up with a reported number of dollars saved per dollar spent so that comparisons can be made with other health and nonhealth programs. Although this is the only logical long-run way to evaluate disparate government expenditures, there are technical and political problems that preclude its use at present. Early studies compared the present value of costs not incurred with the individual's life earning power. Such a method obviously discriminates against the older worker and against persons not in the work force, so it has had limited relevance for an economy with great wealth and unemployment. Moreover, we have yet to account effectively for qualitative values associated with research, training, and personal suffering. As a result, we are a long way from utilizing suitable objective functions for benefit-cost analysis or even cost-effectiveness studies.

Up to this point this chapter has emphasized some of the problems of applying relatively sophisticated tools to health problems. This does not mean that we cannot or should not attempt, especially in an academic setting, to improve continually on our ability to cope with decision-making problems in this environment. At the same time that the work in the health field goes ahead with the benefit of elementary system analyses, experiments must be run to integrate our knowledge of quantitative methods and behavioral science to achieve greater sophistication in analysis.

A study by students in the Harvard Interfaculty Program in Health and Medical Care illustrates the pleasures and pains of conducting such an experiment in order to adapt standard models to the needs of medical decision-makers.[6]

[6] This study was conducted by Joel Kavet, doctoral candidate in the Harvard School of Public Health, and David M. Kelly and Frederick M.

The study was conducted for and with the operating room supervisors of a large teaching hospital. Its purpose was to assist the supervisors in evaluating their rules for assigning and training operating room personnel. The assignment problem typically is approached through one or more variants of the linear programming models. It was considered important to the hospital because the operating room staff was the resource that seemed to be constraining the quantity of surgery.

The hospital staff, especially the OR Supervisor and the OR Head Nurse, participated extensively in the study. The nursing shortage was acute throughout the hospital. Many beds were idle for lack of staff in a hospital that normally ran close to the 100 percent occupancy level. On a typical day only six of the eight operating rooms might be used because of the shortage of operating room staff. All emergencies were handled and this amounted to 10 to 15 percent of the total workload. The students concerned themselves only with the remaining, controllable 85 to 90 percent of the surgery. Inasmuch as many surgeons held multiple appointments, the operating room management felt it might have greater than normal maneuverability in controlling the output of the surgical suite. Surgery not performed at this prestigious hospital, if necessary, would be performed elsewhere within a reasonable period of time.

As usual, the initial step was to define the problem and reduce it to a tractable state. The assignment problem can be a nasty one to compute. The staffing of the operating rooms is especially knotty because the time required to perform an operation is uncertain and is a function of the skill of the individuals assigned. In most formulations it also is an integer linear programming[7] problem and this complicates

Whitmeyer, M.B.A. and D.B.A. candidates, respectively, Harvard Graduate School of Business Administration. This work was presented in Interfaculty Program Seminars conducted by Professors M. S. Feldstein and R. E. Berry of the Economics Department and C. P. McLaughlin of the Graduate School of Business Administration.

[7] The linear programming problem can be expressed succinctly as: Find the maximum value of $Z = \sum_{j=1}^{n} c_j x_j$ where $j = 1, \ldots, n$ and subject to a series of constraints, also linear and of the form $\sum_{j=1}^{n} a_{ij} x_j \leqslant b_i$ and $x_j \geqslant 0$. The values of the x_j variables are unknown and are manipulated according

things considerably. The students worked closely with the supervisors to reach a formulation that was both manageable and relevant. The supervisors agreed that they were interested not in the assignment of individuals to specific rooms, but in decision rules that would give the best results over time. They were willing to improvise around the random occurrence of vacations, illness, and emergencies, and the variations in the time for procedures due to unforseen complications or surgeon differences. It was understood that operations must be scheduled daily in integer units and that the staff on duty would be limited to full or half-time equivalents of personnel. The study itself concentrated on the needs for proper staffing on an annual basis to meet the overall needs of the hospital.

Three basic types of information were available: the surgical procedures previously performed, the nursing personnel currently available, and their current wage rates. The salary data was used, but was of limited value since hospital pay scales reflect educational background and seniority, not proficiency. The study, therefore, relied on the quantified judgments of the supervisors to evaluate the personnel on hand. The nursing staff consisted of registered nurses, graduate nurses (usually foreign trained), and surgical technicians, all of whom could effectively, if not legally, fulfill all of the functions of the scrub and circulating nurse positions. One of each position was needed for 90 percent of procedures. The supervisors felt that they could classify the nursing personnel into four skill categories based on proficiency, which was the way that they already were being assigned, even though a more skilled technician might make thirty-five dollars a week less than a less experienced registered nurse. Given the four classifications, it was possible to compare alternative assignments of personnel in pairs (one each serving as scrub nurse and circulating nurse) with different combinations of skills, i.e., two Class 1, the highest skill, versus one Class 1 teamed with a Class 4, the least skilled.

Just as the supervisors were willing to classify personnel,

---

to mathematical formuli to yield a proved maximum (or minimum) of the objective function Z. This procedure is outlined in terms relatively understandable to the layman in Baumol (1965). In integer linear programming the values of x_j must be integers (whole numbers), a set of conditions which complicates things no end.

they also were willing to classify surgical procedures by type. Here six categories based on complexity appeared adequate for an initial evaluation of the approach. The four classes of personnel yielded a set of ten possible skill combinations each for the six classes of operations, or a total of sixty possible assignments. Some feasible assignments were so inappropriate that they were dropped from the formulation, reducing the alternatives considered to forty-six.

The remaining major problems were to evaluate each assignment for the objective function and to formulate the constraints. The latter was relatively simple. The number of personnel hours of each class of skill available was known, and so was the historical number of hours devoted to each class of procedures. This, of course, was a function of the assignments previously made while short of nursing personnel, but one of the objectives of the study was to see what would happen when these constraints were lifted.

The objective function was expressed partly in terms of the wage costs of personnel, but the supervisors felt that this was insufficient. After all, operating room staff were in short supply and they would take and keep all that they could get. The question was how to use them and how much effort to put into training them. It was decided, therefore, to build and then use as an objective function a preference function which included wages, but was strongly weighted for the assignment preferences of the OR supervisors, which in turn were related to their subjective evaluation of the impact of specific team assignments on quality and on labor utilization.

The preferences of the supervisors were evaluated by determining the indifference points at which 40 hours of combination of skills, say a Class 1 and a Class 3, could be substituted without a feeling of loss or gain for X hours of another combination. For example, for a specific class of surgery the supervisors would be equally happy to get at equal cost the amount of time shown in Table 1. These evaluations reflect the supervisors' preferences for the more skilled personnel. The adjusted value column in Table 1 represents the weighted value that was subtracted from the average wage costs for a pair of nurses to reflect these perferences in the objective function of the linear programming formulation. Thus, if the salary of a nursing hour of

Table 1. Time-Cost Evaluation of Operating Room Personnel Skills.

Skill Combination	Hours	Adjusted Value [(40 Hrs)/Hrs] × 10
1 and 1	32	2.50
1 and 2	34	1.78
1 and 3	34.5	1.60
1 and 4	36	1.11
2 and 2	38	0.52
2 and 3	40	0.00
2 and 4	45	−1.11

skill level 1 and 1 was \$6.40, the effective cost used in the linear programming model would be \$6.40 − 2.50, or \$3.90. If a team of 2 and 4 was assigned at the average cost of \$5.78, the objective function for that team would be \$5.78 − (− 1.11), or \$6.89. With this information it was possible to formulate test assignment problems to evaluate the arbitrary weightings and the decision rules of the supervisors.

With this analysis completed it was possible to develop a linear programming matrix like Table 2, feed it to the computer program for solution, and evaluate the results. The original formulation allows a surplus of nursing personnel, which was the opposite of the true situation, but successive runs were made reducing the availabilities and seeing what rules would apply. The formulation strongly reflected the nursing supervisors' preferences for skilled personnel, assigning all Class 1 and 2 first. It also indicated that, if the preference weightings were accurate, and personnel of all types were short, then the supervisors would be willing to pay at least fifty cents more per hour to new Class 1 and 2 nurses to attract them. It is interesting to note, however, that the 1 and 1 combination, while of the greatest value, was applied to only a minor portion of one class of surgery, because the rest of the Class 1 hours were required to pair with Class 2 and Class 3 nurses in order to fill all requirements.

After the initial tests, the requirements for surgery were increased stepwise, with the result of including more Class 3 personnel and abandoning the 1 and 1 combinations. For example, as the amount of Class D surgery was doubled, all Class 1 personnel were teamed with Class 3 and 4 person-

Table 2. Linear Programming Matrix for Surgical Suite Staffing Model.

Type of Surgery	A								
Skill	1	1	1	1	2	2	2	3	3
Group	1	2	3	4	2	3	4	3	4
Hours Available Constraints									
Class 1	2	1	1	1					
Class 2		1			2	1	1		
Class 3			1			1		2	1
Class 4				1			1		1
Surgery Needed Constraints									
Type A	1	1	1	1	1	1	1	1	1
Type B									
Type C									
Type D									
Type E									
Type F									
Objective Function (Minimize)	3.00	4.35	4.63	5.34	4.75	4.67	6.25	6.70	9.50

Type of Surgery	B							
Skill	1	1	1	1	2	2	2	3
Group	1	2	3	4	2	3	4	3
Hours Available Constraints								
Class 1	2	1	1	1				
Class 2		1			2	1	1	
Class 3			1			1		2
Class 4				1			1	
Surgery Needed Constraints								
Type A								
Type B	1	1	1	1	1	1	1	1
Type C								
Type D								
Type E								
Type F								
Objective Function (Minimize)	3.07	2.80	3.55	5.10	5.34	5.78	6.73	6.80

Type of Surgery	C						
Skill	1	1	1	1	2	2	2
Group	1	2	3	4	2	3	4
Hours Available Constraints							
Class 1	2	1	1	1			
Class 2		1			2	1	1
Class 3			1			1	
Class 4				1			1
Surgery Needed Constraints							
Type A							
Type B							
Type C	1	1	1	1	1	1	1
Type D							
Type E							
Type F							
Objective Function (Minimize)	3.90	4.35	4.45	5.41	5.34	5.78	7.35

Type of Surgery	D				
Skill	1	1	1	2	2
Group	1	2	3	2	3
Hours Available Constraints					
Class 1	2	1	1		
Class 2		1		2	1
Class 3			1		1
Class 4					
Surgery Needed Constraints					
Type A					
Type B					
Type C					
Type D	1	1	1	1	1
Type E					
Type F					
Objective Function (Minimize)	4.98	5.02	5.53	5.86	7.45

Type of Surgery	E							
Skill	1	1	1	1	2	2	2	3
Group	1	2	3	4	2	3	4	3
Hours Available Constraints								
Class 1	2	1	1	1				
Class 2		1			2	1	1	
Class 3			1			1		2
Class 4				1			1	
Surgery Needed Constraints								
Type A								
Type B								
Type C								
Type D								
Type E	1	1	1	1	1	1	1	1
Type F								
Objective Function (Minimize)	3.90	4.02	3.94	4.74	4.75	4.67	6.25	6.60

Type of Surgery	F									
Skill	1	1	1	1	2	2	2	3	3	Limiting
Group	1	2	3	4	2	3	4	3	4	Value
Hours Available Constraints										
Class 1	2	1	1	1						$\leqslant$22000
Class 2		1			2	1	1			$\leqslant$16500
Class 3			1			1		2	1	$\leqslant$22000
Class 4				1			1		1	$\leqslant$ 1650
Surgery Needed Constraints										
Type A										$\geqslant$ 6073
Type B										$\geqslant$ 2033
Type C										$\geqslant$ 5517
Type D										$\geqslant$10508
Type E										$\geqslant$ 1060
Type F	1	1	1	1	1	1	1	1	1	$\geqslant$ 592
Objective Function (Minimize)	4.98	4.85	4.77	5.41	5.05	5.26	5.73	5.70	7.07	

nel, and most Class 2 nurses also were teamed with 3s and 4s. This is not an intuitively obvious answer where the 1 and 1 combinations are so highly valued. These results also indicated that there was considerable value in upgrading Class 3 and Class 4 personnel. A second series of experiments ranging the right hand side of the constraint equations could be conducted to indicate which types of surgery would be performed and which would be turned away, if the basis of evaluation was solely that of the OR supervisors.

The trained operations researcher will undoubtedly be concerned about the funny money used for the objective function, the implicit assumptions made about the structure of the supervisors' preference functions, the interpretations that apply to the shadow prices from the solution, and the sensitivity of the results to the arbitrary weightings used. On the whole the study did, however, represent a direct and honest effort to deal with the problems as the decision-makers defined it. Considerable ingenuity was required to formulate the problem, design the successive experiments, and painstakingly elicit the preferences.

The selection of the OR supervisor as the viewpoint of the model may not have been the most appropriate one, but such errors may be unavoidable in health. Theoretically, one would like to build the model from the point of view of some decision-maker who weighs all the considerations and seeks an efficient total system. There is no such position in most health organizations, and one ends up supporting merely the ends of specific subunits. For example, the model presented in Table 2 ignores social and revenue aspects of the problem. Both beds and operating rooms were idle for lack of nursing and OR staff, so it might have been desirable to leave even more operating rooms idle and assign the RNs elsewhere. The analysis presented above also begged the question as to which class of surgery should be curtailed owing to a shortage of personnel. This would depend in turn on a total, hospital-wide determination of relevant dollar costs and revenues and sociomedical value. Unfortunately, such an analysis probably would upset the classification of the surgical procedures, because the incomes generated may bear no relationship to the nursing skills required; in fact, it would be most surprising if they did. The pricing policies of hospitals seldom relate to anything except the ability or willingness of patients or insurers to pay.

This project illustrates one way to overcome the complications presented by qualitative factors in the evaluation of services and by lack of a central decision-making authority in the organization. Many of the questions that could be raised about this study really relate to the major problem of developing an administrative authority in a health organization, a philosopher king, to deal with the medical system as a whole and to enhance its sole purpose—patient care. This is the greatest need today in the health field.

Earlier in this chapter I stated that I agreed with Flagle that the real hope for improvement was the education of the young. My experience with professional students at the Harvard School of Public Health makes me optimistic about the feasibility of educating these men. Yet it will be a long time before they are available in significant numbers and work their way up seniority-conscious medical ladders.

A supplementary approach would be the education of the old—purportedly and impossible task, but one which can be accomplished with amazing speed by self-motivated individuals. How can the medical professional or administrator, now out of school, master the conceptual material he needs if he is to act authoritatively and gain leverage on a health organization? If he has the motivation and is not prone to symbol shock and a math block, he can start mastering concepts on his own, one at a time.

To the man who wants to teach himself enough to become involved as an evaluator of or a participant in systems studies, I would recommend the basic text, McMillan and Gonzalez, *Systems Analysis*, Revised Edition (1968). This book has the strong advantage of teaching elementary computer programming skills along with the theory and applications of probability, queuing, feedback, planning models, simulation, and linear programming. A man who can find a little computer time will be drawn onward into the assignments by the novelty and continuous feedback of the computer assignments. Also his willingness to obtain small amounts of computer time is probably a good test of his motivation. The most serious drawbacks of the book are its emphasis on computers, its emphasis on business applications, and its omission of classical statistical and economic models. As I have indicated in my discussion of the kidney project, computer models often can be dispensed with in health studies, so programming is not a basic requirement of the analyst. Yet it undoubtedly will prove handy in our future world and it is a rapid, thoroughly ego-deflating way to instill an understanding of rigorous, analytical thought. The health-oriented student can omit the intensive treatments of the inventory systems theory in Chapters 5, 7, and 8, viewing them solely as vehicles for the teaching of other integrated material.

Once he has mastered the materials in this or some other basic text, the administrator can go on to the more advanced texts referenced by the authors and to the literature that relates these approaches to the problems of medical care. A set of references for the health applications of these systems techniques has been provided in a separate paper on the literature of systems and health. Table 3 outlines the topics of the book and the medically oriented papers that could be coordinated with them in a course of study. This material, together with any one of the many good texts on classical statistics and a book on medical economics—probably Klarman (1965)—can provide an introduction to the conceptual skill required for representative systems or operations research studies of health activities.

The future of systems analysis in health looks good. Costs are rising, resources are limited, and people inside and outside the health field are committed to increased effectiveness. Time and events will mold men to take on the task that needs doing. There is a power vacuum and it will be filled. It has been the purpose of this chapter to outline the background and problems of the systems analysis movement, so that it can be understood and furthered responsibly. Structural problems have been emphasized, not because they are overwhelming, but because their effects can be minimized. The projects described here suggest a process for the analysis and some ways in which the structural problems can be faced. A potential self-education program for health professionals has been outlined that could provide the conceptual skills to achieve professional acceptance and more importantly, results.

Problems worthy of attack
Prove their worth by hitting back.
Piet Hein, *Grooks*, The M.I.T. Press, 1966.

Table 3. Concepts Applied to the Health Area—Examples.

Subject	Application Type	References
Systems and models	All types	Flagle (1962, 1967) Horvath (1966, 1968)
	Hospitals	Flagle (1960) Smalley and Freeman (1966)
	Environmental health	Harrington (1966)
Probability concepts	Diagnosis	Lincoln and Parker (1967) Tsao (1967) Warner *et al.* (1961)
	Treatment	Kendall (1945) Lechat and Flagle (1965) Scheff (1963)
	Epidemiology and ecology	Bailey (1967) Bartlett (1961)
Queuing and simulation	Clinics	Bailey (1952) Fetter and Thompson (1966)
	Hospital services	Thompson, Fetter, *et al.* (1963)
	Private practice	Fry (1964)
Planning models	Surgery	Smalley and Freeman (1966)
Matrix methods—linear programming	Diets	Balintfy in Smalley and Freeman (1966)
	Facilities planning	Feldstein (1967)
	Environmental health	Harrington (1966)
Markov processes	Hospital census	Balintfy in Smalley and Freeman (1966)
Feedback	Medical science	Gann (1963) Machin (1964)
	Medical care	Harvey (1965)

References

Ackoff, R. L.
(1956), "The Development of Operations Research as a Science." *Operations Research, 4,* 265–266.
Affel, H. A., Jr.
(1964), "System Engineering." *International Scence and Technology,* 3 (November), 18–26.
Bailey, N. T. J.
(1952), "Studies of Queues and Appointment Systems in Hospital Outpatient Departments with Special Reference to Waiting Times." *Journal of the Royal Statistical Society* (Series B), *41,* 185–198.
——— (1967), *The Mathematical Approach to Biology and Medicine.* New York: Wiley.
Baker, N. R.
(1967), "Toward an Analytical Framework for Service Operations." Presented at 14th International Meeting on The Institute of Management Sciences, Mexico City, August.
Bartlett, M. S.
(1961), "Monte Carlo Studies in Ecology and Epidemiology." *IV, Proceedings of the 4th Berkeley Symposium on Mathematics, Statistics and Probability,* Berkeley: University of California Press, pp. 39–55.
Bauer, R. A. (ed.)
(1966), *Social Indicators.* Cambridge: M.I.T. Press.
Bauer, R. A.
(1967), "Societal Feedback." *Annals of the American Academy of Political and Social Science, 373,* 180–192.
Baumol, W. J.
(1965), *Economic Theory and Operations Analysis.* Englewood Cliffs: Prentice-Hall. 2nd ed.
Bellman, R.
(1964), *Challenges of Modern Control Theory.* Report RM–3956–PR, Santa Monica: RAND Corporation.
Biderman, A.
(1966), "Social Indicators and Goals." In Bauer, 1966.
Boguslaw, R.
(1965), *The New Utopians.* New York: Prentice-Hall.
Boulding, K. E.
(1966), "The Ethics of Rational Decision." *Management Science, 12,* B–161—169.
Cyert, R. M., and J. G. March
(1963), *A Behavioral Theory of the Firm.* Englewood Cliffs: Prentice-Hall.
Donabedian, A.
(1968), "Evaluating the Quality of Medical Care." *Health Services Research I (The Milbank Memorial Fund Quarterly) 44,* 166–206.
Ebert, R. H.
(1966), "The Role of the Medical School in Planning the Health Care System." Delivered at the Annual Meeting of the Association of American Medical Colleges, October.
Edgecumbe, R. H.
(1965), "The CASH Approach to Hospital Management Engineering." *Hospitals,* 39 (March 16), 70–74.
Feldstein, M. S.
(1967), *Economic Analysis for Health Service Efficiency.* Amsterdam: North Holland.

Fetter, R. B., and J. D. Thompson
(1966), "Patients' Waiting Time and Doctors' Idle Time in the Outpatients Setting." *Health Services Research, 1* (Summer), 66–90.
Flagle, C. D.
(1960), "Operations Research in a Hospital," Chapter 25 in C. D. Flagle, W. H. Huggins, and R. H. Roy (eds.), *Operations Research and Systems Engineering.* Baltimore: Johns Hopkins Press.
——— (1962), "Operations Research in the Health Services." *Operations Research, 10,* 591–603.
——— (1967), "A Decade of Operations Research in Health." In F. Zwicky and A. G. Wilson, *New Methods of Thought and Procedure,* New York: Springer-Verlag, pp. 33–45.
Fry, J.
(1964), "Appointments in General Practice." *Operational Research Quarterly, 15,* 233–237.
Gann, D. S.
(1963), "Systems Analysis in the Study of Homeostasis with Special Reference to Cortisol Secretion." *American Journal of Surgery, 114* (July), 95–102.
Gilmore, J. S., J. J. Ryan, and W. S. Gould
(1967), *Defense Systems Resources in the Civil Sector: An Evolving Approach, an Uncertain Market.* Denver: Denver Research Institute.
Harrington, J. J.
(1966), "Environmental Hazards. Operations Research—A Relatively New Approach to Managing Man's Environment." *New England Journal of Medicine, 275,* 1342–1350.
Harvey, N. A.
(1965), "Cybernetic Applications in Medicine." *New York State Journal of Medicine, 65,* 765–772, 871–875, 995–1002.
Horvath, W. J.
(1966), "The Systems Approach to the National Health Problem." *Management Science, 12,* B–391—395.
——— (1968), "Organizational and Management Problems in the Delivery of Medical Care," *Management Science, 14,* B–275—279.
Howard, R.
(1960), *Dynamic Programming and Markov Processes.* New York: Wiley.
Jackson, R. R. P.
(1964), "Design of an Appointments System." *Operational Research Quarterly, 15,* 219–232.
Kendall, D. G.
(1945), "Mathematical Models of the Spread of Infection." In *Mathematics and Computer Science in Biology and Medicine,* London: Mathematics Research Council. Pp. 213–215.
Kershner, R. B.
(1960), "A Survey of Systems Engineering Tools and Techniques." In C. D. Flagle, W. H. Huggins, and R. H. Roy (eds.), *Operations Research and Systems Engineering,* Baltimore: Johns Hopkins Press. P. 141.
Klarman, H. E.
(1965), *The Economics of Health.* Columbia University Press.
Kuhn, T. S.
(1962), *The Structure of Scientific Revolution.* University of Chicago Press.
Lechat, M. F., and C. D. Flagle
(1965), "Allocation of Medical and Associated Resources to Control Leprosy." Chapter 9 in N. N. Barish and M. Verhulst (eds.), *Management Sciences in Emerging Countries,* Oxford: Pergamon Press.

Levin, R. I., and C. A. Kirkpatrick
(1966), *Planning and Control with PERT/CPM.* New York: McGraw-Hill.
Levine, S., and P. E. White
(1961), "Exchange as a Conceptual Framework for Study of Interorganizational Relationships." *Administrative Science Quarterly, 5,* 583–601.
Lincoln, T. L., and R. D. Parker
(1967), "Medical Diagnosis Using Bayes' Theorem." *Health Services Research, 2,* 1, 34–45.
Litchfield, E. H.
(1956), "Notes on a General Theory of Administration." *Administrative Science Quarterly, 1,* 1, 3–29.
Lortie, D. C.
(1958), "Anesthesia: From Nurse's Work to Medical Specialty." In E. G. Jaco (ed.), *Patients, Physicians, and Illness,* Glencoe: Free Press. 405–412.
McDonough, J. J.
(1968), "Planning Patterns and the Implications for Management Control: A Study of Planning, Programming, and Budgeting at the U.S. Public Health Service." Unpublished doctoral dissertation, Harvard University Graduate School of Business Administration.
Machin, K. E.
(1964), "Feedback Theory and Its Application to Biological Systems." *Symposia for the Society for Experimental Biology, 18,* 421–445.
McMillan, C., and R. F. Gonzalez
(1968), *Systems Analysis: A Computer Approach to Decision Models.* Homewood, Ill.: Irwin. Revised ed.
Marschak, T. A.
(1964), *The Role of Project Histories in the Studies of R & D.* Santa Monica: RAND Corporation, Paper P–2850.
Morris, W. T.
(1967), "On the Art of Modeling." *Management Science, 13,* B–707—717.
Naylor, T. S., J. L. Balintfy, D. S. Burdick, and K. Chu
(1966), *Computer Simulation Techniques.* New York: Wiley.
Packer, A. H.
(1968), "Applying Cost-Effectiveness Concepts to the Community Health System." *ORSA Journal, 16* (March-April), 227–253.
Page, T. L.
(1960), Chapter 6 in C. D. Flagle, W. H. Huggins, and R. H. Roy (eds.), *Operations Research and Systems Engineering,* Baltimore: Johns Hopkins Press.
Peterson, O. L., L. P. Andrews, R. S. Spain, and B. G. Greenberg
(1956), "Analytical Study of North Carolina General Practice, 1953–1954." *Journal of Medical Education, 31* (12), Part 2, 1–165.
Pett, L. B.
(1965), "Operational Research and Health Services." *Canadian Journal of Public Health, 56* (November), 457–461.
Report of the Committee on Chronic Kidney Disease (1967). Prepared for the Bureau of the Budget, Washington, D.C., September 14. Frequently referred to as the Gottschalk Report.
Rosenbloom, R. S.
(1965), "Information Requirements for Development Decisions." In J. Spiegel and D. Walker (eds.), *Information Systems Sciences,* Washington, D.C.: Spartan Books. Pp. 391–401.
Saunders, B. S.
(1964), "Measuring Community Health Levels." *American Journal of Public Health, 54,* 1063–1070.

Saxberg, B. O., and J. W. Slocum, Jr.
(1968), "The Management of Scientific Manpower." *Management Science: Application, 14,* B-473—489.
Scheff, T. J.
(1963), "Decision Rules, Types of Errors and Their Consequences for Medical Diagnosis," *Behavioral Science, 8,* 97–107.
Scott, W. R.
(1966), "Some Implications of Organizational Theory for Research on Health Services." *Milbank Memorial Fund Quarterly, 44,* 4, Part 2 (October), 35–59.
Smalley, H., and J. Freeman
(1966), *Hospital Industrial Engineering.* New York: Reinhold.
Smith, H. E.
(1958), "Two Lines of Authority: The Hospital's Dilemma." In E. G. Jaco (ed.), *Patients, Physicians, and Illness.* Glencoe: Free Press. Pp. 468–477.
"Systems Analysts Are Baffled by Problems of Social Change" (1968), *New York Times,* March 24, p. 28.
Tagiuri, R.
(1964), "Value Orientations of Managers and Scientists." In C. D. Orth III *et al.* (eds.), *Administering Research and Development,* Homewood, Ill.: Irwin.
Taylor, F. W.
(1911), *Principles of Scientific Management.* New York: Harper.
Thompson, J. D., R. B. Fetter, C. S. McIntosh, and R. J. Pelletier
(1963), "Predicting Requirements for Maternity Facilities." *Hospitals, 37* (February), 45–49, 132.
Tsao, R. F.
(1967), "A Second Order Exponential Model for Multidimensional Dichotomous Contingency Tables, with Applications in Medical Diagnosis." IBM Cambridge Scientific Center Report 320–2014, August.
U.S. Public Health Service, HEW (1967), *Kidney Disease: Program Analysis.* Prepared under the direction of Office of Program Planning and Evaluation, Office of the Surgeon General, Washington, D.C. Frequently referred to as the Burton Report.
Vollmer, H. M., and D. L. Mills
(1966), *Professionalization.* Englewood Cliffs: Prentice-Hall.
Warner, H. R., A. F. Toronto, L. G. Veasey, and R. Stephenson
(1961), "A Mathematical Approach to Medical Diagnosis." *Journal of the American Medical Association, 177,* 177–183.
White, K. L.
(1968), "Research in Medical Care and Health Services Systems." *Medical Care, 6,* 2 (March-April), 95–100.

Daniel Howland

11. Toward a Community Health System Model

Rising costs and demands for health services pose many difficult resource allocation problems for health system planners. Many of the most pressing problems arise from the fact that costs per patient day and hospital admissions are rising steadily, as shown in Figure 1. These trends result in part from social legislation enacted to ensure that health services are provided for a growing population, and in part from advances in health system capability.

There are two alternatives for dealing with these trends. The first is to reduce costs by reducing services. The second is to manage health systems in such a way that the highest possible level of care is assured within resource constraints. It is very unlikely that the latter course, which is the one we are now embarked on, will result in lowered costs. As system capability increases, so will the pressures to use it. Since the first alternative is basically unacceptable in our society, Medicare, Blue Cross, and other third-party payment plans have been devised to spread the risks and benefits of health system capability.

The combination of increasing costs and demands is having two important consequences. First, medical services are increasingly regarded as a right, rather than a privilege, a fact with interesting political implications. Second, there is a growing realization that the delivery of health services is a system rather than a component problem. The nurse, patient, and physician must be viewed as interacting components of a health system rather than as independent entities.

Because of the need to plan in a system context to ensure that the social legislation which has been enacted will lead to desired goals, new ways of managing health systems are needed. The new management techniques, growing out of wartime operations research and postwar systems analysis, have evolved into planning-programming-budgeting systems

This investigation was supported in part by a Public Health Service Grant (NU 00095) from the Division of Nursing, Bureau of Health Manpower. It is part of a long range program in Systems Research conducted by the Adaptive Systems Research Group, College of Administrative Science, The Ohio State University, Columbus, Ohio.

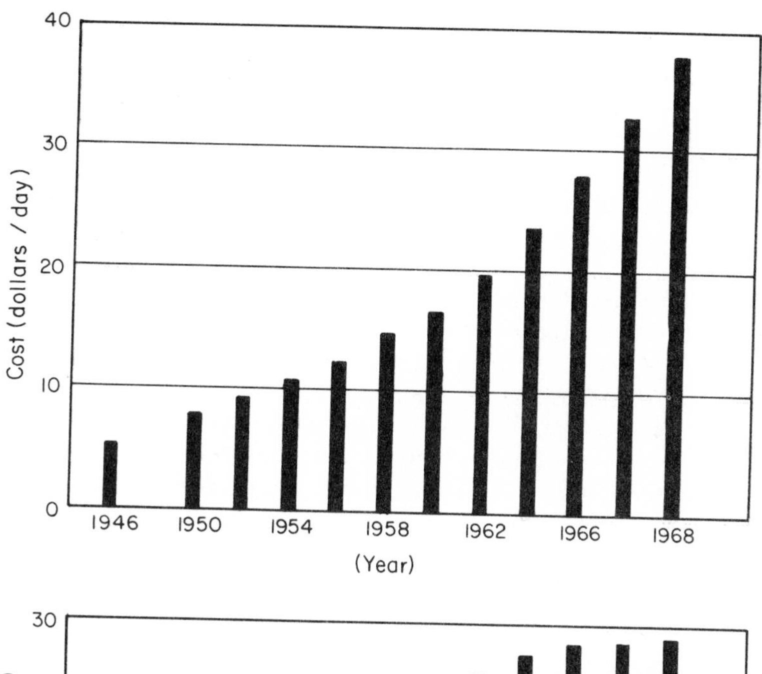

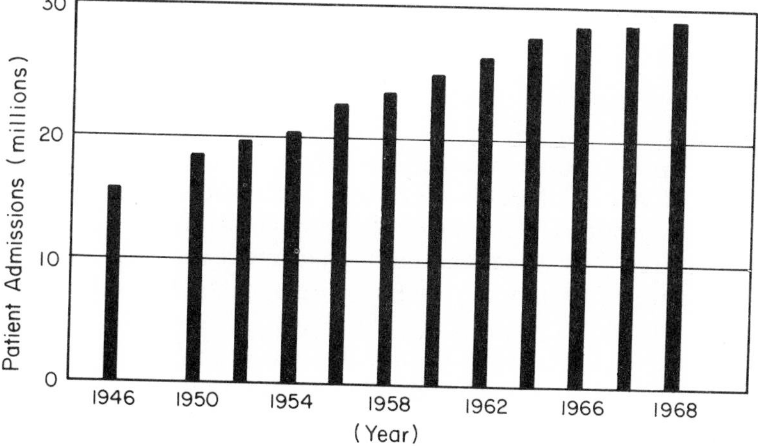

Figure 1. Trends in costs and demands for hospital service.

which are devised to relate programs and budgets over time (Hitch 1963). The requirement for planning has a salutary effect. The mere fact it is required forces managers to look ahead and develop long-range plans which, hopefully, will reduce the requirement for day-to-day crisis management. In addition, the development of programs and budgets for the future helps to ensure continual monitoring of system performance. This may alert the planner to the need to revise his plans in time to modify them if actual and desired system performance is diverging.

Although there can be no quarrel with the planning objectives, there has been considerable criticism with both the methods and the results. Many of the problems have been explored by Senator Henry M. Jackson's Subcommittee on National Security and International Operations (U. S. Congress 1968). Regardless of what one thinks of the methods, however, planning problems are growing in complexity, and ways of solving them are growing in urgency. Medical practitioners, planners, and patients demand assurance that they are getting the best possible patient care in return for the resources invested in health systems (Crystal and Brewster 1966). For this reason, methods for managing health systems which meet the planner's needs and the critic's objections must be developed. The methods which are currently being used will be reviewed briefly, some of the difficulties encountered in their use will be described, and an alternative suggested.

I. The Planning Methods

As noted above, the evolving methods for managing health systems have their roots in the operations research efforts of World War II. These methods are being used in government as the result of a presidential directive of 1965 (U.S. Congress, 1965) to all government departments instructing them to adopt the planning methods used in the Department of Defense.

Operations research originated as an organized activity in England when scientists from many disciplines were drawn into the war effort to offer advice to hard-pressed military planners (Blackett 1962). Their first notable success was the development of plans for integrating newly developed radar into the air defense system. Localization of enemy bombers and accurate target predictions made it possible to concentrate the British fighters, thus effectively increasing defense force capability. Other studies followed. One of the most famous is the work of the RAF Coastal Command against submarines. A mathematician, flying on patrols and collecting operational data, was able greatly to improve force effectiveness by recommending a change in the depth at which depth charges went off (Air Ministry 1963). He also noted some of the psychological problems of monitoring a radar scope. As a result of his observations, a series of experiments on monitoring and vigilance was initiated by the Applied Psychology Unit at Cambridge (Mackworth 1961). Mackworth's results seem to have had little impact on the design of patient monitoring systems, but the findings, such as the facts that there may be a severe drop in vigilance after thirty minutes, and that the decrement is related to the task, might be of interest to the designers of patient monitor systems (Howland and Wiener 1963).

Although a wide range of military problems was investigated, all the studies had one thing in common: they were based on observation and measurement of the performance of forces in being. The objective of the studies was to decide how to use available forces effectively. Because observation and measurement were possible, the classical methods of the empirical sciences were used to develop models for evaluating system performance (Kimball and Morse 1951). Policy decisions were formulated on the basis of empirical evidence.

Following the war, the situation changed. No longer was the management problem that of using forces in being; managers were now required to design forces for the future. Observation and measurement were impossible for unbuilt systems, and many of the factors which had been parameters in World War II operations research studies were now variables (Hitch and McKean 1960). Simulation was necessary to decide what kinds of forces to develop for the future.

Analysis for the future is complicated by many factors (Quade 1965). Among the most difficult are the uncertainties about the environment and technological development. Another difficulty is cost assignment. Cost, in the dollar sense, was of little concern to the commander trying to decide how best to use the forces at his disposal. Costs, however, are a major concern to the planner attempting to decide on the most economic force structure to meet unclear future requirements.

The difficulties of future planning led economists and others at the RAND Corporation to develop techniques of economic analysis to generate information for the selection of complex systems. Charles J. Hitch, who joined the government as comptroller under Secretary of Defense Mc-

Namara in 1961, led in the development of methods for applying the concepts of classic economic theory to the solution of systems design problems. His book, written in collaboration with Roland N. McKean, remains one of the most important in the field (Hitch and McKean 1960).

Basically, the approach is an application of the concepts of microeconomic theory to the solution of system trade-off problems. The selection of a particular system is based on cost and effectiveness criteria—the marginal utility of adding another increment to the force. The steps in such an analysis (Hitch and McKean 1960, p. 118) may be summarized as follows. (1) Specify the aims or objectives which must be accomplished. The fundamental importance of choosing the right objective is stressed; "if this decision is wrongly made, the whole analysis is addressed to the wrong question." (2) Develop alternative systems, complexes of "men, machines and tactics for their employment needed to accomplish the objectives." (3) Assign costs to the alternative systems. These are the costs incurred by utilizing resources. Costs are negative values in the analysis, and are represented by what has to be given up in any specified trade-off. (4) Select or develop models of the alternatives, or systems, "to trace the relations between input and outputs, resources and objectives, for each of the systems to be compared, so that we can predict the relevant consequences of choosing any system." (5) Select a criterion, or test to choose between systems. In principle, one would choose the "optimal" system; the one which, in economic terms, "yields the greatest excess of positive values (objectives) over negative values (resources used up, or costs)."

How do we do all these things? How do we specify aims and objectives and deal with conflicts between them? How are the concepts for alternative systems generated? How, and to what, do we assign costs? Specifically, what are the aims and objectives of health systems? How does one measure health system effectiveness? If we measure "effectiveness" in terms of saving lives, we must assign a value to life. But, say Hitch and McKean (1960, p. 185), "there is no generally acceptable method of valuing human lives." How then can the cost-effectiveness methods be made to work? If not the cost of life, or health, what effectiveness criteria can we use? Do we end choosing systems in terms of their dollar costs, or their capability for alleviating human suffering? How, for example, would we translate the effectiveness of a heart transplant into dollars? If we use the methods of economic analysis, are we restricted to a consideration of those system variables which can be measured and to which costs can be assigned? Critics of the methods point to the diplomatic repercussions in England of the cost-effectiveness decision to cancel the Skybolt program. This incident is cited as an example of the consequences of omitting factors which are difficult to measure, such as political considerations, from the analysis. Other critics suggest that, since effectiveness is hard to measure, cost is really the criterion for system selection.

If we examine the problems of designing health systems, the methods which have been developed to solve them, and the criticisms of the methods, it appears that the root of the problem is the *model* upon which the analysis is based. The model, if it is to be of any help to the planner in tracing "the relations between input and outputs, resources and objectives, for each of the systems to be compared, so that we can predict the relevant consequences of choosing any system" (Hitch and McKean 1960, p. 118) must be descriptive of the system for which plans are being made. Good management depends on good models.

II. The Models

Since the planner must understand the system for which he is making plans well enough to ensure that his resource allocation decisions will result in goal achievement, the first step in analysis is to select or develop models to describe system performance. These models can then be used to generate the data required for analysis. The existing system is only one alternative. The behavior of the others can be assessed only by simulation with a model.

Usually not one but many models must be used to analyze a system. These models have different purposes and are constructed differently. They fall into two general classes, descriptive and prescriptive, and may be developed by formal, empirical, or combined methods (Dorfman 1960; Flagle 1963).

In order to determine the characteristics of the various models needed, and to relate them to avoid the dangers of suboptimization (Hitch 1953), it may be helpful to partition the system into a number of functional levels, as shown in Figure 2 (Howland 1964).

One of the principal differences between system levels is the degree to which resources are variables or parameters. At the lowest, tactical level, for instance, the decision-maker chooses among the resources at hand. He functions in an immediate time frame and can use only the resources which are immediately available. The anesthesiologist, for example,

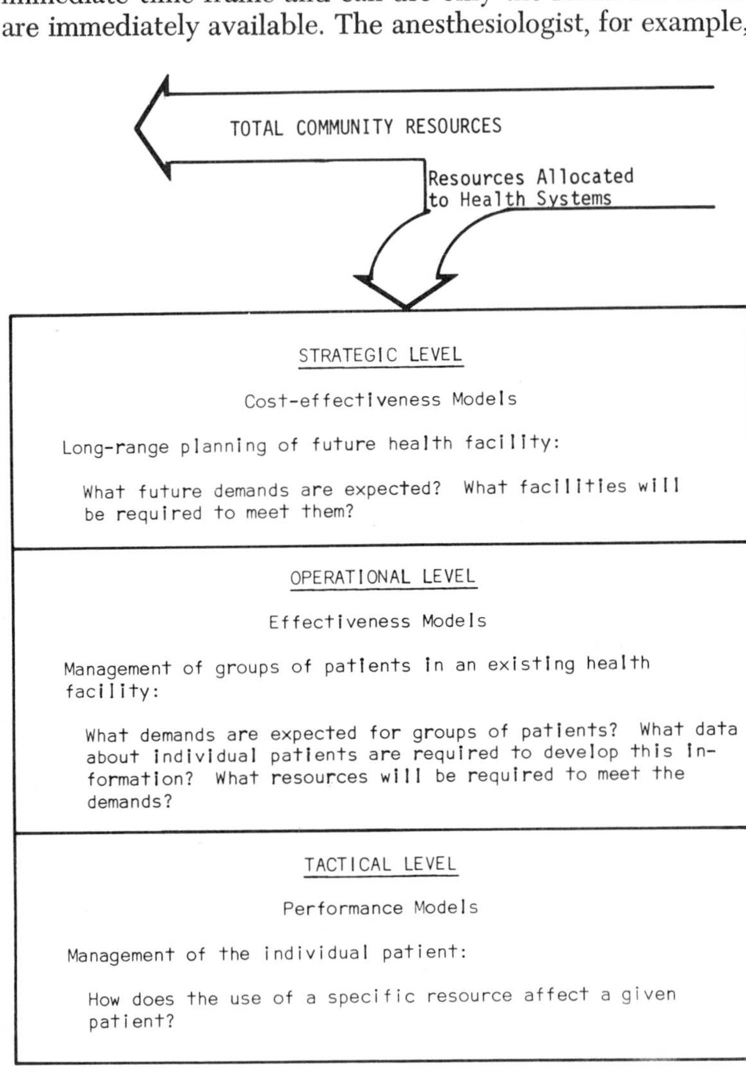

Figure 2. The functional levels of a health system.

must work with the resources provided by the hospital. In addition, at the tactical level, the physician is concerned with individual patients. This means that his decisions about medications, therapy, and the like must be based on the individual responses of a specific patient, not on the expected response of patients in general. It therefore follows that any model used to understand organzational performance at this level must describe individual patient behavior. This requirement suggests the need for adaptive, rather than predictive, system models.

At the next, or operational, level the planner works with different information and in a different time frame. Resources which are parameters at the tactical level may now be variables. The problem at this level is to organize available resources for the immediate future. The nursing supervisor, for example, must decide how to staff her nursing unit with the personnel at her disposal. At this level, planning factors may include the fact that Dr. X, whose specialty is procedure Y, is on vacation, and that it would be wise to postpone elective surgery until he returns.

Planning at the operational level may be based on statistical, or expected value information, but the numbers from which the statistics are computed must be generated at the tactical level. The decisions made at the operational level depend on group, rather than individual, behavior. For example, the scheduling of laboratory tests, and the use of facilities such as x-ray, are based not only on the needs of the individual patient, but also on system capabilities and limitations. For the individual, waiting his turn in the corridor, the scheduling procedures may seem inhuman. The system management problem is one of trading off individual demands against system capability. At the operational level, the interaction of the individual and the system is a major problem.

Much of the analytical work on health systems has taken place at the operational level. Models which describe various aspects of system behavior, such as the queue in the doctor's office or outpatient department (Flagle 1962; Flagle and Young 1966), or menu planning (Balintfy 1964), have been used to make recommendations regarding various aspects of system management. Prescriptive, rather than descriptive, models have been used for analysis. They provide guidance on what *ought* to be done to some specified criterion, such as waiting time or menu cost. The decision criterion is no longer individual, as it was at the tactical level. The relationship between these two levels can be conceptualized in terms of actuarial statistics; mortality curves are developed by aggregating data from individuals. They can be expected to predict, within limits, the probability of death at any age for a group. They cannot, however, be used to predict the death of individuals in the group. This is the concern of the tactical level model. Model building at the operational level is based to a large degree on available mathematical theory such as probability and statistics, matrix theory, or differential equations. Workers at this level have been more successful in the application of existing mathematics to specific problems than in the development of new theories and concepts.

At the top, or strategic, level planners work in an even more remote time frame. Many factors which are parameters at both the operational and tactical levels, such as physical plant, are variables here. Decisions may be made regarding the construction of new facilities. The size and location of facilities, and the kind of service to be provided, are variables. A major decision-making task at this level is to gauge trends in demands and assess the level of community resources which will be allocated to health systems.

Conceptualizing health systems in this way has at least two advantages. First, it provides for an examination of criteria at the various levels and, hopefully, tends to reduce the danger of suboptimization, or the tendency for system behavior to be efficient at one level at the expense of operations at others (Hitch 1953). The surgeon, for example, who makes unexpected and unusual demands on the operating room supervisor may be doing the best for his patient, but his actions may result in additional problems for others. As another example, the physician who utilizes all his resources in a vain attempt to save one seriously injured patient might, if he had been willing to spread the same resources around, have saved a number of the less seriously injured. Recognition of this fact has led to the assignment of a "sorting" officer in some military hospitals to decide which patients can benefit from available resources. The second major advantage of this partitioning scheme is that attention is focused on the problem of providing top-level planners with a way of assessing the consequences of their design decisions at the tactical level.

Having conceptualized a health system in terms of three interacting levels, the systems researcher must decide where to begin his research. Although most systems analysis starts at the operational and strategic levels, we have elected to start at the tactical level in an attempt to understand how the system deals with the individual patient. We elected to start our investigation here because, judging from the experience with military systems, serious problems can result from attempts to conduct strategical planning studies without understanding tactics.

III. Health Tactics

Since our research is focused on the individual patient at the tactical level, a measure of tactical effectiveness and a model relating this measure to resource utilization decisions are required. The measure of effectiveness that we have developed is based on Cannon's concept of "homeostasis" (Cannon 1932). This concept derives from the observation that the healthy organism is able to maintain "constant condition," or steady states in the body. "The coordinated physiological processes which maintain most of the steady states in the organism are so complex and so peculiar to living beings—involving, as they may, the brain and nerves, the heart, lungs, kidneys and spleen, all working cooperatively—that I have suggested a special designation for these states, 'homeostasis'. The word does not imply something set and immobile, a stagnation. It means a condition—a condition which may vary, but which is relatively constant" (Cannon, 1932, p. 24). Although the word *homeostasis* is somewhat old-fashioned, it does not appear to differ much in meaning from the more stylish concept of *dynamic equilibrium.*

The basic ideas which Cannon developed stemmed from Bernard's pioneer work of the midnineteenth century (Bernard 1865). Bernard wrote about the "free and independent life" of the higher organisms, noting that this kind of life is possible only if the organism can adapt to its environment. This it does by "preserving constant the conditions of life in the milieu intérieur." Adaptive organisms can lead the "free and independent life" because they have the capability of adjusting their physiological subsystems, that is, their resources, to cope with a wide range of disturbances impinging on them from the external environment.

If we think of health in terms of the individual's capability for leading a "free and independent life," we can define "patients" as members of society who are unable to perform the necessary homeostatic functons unaided. Health systems can be defined as the organizations designed to perform this function for the individual within resource constraints. Using these concepts, "patient care" can be measured in terms of the degree to which the system is successful in maintaining the patient in a state of dynamic equilibrium, of holding patient variables within the limits prescribed by the responsible physician for freedom and dependence (Howland and McDowell 1964).

Having defined our "patient care" measure of effectiveness as the degree to which the health system is able to assist the patient to behave homeostatically, we are faced with the problem of the terminal patient. How do we fit him in? At some point, for each of us, the free and independent life is no longer possible. We deal with the terminal patient by considering only those variables which the responsible physician wishes to hold within limits. In the case of the terminal cancer patient, for example, the amount of diseased tissue may be a variable over which control can no longer be exerted, but it may be possible to regulate the level of pain. So limits are set for pain, resources are expended to maintain the patient within these limits, and other variables are uncontrolled.

IV. Adaptive Systems and Cybernetic Models

If we think of "patients" as people whose homeostatic mechanisms are impaired, and "hospitals" as organizations which attempt to assist them in reestablishing their capability for coping with their environment, we find that cybernetic models are useful for modeling and understanding the type of adaptive behavior exhibited by the patient in the health system environment.

The word *cybernetics* was derived by Norbert Wiener from the Greek word meaning "steersman." He coined the word to describe the ideas he was developing in the design of fire control systems for the Navy in World War II. This work was based on servo theory, to which he made many notable extensions (Wiener 1948). He noted the similarity between the behavior of the systems he was designing and many human organisms and organizations. Cannon (1932, p. 308) also drew parallels between organisms and organizations and asks: "might it not be useful to examine other forms of organizations—industrial, domestic or social—in the light of the organization of the body?"

Wiener (1954) foresaw the possible misuse of the concepts and his later book, *The Human Use of Human Beings*, describes some of his concerns for the implications and dangers of cybernetics. Ashby, a British physician, has been concerned with developing cybernetic concepts to describe the behavior of a wide range of adaptive systems which he views as being "open to energy but closed to information and control—systems that are information tight" (Ashby 1957, p. 4).

In spite of the relevance of the concepts, there has been relatively little interest in their development in this country; the word "cybernetics" has, in fact acquired unpleasant connotations (Pierce 1961). If one speculates on this lack of popularity, one major reason appears to be that cybernetic models have not been developed to the point where they can be used to solve immediate problems, as the queuing theory or linear programming models can. Much fundamental work is required to develop the methodology of cybernetic modeling. The support of basic methodological research, however, is not popular in our pragmatic society. It is much easier to find support for methods for developing "quick and dirty" solutions to immediate problems. The second reason for lack of popularity stems from the first: the methods are not further developed because they are difficult. In order to deal with the complexity of the real world, the kind of simplifying assumptions which are necessary to make mathematical models tractable assumes the major problem, dealing with complexity, away. Under these circumstances, the model may generate information which answers the wrong question (Kimball 1957). Because of the methodological problems of developing cybernetic models our research has dual objectives: (1) to develop methods for modeling adaptive systems, and (2) to use the models to develop information which can be used by system managers to aide them in making resource allocation decisions.

V. A Cybernetic Model of an Adaptive System

Having elected to view health systems as adaptive, and to use cybernetic concepts to model them, how do we proceed? Model building is a circular process, and the loop can be entered anywhere. We entered with a regression model (Howland 1961):

Patient care = $A_1X_1 + A_2X_2 + A_3X_3 + A_4X_4$, where

X_1 = sociological factor.
X_2 = psychological factor.
X_3 = physiological factor.
X_4 = physical factor, and
A_1–A_4 = Respective weight, determined by expert opinion.

The model proved to be unworkable because no measure of patient care was available. As a result, this model was rejected and alternatives sought. Further observations of the hospital system were made, its adaptive characteristics were observed, and cybernetic concepts were selected to describe it. We are now collecting the data needed to modify and test the cybernetic model. The procedure is shown in Figure 3. Data describing the interactions of patients with the hospital environment are collected by nonparticipant nurse observers. The data are coded, key punched, and analyzed to display relationships between patient behavior and system resource utilization.

The cybernetic model which guides us in our data collection and analysis is shown in Figure 4. Referring to this figure, the *state processor* represents the patient. It is the information source which emits messages describing patient condition. These messages trigger action by the regulator and controller. Messages from the patient are the values of the physiological, psychological, or other variables which the regulator wishes to hold within the limits specified by the controller. The monitor serves a measuring and estimating function. Patient condition is measured in a variety of ways, ranging from visual observation to the use of complex electronic devices. Patient state information is relayed to a comparator, which compares actual and desired states and forwards difference information to the regulator. Mes-

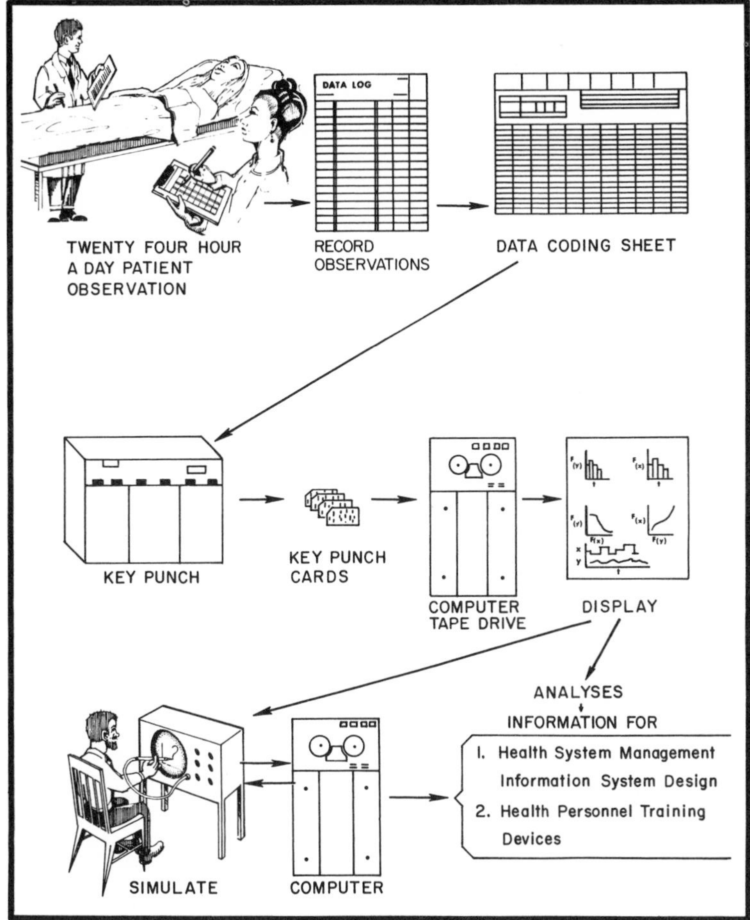

Figure 3. The research process.

sages from the controller to the comparator specify the limits of the essential variables which are to be maintained, and the comparator, in turn, forwards difference information to the regulator. The regulator uses system resources to change the values of the patient state variables in the direction indicated by the comparator. If, for example, blood pressure were rising, a vasopressor would be applied to lower it. Or, if the patient reported pain, a pain reliever would be used to reduce the value of this variable. The environment is the source of disturbances which tend to drive the patient's essential variables out of limits. These dis-

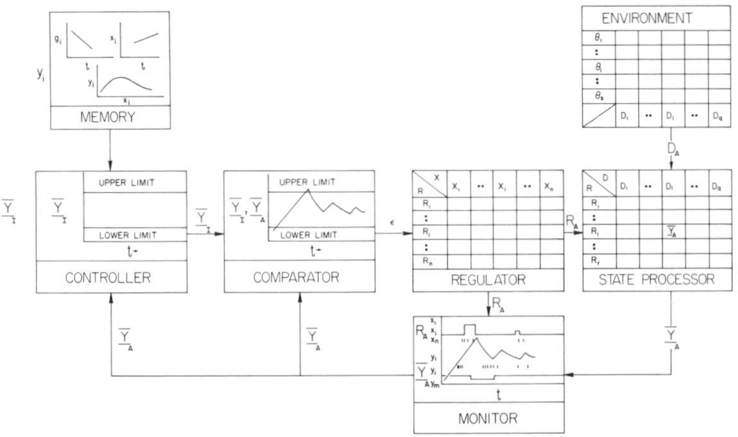

Figure 4. Cybernetic models of adaptive systems.

turbances may come from the external environment, the surgeon, noise, family, other patients, or other factors. They may originate in the internal environment as a result of physiological or psychologcal condition such as tissue damage, an infection, or emotional stress.

It was noted earlier that this model was designed to describe the adaptive behavior of the health team in response to the needs of the individual patient. Since patients are similar in many respects, the similarities (expected values of the patient variables) may be used to assist the controller in setting limits. Expected patient response information is stored in the memory. A simulation study of the anesthesiologist's response to changes in patient state information was conducted (Silver 1965), to find out what information the anesthesiologist required to make his resource utilization decisions. It was found that the anesthesiologist's tactics were related to training and experience. These differences were explained in terms of the memory. Highly trained and experienced physicians asked for more complex information, but were able to make their medication allocation decisions with less patient information than the less experienced nurse anesthetist.

One characteristic must be noted in the cybernetic model: with the exception of the patient, represented by the state processor, the boxes in the diagram represent system tasks, not people. Any member of the health team may be performing one or more of the tasks of controlling, comparing, regulating, or disturbing. One of the trade-offs in system design is the degree to which mechanical or electronic devices can be substituted to perform tasks.

The arrows connecting the boxes represent communication channels. Identification of the messages which flow through these channels and the effect of information on resource allocations and changes in patient state present interesting research questions.

VI. Data Collection and Analysis

The collection and analysis of the data required to develop and test this model presents a number of difficult problems, not the least of which is finding the money to do it. We have selected abdominal hysterectomy patients for study. This decision solves a number of sampling problems, such as homogeneity of sex, age, and diagnosis.

Dr. William E. Copeland, the surgical member of our team, selects the patients for our study, and ascertains their willingness to participate. If they agree, they are met by one of our registered nurse-observers as they are admitted. The observers do not participate directly in providing care. They collect data during four-hour shifts from the time the patient is admitted until she is discharged. During this time they attempt to record every patient-system interaction, that is, every utilization of a resource, every measurement of patient state and communication. They are instructed not to interpret what they observe, but merely to record it. The form which is used to convey these data is shown in Figure 5.

Once the data have been collected, they must be coded and punched on IBM cards and eventually put on tape. A detailed coding scheme has been developed (Pierce, Brunner, and Larabee 1968). Observers who are not on the team actually making the observations at any given time act as data coders. We have found that experience with data reduction greatly increased their effectiveness as observers. Once the data have been coded and punched on IBM cards (Figure 6), they may be analyzed in a number of different ways. According to our theory, patient demands for resources should decrease as their own homeostatic capability improves. We would therefore expect the use of resources (x)

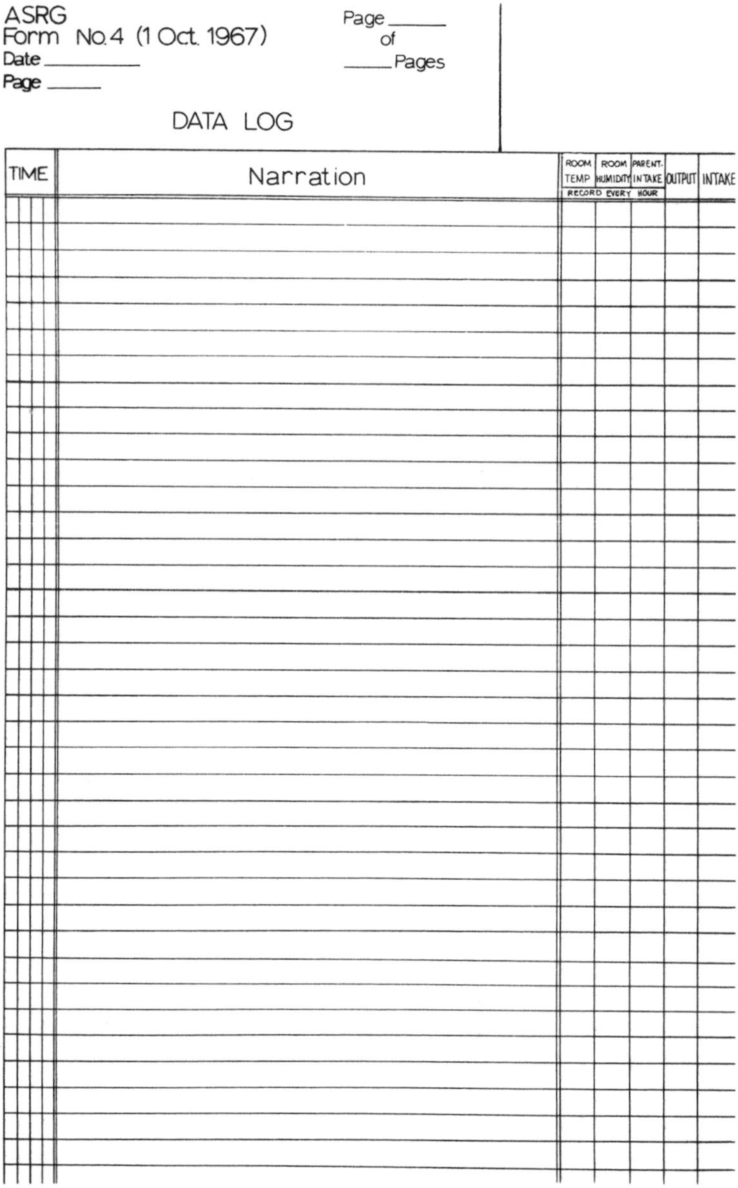

ASRG
Form No. 4 (1 Oct. 1967)
Date ______
Page ______

Page ______ of ______ Pages

DATA LOG

TIME	Narration	ROOM TEMP	ROOM HUMIDITY	PARENT. INTAKE	OUTPUT	INTAKE
		RECORD EVERY HOUR				

Figure 5. Data log sheet.

to rise sharply during the day of surgery, and then decline as the patient assumes more and more of the regulatory function herself. It can be seen that either the slope or the

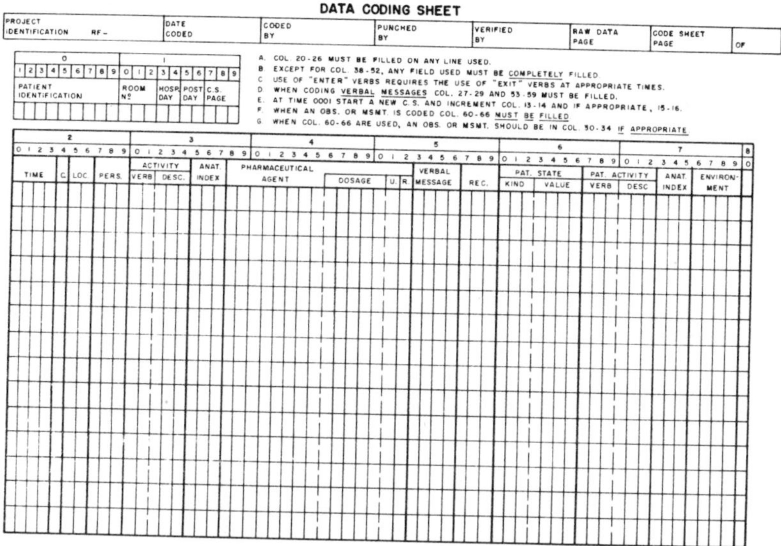

DATA CODING SHEET

PROJECT IDENTIFICATION RF–	DATE CODED	CODED BY	PUNCHED BY	VERIFIED BY	RAW DATA PAGE	CODE SHEET PAGE	OF

PATIENT IDENTIFICATION (0: 1–9)	ROOM Nº (1: 0–2)	HOSP. DAY (1: 3–4)	POST DAY (1: 5–6)	C.S. PAGE (1: 7–9)

A. COL. 20-26 MUST BE FILLED ON ANY LINE USED.
B. EXCEPT FOR COL. 38-52, ANY FIELD USED MUST BE COMPLETELY FILLED.
C. USE OF "ENTER" VERBS REQUIRES THE USE OF "EXIT" VERBS AT APPROPRIATE TIMES.
D. WHEN CODING VERBAL MESSAGES COL. 27-29 AND 53-59 MUST BE FILLED.
E. AT TIME 0001 START A NEW C.S. AND INCREMENT COL. 13-14 AND IF APPROPRIATE, 15-16.
F. WHEN AN OBS. OR MSMT. IS CODED COL. 60-66 MUST BE FILLED.
G. WHEN COL. 60-66 ARE USED, AN OBS. OR MSMT. SHOULD BE IN COL. 30-34 IF APPROPRIATE.

TIME	C.	LOC.	PERS.	ACTIVITY VERB	ACTIVITY DESC.	ANAT. INDEX	PHARMACEUTICAL AGENT	DOSAGE	U.	R.	VERBAL MESSAGE	REC.	PAT. STATE KIND	PAT. STATE VALUE	PAT. ACTIVITY VERB	PAT. ACTIVITY DESC	ANAT. INDEX	ENVIRON-MENT

RF 1651, FORM #12 (20 JUNE 1968)

Figure 6. Data coding sheet.

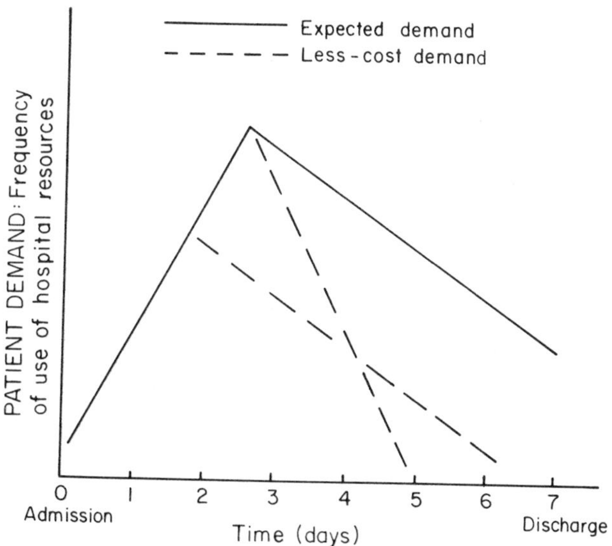

Figure 7. Patient demand for resources as a function of time.

maximum point of the curve would have to be lowered in order to reduce the cost of patient care, as shown in Figure 7.

We are interested in knowing who spends time with the

patient, what tasks they perform, and how the patient responds. We would expect registered nurses to spend a lot of time with patients during the first part of the hospitalization, but that other, less well-trained personnel would take over the tasks initially performed by the registered nurse as the patient's condition improved. Preliminary findings support this expectation. The problem of determining what resources have been used and how patients have responded is more difficult. Data for a typical patient, obtained during surgery, are shown in Figure 8. These curves were plotted manually, but programs are being developed to draw them by computers.

VII. System Simulation

Our data can be used to describe what is happening, but a simulator is needed to describe the behavior of alternative, unbuilt systems. Silver's (1965) paper and pencil simulator was developed to determine how the anesthesiologist responds to changes in patient states in surgery. As a result of our experience with this simple simulator, we are constructing a more flexible device which will allow us to study the information requirements of the regulator. This work is very much in the preliminary design stage.

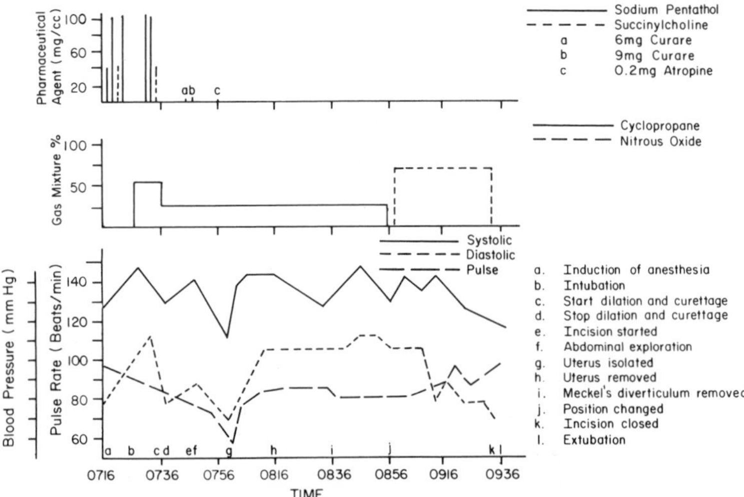

Figure 8. Patient response to resource utilization in surgery.

VIII. Conclusions

Our long-range objective is to develop a set of models relating community health system design decisions to their consequences for patients. Our research strategy has been to focus on the impact of the health care system on the individual patient as a necessary prerequisite to system planning at higher levels. Strategic decisions are difficult to make unless tactical behavior is understood.

Our work to date has substantiated our view of the adaptive nature of the system. Many decisions are made routinely for all patients, but many are made in response to patient behavior. Our cybernetic model focuses attention on the requirements for the information feedback which is essential for dealing adaptively with the indivdual patient. We believe that the presence or absence of feedback information can drastically change system effectiveness. The resources to deal with a specific problem may be available, but the information that is needed to use them effectively may be missing. We are, therefore, focusing our attention on the problems of information acquisition and display for decision-making. We believe that such a decision-information analysis is a necessary prerequisite for information system design. As Ackoff (1967) has pointed out, the tendency to automate what exists should be avoided in the design of information systems. The design of such systems should be based on detailed information on the decisions which must be made, and the information required to make them. We believe that there will be increased interest in system simulation to study the impact of information in various parts of the system on overall system performance.

Returning to Cannon's basic concepts, the key to survival of organizations as well as individuals by homeostatic coping with disturbances from the environment is information. Finally, the cybernetic concepts provide a conceptual framework for modeling and understanding the adaptive behavior of systems.

References

Ackoff, R. L.
(1967), "Management Misinformation Systems." *Management Science, 14* (December), B-147—156.
Air Ministry (1963), *The Origins and Development of Operational Research*

in the Royal Air Force. Air Publication 3368. London: Her Majesty's Stationery Office.
Ashby, W. R.
(1957), *An Introduction to Cybernetics.* New York: Wiley.
Balintfy, J. L.
(1964), "Menu Planning by Computer." *Communications of the ACM, 7* (April), 255–259.
Bernard, C.
(1865), Introduction to *L'Étude de la médecine expérimentale.* Paris: J. B. Ballière.
Blackett, P. M. S.
(1962), *Studies of War.* New York: Hill and Wang.
Cannon, W.
(1932), *The Wisdom of the Body.* New York: Norton.
Chapman, R. L., and K. L. Kennedy
(1956), "The Background and Implications of the Systems Research Laboratory Studies." In G. Finch and F. Cameron (eds.), *Air Force Human Engineering Personnel and Training Research.* Washington D.C.: National Academy of Sciences, National Research Council. Pp. 65–73.
Crystal, R. A., and A. W. Brewster
(1966). "Cost Benefit and Cost-Effectiveness Analysis in the Health Field: An Introduction." *Inquiry, 3* (December), 3–13.
Dorfman, R.
(1960), "Operations Research." *American Economic Review, 50* (September), 575–623.
Flagle, C. D.
(1962), "Operations Research in the Health Services." *Operations Research, 10* (September-October), 591–603.
——— (1963), "Operational Research in the Health Services." *Annals of the New York Academy of Sciences, 107* (May), 748–759.
———**, and J. P. Young**
(1966), "Application of Operations Research and Industrial Engineering to Problems of Health Services, Hospitals, and Public Health." *Journal of Industrial Engineering, 17* (November), 609–614.
Hitch, C. J.
(1953), "Sub-Optimization in Operations Research." *Operations Research, 1* (May), 87–99.
——— (1963), "Plans, Programs and Budgets in the Department of Defense." *Operations Research, 11* (January-February), 1–17.
———**, and R. N. McKean**
(1960), *The Economics of Defense in the Nuclear Age.* Cambridge: Harvard University Press.
Howland, D. (ed.)
(1961), *The Development of a Methodology for the Evaluation of Patient Care.* Report No. 940–6 of the Systems Research Group. Columbus: Ohio State University.
Howland, D.
(1964), "A Model for Hospital System Planning." In G. Kreweas and G. Morlat (eds.), *Proceedings of the Third International Conference on Operations Research.* Paris: Dunod. Pp. 203–212.
———**, and N. Wiener**
(1963), "The System Monitor." In D. N. Buckner and J. J. McGrath (eds.), *Vigilance: a Symposium.* New York: McGraw-Hill. Pp. 217–223.
———**, and W. McDowell**
(Winter, 1964), "The Measurement of Patient Care: A Conceptual Framework." *Nursing Research, 13,* 4–7.

Kimball, A. W.
(1957), "Errors of the Third Kind in Statistical Consulting." *Journal of the American Statistical Association,* 52 (June), 133–142.
Kimball, G., and P. M. Morse
(1951), *Methods of Operations Research.* New York: Wiley.
Mackworth, N. H.
(1961), "Researches on the Measurement of Human Performance." In H. W. Sinaiko (ed.), *Selected Papers on Human Factors in the Design and Use of Control Systems.* New York: Dover. Pp. 174–331.
Pierce, J. R.
(1961), *Symbols, Signals and Noise.* New York: Harper.
Pierce, L., N. Brunner, and J. Larabee
(1968), *Data Reduction Procedure Manual,* Adaptive Systems Research Group, The Ohio State University, Columbus, Ohio. In progress.
Quade, E. S. (ed.)
(1965), *Analysis for Military Decisions.* Chicago: Rand McNally.
Silver, A. N.
(1965), "An Investigation of Informational Factors upon the Performance of the Human Regulator." Unpublished doctoral dissertation, Ohio State University, Columbus, Ohio.
U. S. Congress (1965), Senate Subcommittee on National Security and International Operations of the Committee on Government Operations, *Hearings, Planning-Programming-Budgeting.* 90th Congress, 1st Session.
——— (1968), Senate Subcommittee on National Security and International Operations of the Committee on Government Operations, *Hearings, Planning- Programming-Budgeting.* 90th Congress, 2nd Session.
Wiener, N.
(1948), *Cybernetics.* New York: Wiley.
——— (1954), *The Human Use of Human Beings.* Garden City, New York: Doubleday. 2nd ed.

Gerald Rosenthal

12. Planning in the Health Care System

The Choice of Policies

This paper presents a discussion of the process of planning and the factors that affect the choice of policies by planners. It does not provide a recipe for "doing" planning. Rather, it discusses some generalizations that follow from viewing planning as a process of intervention by means of planning policies into the activities of an operational system (or subsystem). Such a view places into clearer perspective the activities that go to make up the planning process; defining the relevant system, specifying the planning objectives, selecting and implementing appropriate policies, evaluating the effects of those policies on the system of interest, and adapting policies to that experience.

While the circularity is essential to effective planning, this paper is primarily directed at a discussion of policy choice and factors which affect the ability of planners to draw on theoretically feasible policies. Such limitations on policy choice reflect attributes both of the planners themselves and of the particular operating system within which changes are desired. The degree of success of planning will depend both on the specification of objectives and the available "menu" of policy choices. The process of evaluation requires identification of the operating system's responses to policies and a comparison of actual responses to desired (or expected) responses. Ideally, evaluation provides the basis for policy adaptation. The emphasis in this paper on the policy choice issues is not a response to importance but, rather, to space constraints.[1]

The Process of Planning

Most of the observations in this paper, although referring to examples of planning for health services, have a degree of generality about the process of planning applicable to any system as well as to the health care system. Basically, the objective of planning is to affect the behavior and/or outcomes of an operating system. The terms *planning* and *op-*

[1] An extensive discussion of the requirements of such an evaluation system for formal planning activities consistent with those described in this paper is to be found in OSTI (1969).

erating are used here in a particular sense.[2] It may be useful to describe the relationship between these terms as an initial step in our discussion. A distinction is made between two separate sets of activities—operations and planning. Operations is the production dimension of the system being considered (e.g., transportation, education, etc.). The elements of the operating system are operators. In the health system, operators would be hospitals, physicians, medical groups, and the like. Most of the analyses of health care systems have concentrated on the relationship among operators within the system. The relationship between hospitals and nursing homes, patients and hospitals, patients and physicians all are examples of operational relationships within the system.

Planning, on the other hand, includes all activities carried out by nonoperators (*or operators outside of their operations sphere*) which have the specific objective of affecting the results of the health care operating system. The elements of the planning system are called *planners*. It is important to note that this definition does not include the activities carried out by operators which are directed at shaping their own future operations in accordance with their own objectives. While traditionally each operator calls these activities "planning," they are, in the context of this analysis, only an extension in time of direct operating activities. The object here is to distinguish between those activities designed to make each operational activity perform *its* chosen tasks better (or longer), and those activities designed to make the results of operations serve different objectives.

If the true objectives of the operators are those of the relevant nonoperators, there may still be a role for the nonoperator, but *by the definition here* such activities would not be called planning. The object of the outside activity would not be to make the operator's activities serve a different purpose but, rather, to make the operators meet their own objectives more effectively. Such activity might be called *consulting*,[3] although much of the activity of "plan-

[2] The meaning of the word *planning*, as used here, is specific and limited. The purpose served by this constrained definition is enablement of meaningful discussion.

[3] This definition is somewhat broader than the term as used in operators' research terminology.

ning" staffs in operating units is of this type. Consulting would consist of providing more technical inputs, expanding the menu of options for the operator, etc. These activities come close to those included in the definition of participatory planning, which is held to change operators' behavior by changing operators' objectives as to the desired end result of operations. However, its value is often argued even in the absence of changes in the operating system's output. This latter circumstance suggests that one behavioral attribute of the operating system desired by planners is participation (of consumers, community, etc.) and pressure from outside the operating system (by planners) to achieve participation is an effort to change the behavior (and, perhaps, the end result) of the operating system.

It should be emphasized that this does not preclude operators acting as planners from generating policies designed to effect operations beyond those with which they are specifically concerned or for which they individually have primary responsibility. For example, many formal planning structures include operators (physicians, etc.) as part of the group. A voluntary association of hospitals may function as a planner although it consists solely as a group of operators. There is no requirement by this definition that these elements are planners in the formal sense of having responsibility for coordinatng or structuring the system. Rather they are planners in that *they are attempting to generate activities and policies which are designed to affect the operating system in areas beyond those where they have a specific requirement for performance.*

There are other activities outside of the operating part of the health care system which will affect the results of operations besides those which have been described here as planning. In order to qualify as a planning activity in a given system there must be some *deliberate* intent to effect that system's operations. Exogenous activities which might interact with health systems operations represent the external effects of decisions relating to operating systems other than health care. From the planner's point of view this spillover from alternative operating systems is a matter to be considered, but such activities are not regarded as planning. Planning activities occur in response to some form of dissatisfaction with the end result of the operating process or as a response to exogenous forces which impinge on the operating system. Dissatisfaction can be described as an inconsistency with the normative notions of the planner or nonoptimization of his objective function. It can take a number of forms—a feeling on the part of the planner that the mix of output is wrong; the quantity is not sufficient, that the distribution of such output is wrong, that the quality is inadequate, that the wrong people are making decisions, or that there is the wrong ratio of inputs to output. The performance of planning must be evaluated in terms of the degree to which it changes the outcome of the operating system in a manner which moves that outcome closer to that desired by the planner.

In summary, planning is defined here as deliberate intervention for change in an operating system by a source not having operating responsibility for the particular activity of the system in which change is desired. Any such source is defined as a planner.

Defining Relevant Operating Systems

The actual process of planning must encompass at least four distinguishable but interrelated activities: system definition, specification of objectives, generation of policies, and evaluation and policy adaptation. It is essential to define the relevant operating system within which changes are desired. For example, within the health planning field the relevant operating system is often defined so as to exclude activities such as nutrition and water supply engineering. Such activities influence the degree to which operating policies of a more narrowly defined health system are likely to be effective. Nevertheless, some criterion for defining the relevant operating system in order to provide as basis for the selection for appropriate planning policies is essential. The relevant operating system at this point in our discussion relates only to the kinds of activities which the planners wish to affect. Issues of the area or subtypes of the health and medical care system, such as the hospital subsystem or the Veterans Administration subsystem, for which the planning is to be undertaken are discussed below. Nevertheless, there is need to define the object of the planner's interest and inquiry.

The definition of the relevant operating system will also provide the basis for distinguishing between operators and planners. If the relevant operating system is very narrowly defined, more activities will fall within the planning definition. For example, if the relevant operating system is the production in a factory, then the operators will consist of workers and foremen. The management of the firm will select policies such that the behavior of these operators yields an end result closest to the objectives of the management.

Let us suppose that the operator's objectives are to maximize wages and minimize work. Management will seek to maximize output and minimize costs. These latter goals are highly dependent on the operator's behavior. The policies selected will include coercive policies (work rules, etc.), stimulative policies (bonuses for performance, incentive wages, overtime pay, etc.) and persuasive policies (company spirit, newsletters, review of work, etc.).[4] With respect to the narrow operating system defined above, management is engaged in a planning activity. If the relevant operating system is the firm, the operators' objectives might be profit maximization and the operators would include management. Planning must emanate from industry control boards, the National Labor Relations Board, trade associations, the government, and other firms in the industry. If the industry as a whole is the operating system, the last group would not be planners but would themselves be operators.

Often, the definition of the operative system is determined by the planners' view of that subset of activities which they believe they are able to influence. For example, much of what has been called health planning has really been primarily hospital planning. This is a reflection of the feeling that the hospitals are more likely to respond to planning policies since they are more subject to outside influences through financing, need for community status, and dependency on outside funds for capital expansion. A constrained view of the operative system limits feasible objectives considerably.

Establishing Objectives

Another major step, highly interrelated with defining the relevant operating system, is establishing the objectives for

[4] A more extensive discussion of policy choices follows.

the system for which planning is desired to be undertaken. There are a number of forms that such objectives can take. For example, they may be quite general, that is, better health, or they might be quite specific, for example, increased supply of physicians. Often more specific goals are predicated on an assumed association with broader objectives. For example, the objective of increasing physician supply is predicated on the presumption that this will generate a greater quantity of medical care, which in turn ought to result in better health. (More medical care may be desired in and of itself because that is what consumers wish without the presumption that this will result in improved health levels.) Whether or not such assumptions are true is a matter of empirical analysis. Nevertheless, they may provide the basis for limiting planning to specific objectives when it is really the general objectives which are of primary interest to the planner.

The definition of planning used here imposes an additional constraint of the form of the specification of objectives. Since planning is a process designed to affect the activities of an operational system, the objectives of planning must be stated in terms of a desired set of changes. This degree of specification is essential if any meaningful evaluation of the effectiveness of policies is to be made. While the relevant operational system can be specified in general terms, the process of policy selection requires relating feasible points of change in that system to the policies which might serve to generate desirable (from the planners' viewpoint) changes. The specification of objectives for policy selection is an identification of those desired changes.

The implications of the planners' objectives for the operating system will often be articulated in a formal "plan." Such a development is not essential to plannng as described here. The formal "plan" is often a descriptive configuration of what the operating systems ought to look like if it is to perform optimally by the planners' criteria. This description may be in physical input terms or in output-service terms. In this case, the plan is a target for the planning process, and policies will be selected to move the operating system toward this normative end state.

Alternatively, the formal "plan" may be a timetable of policies. In this case, the "plan" is directed toward the planning process and serves to provide an analytic framework for evaluating the planners' performance.

In any case, the development of a formal plan may serve to coalesce planning action by coordinating and organizing the planning activity. However, experiences suggests that "plan" development often serves as a substitute for effective (change-generating) planning activities. It may, however, provide an operational focus for the planners' objectives.

Objectives may be directed in the form of absolute levels of medical care. For example, to provide medical care to the extent that all people desire it or need it is an absolute objective. On the other hand, the objectives may be stated terms of maximization, utilization of the resources in an operating system in such a manner as to yield maximum benefit in terms of available health services (or any other agreed-on terms). Selecting policies to serve objectives once the objective has been defined is essentially a form of benefit maximization or cost minimization—a part of the traditonal analytic structure of economics. The empirical problems of quantification, while acute, do not diminish the potential utility of the analytic framework.

There are often multiple objectives on the part of the planners, each of which conflicts somewhat with others. For example, the objectives in health care of high quality, high levels of output, and cost minimization represent an often conflicting set of objectives. Multiple objectives, if they are truly nonidentical, will require that a different policy be generated to optimize each objective (Tinbergen 1952). If the activities of a planning group are limited, certain objectives will often have to be sacrificed for others. Nevertheless, the maximization models which incorporate the offsetting influences of achievement of inconsistent objectives can often serve to illuminate this problem and aid in the selection of appropriate policies.

Policy Selection and the Operating System

The two major initiating processes, the establishment of performance objectives for a system and the designation and definition of the relevant operating system, provide the basis for the third and major stage of the process of planning: the selection and implementation of policies. Such policies ought to be based on analysis and evaluation of the operating system both to determine its appropriateness as a locus for achievement of the planners' objectives and to understand the potential impact of planning policies given the operators' objectives and the organization of the operating system. The object is to select *planning policies* which are most likely to interact with an ongoing operating system to change its performance in a way that serves the normative objectives of the planner (i.e., to result in a new set of system attributes closer to the planner's ideal than would have occurred in the absence of the policy).[5] The objective must be present whether or not the policy is effective. It is conceivable that certain planning policies will have a neutral or undesirable effect on operations (i.e., stimulate no change or undesired changes). However, the intent of impact must be present.

Given the existence of more than one source of planning policies (many planners), it cannot be presumed that the end result of all planning activities will yield a consistent or universal set of policies, any more than it would be assumed that all planners' objectives are identical. While it is essential that the planning be deliberate, in the sense of intending to affect operations, it is not essential that it be consistent with other planning activities. There is considerable evidence that inconsistency is likely to be the case and that "normative myopia" will occur even for diverse policies emanating from a single planning source.

Planning rules are prescribed arrangements external to operations which affect the way in which planners develop policies and respond to the stimulus of observed inconsistency with the results desired for the operating system. The resources devoted to health and medical care will be organized and structured by means of *operating rules.* In the absence of planning, this base-line organization of the health care system is a result of the interactions of the operators as they serve their individual objectives in the operating system.

It is unrealistic, of course, to think of a state in which there is an absence of planning as here defined. Nevertheless, it is

[5] What are referred to in this paper as planning policies have been referred to in other circumstances as instruments of planning. Planning policies *are* the instruments of planning, and for the most part these terms can be used interchangeably.

useful to distinguish between operating rules, which could be generated internally through the system, and those rules adopted in response to planning policies. An analysis of internal market structures in the absence of outside influences specifically directed at consumer market relationships would be an analysis of operating rules. Theoretical models of perfectly competitive markets are attempts to infer such rules under certain specific operating conditions. Fair labor standards laws and antitrust laws are examples of planning policies directed at making the operating system yield results more in a line with "the public interest" as defined by the "planners" responsible for generating those policies. In the health care area, licensing requirements and accreditation procedures are policies designed to affect operations.

As a result of planning policies, new operating rules, or *operating policies,* will be developed. The object of these operating policies will be to maximize the operators' objectives in light of changes which occur as the result of planning activities. In many cases, the mere formalization of a planning process may result in new operating policies prior to any specific policy generation by the planners. Operating policies may be new, or they may be adaptations of old operating rules which will minimize the impacts of the planners on the operating system. An example of this, outside of the health field, would be reductions in output or a shift to more capital intensive production in response to a minimum wage law. Within the health field many shifts in records-keeping and expenditure on skilled personnel within the nursing home field and the hospital occurred as a result of the Medicare legislation, which was designed to affect the behavior of the health care operating system. These new arrangements for record-keeping and the like represent operating policies in response to planning policies generated through the system.

The presumption of operators' defensive (change minimizing) response to planning activities is essential to the full understanding of the impact of planning policies in the system. This follows from the fact that the performance of the operating system is performed to maximize the objectives of the operators in that system within the existing planning context at any point in time.[6] The addition of new planning

[6] This assumption is equivalent to an assumption of rationality on the part

policies is likely to generate a response which represents a minimum shift from a previously held position to that position which is best with respect to the operators' objectives, given the constraining influence of the new planning policies and the operating limitations noted in footnote 6. To the extent that the planning policies would serve as a stimulus for the realization of objectives which are already in existence in the system, such response may be less noticeable. Formal planning activities might bring forth new objectives of the operators or affect the relative importance of existing objectives.[7] However, the planning activities usually press new objectives on top of those of the operators. The immediate objective of planning policies is to yield new operating policies which will result in operators' behavior more consistent with the normative notions of the relevant planning source.

Planning Policies—The Range of Policy Choices

The actual policies can take a number of different forms, but they can generally be arrayed on a continuum on which five types can be denoted. They can be roughly described as (1) prohibition, (2) restriction, (3) persuasion, (4) stimulation, and (5) coercion. Each form has a specific type of potential impact and may have more relevance in dealing with certain perceived deficiencies in operations than others. In addition, certain types of policies are more relevant (or feasible) for certain types of planners than others. These policies are instruments of planning. The choice of the appropriate instrument of planning or planning policy then becomes the task of planning.

A *prohibitive policy* is one that forbids certain action or behavior by operators. Typical of such prohibitive policies are abortion laws, which forbid the use of resources for certain kinds of activities normally within the control of a health system. Regulations which forbid unlicensed people to prescribe drugs are also prohibitive policies.

A *restrictive policy* is one which, while not prohibiting or

of the operators. They are not assumed necessarily to be maximizing their own objectives. Ignorance, inadequate resources, etc., may all preclude optimization without jeopardy to the argument of minimum change in response to policies.

[7] Business concern with hiring the "hard-core unemployable" in the absence of subsidy is an example of a shift in operators' objectives.

forbidding actions, makes such action more costly to the operators and, therefore, less likely to occur. In more direct terms, restrictive policies are those which impose penalties (additional costs) on certain forms of behavior. An example would be a ruling that, while hospitals need not have pathologists on their staff, hospitals without such employees will not be approved for Medicare payments. This restriction makes the cost of not having a pathologist considerably higher than cost figures might show. It is therefore more likely that operators will be responsive to the planners' desire for adding pathology services to the output of medical care facilities.

Thus prohibitive and restrictive policies are essentially negative policies, that is, they are directed at eliminating or reducing certain kinds of activities. *Persuasive policies* are essentially policies that do not involve direct intervention in the operating system. Policies of moral suasion and generation and stimulation of public opinion are designed to influence the operator's behavior either by making known to him that of which he was previously unaware, or by stimulating other groups (such as consumers of his output) to take action which will result in changes in the operating system. Persuasive policies often serve as "veiled threats." An appeal to altruism is made, but the suggestion is at least implied that unsuccessful appeals will result in further constraints on operations which might be less desirable than voluntary changes in operating rules made by the operators themselves. Policies of persuasion represent a considerable amount of the output of what passes for health planning in the United States.

There is another aspect of persuasive policies which merits attention. As was noted earlier, the mere existence of a formalized planning structure may have a catalytic impact on the operation of the system without the specific generation of policies designed to effect the system. The nature of this catalytic impact is likely to operate in two directions. First, the formal planning activities provide a forum for the pooling of information and the generation of new information which may lead operators to change behavior associated with given sets of objectives. For example, a broad scale view among hospital administrators of the economic returns from pooled facilities might yield an organizational structure of hospital services quite different

from that which occur if each individual institution were making its decisions by itself. This could occur even if there were no change in the individual's hospital's objectives with regard to, say, profit in the case of a proprietary institution.

A second response could be the adaptation of an operator's objectives to those of the group in which planning is taking place, without the generation of specific planning policies. The exposure provided in the formal planning body and the relatively public nature of decision-making may actually cause individual operating institutions to change the objectives which they are likely to serve. A move to make the community objectives more significant in the hospital's decision-making process than physicians' objectives might be an example of this kind of transfer.

The point to be made here is that these adaptations do not reflect the impact of specific planning policies and do not represent minimizing responses to changes in the environment within which the planner and the operator act. Rather they represent the impact of information and exposure and formalized planning activities on the operating objectives and operating policies within the operating system itself. These are not truly persuasive policies in a direct sense, because they may not represent deliberate attempts to adapt an operator's behavior on the part of the planner. Nevertheless, they represent a significant, often the most significant, area of impact of formal planning structures, and as such they are inherent in the nature of the planning activity.

Aside from the negative and neutral policies described above, there are a number of positive policies which can be suggested. A *stimulative* policy is one which, while not requiring certain action, makes such action more consistent with the operators' objectives and therefore more likely to occur. Typical of these kinds of policies are grants-in-aid for medical facilities construction, incentive payments for efficiency within the reimbursement structure of the hospital system, and scholarships for medical students. In each case the individual is free to make all the operating choices he previously made, but some additional benefits or reduced costs are offered for the selection of certain courses of action felt by the planner to be preferable. The stimulative policy is the other major instrument of planning within our medical care system.

At the opposite extreme from prohibitive policies, *coercive*

policies require certain actions or behavior by operators. Typical of these regulations are laws requiring annual tuberculosis tests for all employees, building and fire safety codes relating to the physical structures of health care institutions, and the requirement that all students entering school must have a smallpox inoculation.

Constraints on Policy Choice

While all the general classes of policies above are potentially available, there are a number of specific constraints on policy choices. In some cases they reflect the nature of the planner while in others they will reflect the nature of the operating system.

AUTHORITY LIMITATIONS In many cases the ability of the planner to deal with the behavior of certain operators within the health system will be limited by the nature of the planning rules themselves. For example, hospital planning councils, while often interested in broader objectives than those of the hospital system, will nevertheless be able to generate policies which affect only certain parts of the system, while other parts of the system, such as nursing homes or mental hospitals, will be excluded from their sphere of influence. The limitation on the authority of the planner will restrict his choice of policy.

CONTROL LIMITATIONS In many cases the planning rules preclude the selection of policies which are prohibitive or coercive. While the planner may be able to generate some policies which will affect the behavior of the operators in the system, he is not in the position to control such behavior, nor can he preclude alternative forms of behavior. Such circumstances are true of all voluntary planning structures and are inherent in the notions of voluntary arrangements developed under the area-wide planning model and most recently implemented under the Regional Medical Program model.

RESOURCE LIMITATIONS In many cases it is possible that policies which would serve the objectives of the planners most effectively cannot be achieved with the resources available within the system. For example, the lack of home nursing care may, in the short run, preclude attempts to stimulate nursing home care as a way of more effectively providing health care services in the absence of the sufficient

hospital facilities. Perhaps more remote, but even more constraining, would be an inadequate level of housing which precludes home care as a viable alternative.

Even when the resource being considered is money, such limitations may preclude the use of various kinds of stimulative policies. When there are alternative sources of funds sufficient to satisfy the operators' objectives, then there may not be sufficient money resources at the discretion of the planner to implement effective stimulative policies. In this case, stimulative policies would be less likely to be selected and planners would have to turn to different types of policies. In addition, the greater the difference between the objectives of the planners and the objectives of the operators in the system, the greater the resources required to stimulate conformance to planners' objectives. In such a case either coercive policies or the threat of such policies may be required to change operators' behavior (or to generate response to incentives which by themselves would not be adequate). The emphasis given to voluntary planning as a way of avoiding coercive policies and the imposition of outside planning objectives on a smaller medical care subsystem reflect this strategy. Resource constraints may be such that the planner cannot afford to stimulate directly an acceptable level of compliance.

POLITICAL LIMITATIONS Political considerations may make it unlikely that policies which would be feasible would be applied. For example, for many years many medical care policies believed to be desirable by the planners and certainly within the authority and control competency of the planners were not undertaken because of the suspicion that such policies would not be feasible due to the political influence of one of the constituencies of affected operators in the system. Such limitations may serve as a real constraint on policy. Certainly the often raised specter of socialized medicine is an attempt to place a sense of political limitation on planners in terms of developing new patterns of production in the operating system.

CERTAINTY LIMITATIONS The degree to which one is uncertain as to the actual impact of policies may serve to constrain their application. The use of coercive and prohibitive policies requires a fairly high degree of certainty that the adverse impact of such policies will not be significant. When such a degree of certainty is not fully substantiable, there is often reluctance to force behavior within the operating system but rather a preference to select policies which provide an "escape valve." Analyses designed to provide better information about the operating system serve to reduce the constraints of uncertainty on policy selection.

INFORMATION LIMITATIONS In addition to increasing the ability to predict results of policies, information about the operating system may actually generate new policy choices. For example, the analytic demonstration of price and insurance elasticity of demand for hospital services provided the basis for using stimulative policies through the market mechanism to provide greater medical care for the aged. If the view that all who need care receive it without regard to economic circumstances were true, legislation such as Medicare could have no significant impact on the use of "needed" services. Information and analysis demonstrating a wide variation in utilization of health services associated with variation in economic circumstances provided the factual basis for the development of policies to improve the utilization of a group of underusers relative to anticipated "need."

INTERACTION WITH OTHER OPERATING SYSTEMS Some policies will not be selected because of potential adverse impact on operating systems other than the one for which planning is being undertaken. These external effects of planning policies were noted earlier. Although not directly the interest of the planner, they may intervene in the selection of appropriate policies in a significant way. For example, the use of a coercive policy requiring a medical education for all competent individuals would be likely, even if it were politically and operationally feasible, to result in a significant adverse impact on a number of other operating systems relevant to society as a whole. These extreme policies, then, really are precluded by the existence of interactions such as shared resources among operating systems.

Some of the implications of these limitations on policy choice can be noted with regard to health planning in the United States. In the fully planned economy, all of the policy tools described above may be brought into play in order to maximize the degree to which the outcome conforms to normative criteria against which the central planning authority compares performance. There is, however, in a planned economy a tendency to rely more heavily on certain types of planning policies than others. Coercive policies and prohibitive policies require degrees of authority and control which make them more likely to be applied in central planning countries than in countries like the United States. In a mixed economy there is a considerable tendency to rely most heavily on stimulative policies of one sort or another.

Within the United States there is a built-in orientation toward reliance on the market and a willingness to allow the preferences of consumers to determine to a large degree the forms of their consumption. Most of the social welfare activities in the United States take the form of redistribution of money income. This is an attempt to enable certain segments of the population to participate more fully in the operation of existing markets. Under certain circumstances the government may become a producer of goods and services, but this is far less likely to be the norm. There are areas where less market reliance is to be found in determining the use of resources; in the area of defense and, at less aggregated levels of government, fire, police protection, and water supply development are conducted at the level of the community as a whole with the little, if any, private consumer activity.

The difference between fully planned economies and mixed economies, such as that of the United States, is perhaps more basic than the pure planning mechanism itself. When decision-making for the use of resources is centralized or placed in the hands of a single planning agency, it becomes possible to establish objectives for activities explicitly and to evaluate the degree to which these objectives are achieved by means of agreed-upon criteria. For example, it becomes possible for a central planning authority to establish that increases in producers goods production relative to consumer goods production is a desirable circumstance and it becomes possible within the political structure of such a country to get a vote of confidence (preclude resistance) for this kind of objective. On the other hand, in a country like the United States, there is rarely a clear-cut criterion on which to establish a unified single objective. Therefore, any policy which requires serving a single objective on the part of everyone in the society has a much larger potential for misallocation than people are in general willing to accept, and therefore a smaller chance of implementation. For one thing, coercive or prohibitive policies require certainty about the disutility of nonconformance with the objectives implicit in these policies. In most cases, there does not exist any mechanism for ascertaining such a universal objective.

What is more likely to occur is that, through the political process, certain forms of behavior will be regarded by many to be desirable without sufficient certainty in the objective to make it mandatory. The object of a stimulative policy is to make operators a little more disposed toward the behavior which is desired than would otherwise be the case in the absence of the policy without forcing them to behave in ways which might turn out to be undesirable. In most simple terms, the potential for mistakes is considerably less under a set of planning policies designed to stimulate various forms of behavior without precluding alternative forms of behavior if the individual operator in the market so wishes. We rely quite heavily on the political process and on the relative popularity or unpopularity of various kinds of incentives to indicate the degree to which they conform to public objectives or not. By these means we are able to incorporate new incentives for new kinds of behavior as such circumstances arrive. It becomes possible in some cases to offset one incentive with strong incentives in an opposing direction. Because of the difficulty of eliminating existing policies, the ability to water down or offset their impact may have considerable utility, given the political process in the United States. For noncentrally planned economies, there is considerable reliance on stimulative policies of one sort or another, and considerably less reliance on coercive or prohibitive policies. Indeed, even restrictive policies are likely to be looked upon with suspicion in the context of the American political and economic structure.

For many restrictive policies there are some stimulative policies which could yield similar behavior. In such a circumstance, the option is likely to be for the stimulative policy. An example might make this clear. One could adopt a regulation that no hospital will be approved for any public medical payment without a certain ratio of nurses to patients. This policy is restrictive because, while not precluding the operating of a hospital with a low nurse-to-patient ratio, it does make it particularly difficult to carry out such an activity. On the other hand, a policy to offer bonuses to those hospitals with higher nurse-patient ratios could be adopted. The latter case, I would argue, is much more likely to occur. The net impact with regard to the ratio of nurses to patients may, indeed, turn out to be the same. However, the overall results of these policies for medical care operations are likely to differ.

It is likely that more total resources will turn up being applied to health and medical care activities as a result of this emphasis on stimulative policies. Providing additional resources wholly from outside provides little incentive to redistribute existing expenditure within the health services system. To illustrate, if you tell someone that he cannot make a decent amount of money without running a certain kind of hospital, for example, one with a very high level of nurses, he will decide either not to run any hospital at all or to run a hospital with more nurses and, perhaps, fewer other things. If, on the other hand, you tell him he can run any kind of hospital he wants but that if he adds more nurses you will give him more money, then he is more likely to do everything he would have done without that incentive and, in addition, respond to it by adding nursing activities.

The strong emphasis on incentives and policies of stimulation has created a circumstance where more resources are going into these activities than might otherwise have occurred. This would be true both in the case where other kinds of policies had been applied to achieve the same types of ends, and in that where no policies had been applied and the activity had been left solely up to the private market. These additional resources may reflect a social judgment that, this is a preferable way of using the resources available to society. On the other hand, it may be a reflection of the nature of the policies that we have applied to implement public policy as compared to other sectors of the economy which are less the subject of public policy activities and planning.

Subsystems Planning and Policy Choices

Two types of subsystems can be described. One kind represents the interaction of a class or classes of operators such as the hospital system or the medical manpower system. The other type of subsystem is exemplified by the regional health model, which describes the interaction of a subset of all operators in the system relevant to a smaller group of potential consumers of output.

While the interest in this paper is primarily in the latter type of subsystem, it should be noted that each of the limitations of policy choices described above will affect planning for both kinds of subsystems. In addition, planning for class-of-operator subsystems is made more difficult by the greater specificity (and limitation) of objectives and the inability to deal with other inputs to the aggregate system on which the relevant subsystem performance may depend. For example, planning for greater supply of hospital facilities has not always resulted in more use of facilities even when the specific objective was reached. Indeed, the result is a reduction in efficiency of the subsystem.

For regional health subsystems, the constraints on policy choices resulting from interaction with (and dependence on) other systems (and subsystems) is intensified. Indeed, even the primary objectives may be different, or at least take different forms from the objectives for the health system as a whole. For example, if one assumes for the moment no difference in the contribution of a physician in location A to the general level of health compared to a physician in location B, then policies generated by region B planning body in an effort to attract physicians from A to B might yield an improvement in health in region B and represent desirable policies. For the entire operating system, however, such policies are likely only to generate an increase in money resources going into the system without any increase in output and represent reductions in efficiency. On the other hand, if there are differences in the marginal contributions of physicians in different subsystems, then the policies and the interpretation of these policies will be quite different. For example, it could be argued that the transfer of one physician from the greater Boston area to the Mississippi Delta or, indeed, the transfer of one physician from an affluent suburb to an inner city ghetto might represent a net increase in the medical services available to the area as a whole. However, to the extent that each of these constitutes a separate operating subsystem, there is no vehicle for generating effective planning policies. Another example would be the recent response to the suggestion that the more affluent suburban communities share their educational facilities with central city school children. While such an activity would most likely represent a net increase in the aggregate education available to our children, the narrower view of each individual community often precludes these policies from coming to fruition.

Defining the Subsystem

Policy choice will be affected by the manner in which the region is defined as well as the authority under which such regional planning body is constructed. It is essential that the region be related in some consistent way and yield some definable end result or output which is of interest to the planner. A number of alternative linkage criteria can be suggested, each of which has some counterpart in contemporary health planning.

AUTHORITY AND RESPONSIBILITY It is possible to define appropriate planning subsystems based on the degree to which the planners have authority and responsibility for providing or affecting the output of health and medical care services. Examples of such regions or operating subsystems would be the VA Health and Medical system and perhaps the Indian Health Service. Here the geographic criteria are not nearly so well defined, but the subsystems are coherent, identical, and linked solely by the identifiable source of fiscal responsibility and authority for provision of services.

POLITICAL CRITERIA Often regions are defined by the political structure of the area. The structure of the Comprehensive Health Planning Act, which operates through state and local governments, is an attempt to coordinate and generate planning policies to stimulate and effect changes in the output of health and medical care services using the political boundaries of the state as the primary definer of the operating subsystem. This enables the use of various kinds of policies which require a high degree of authority and control, but which already exist under legislation which grants such powers to these political entities.

ECONOMIC CRITERIA It is possible to define regions or operating subsystems in terms of various economic criteria. For example, much economic analyses of the production and distribution of hospital and medical facilities services show significant economies of scale up to between 250 and 500 beds. For certain individual types of health and medical care services, the economies of scale may suggest that most efficient operation is achieved only at a rate of utilization which requires a fairly large population base. For example, open-heart surgery represents a form of medical service which is very costly and which ought to be utilized relatively intensively in order to make the most efficient utilization of the capital and manpower investment required. However, epidemiologically the need for such services arises fairly infrequently within a population, and therefore this kind of activity may require a fairly large geographic catchment area.

One may seek to define an operating subsystem by defining a set of services which are relevant, and by looking for a region which will enable the most efficient use of such services. The economic criteria can be adapted. For example, as part of a research project on the demand for medical care facilities, models were developed by Mr. John Carr which were designed to equate the increasing geographic areas required for given population density to make efficient application of scale economies and the cost associated with additional travel time and relative inaccessibility of services. For some services, such as emergency services, the cost of inaccessibility is very high. The accessibility requirement is considerably less for services rarely provided without considerable scheduling time and referral from some other part of the operating system. For each service, there is an appropriate point of balance between the cost associated with reduction in scale and the cost associated with reduction in accessibility. From this, an appropriate geographic distribution of services can be derived which essentially describes an operating subsystem which is optimally efficient in a cost-benefit sense.

SOCIAL CRITERIA It is possible to designate operating subsystems on the basis of various social criteria. The concept of neighborhood planning and neighborhood health centers incorporates the view that there exists a social entity which has geographical dimensions called "neighborhood" which can plan for health services in a meaningful way. Ethnic criteria for certain kinds of operating subsystems, such as Catholic hospitals, might also fall into this category.

GEOGRAPHIC CRITERIA It is possible to define operating subsystems strictly in geographic terms because of travel and accessibility patterns. For example, the eight areas within the California Regional Medical Program have rather peculiar geographic shapes. However, when they are laid against a relief map of the state of California, it is evident that some regions achieve their shape primarily because of the existence of a rather large chain of mountains running diagonally up the center of the state, thereby effectively insulating large parts of the population from the medical centers which would be closest to them in distance but which are far away in time because of geography. In this way, some natural geographic catchment areas were developed. Indeed, the notion of an Appalachia region for planning purposes reflects, to some extent, purely geographic criteria as well as some observable net deficiency in terms of available services relative to other areas.

Each of these criteria for defining operating subsystems is likely to yield different geographic regions, and each basis for defining such subsystems is likely to influence the potential for fruitful policy selection and for the achievement of particular objectives.

There are some general kinds of observations about the nature of policy choice which can be made when planning is being undertaken for a subsystem. Medical manpower is a useful example. For the country as a whole it may be reasonable policy to stimulate the production of additional physicians. For an individual suboperating system, however, policies to generate additional physicians may or may not prove to be effective. For example, the state of Iowa, which is for some purposes a single planning region, is a net exporter of M.D.'s to the rest of the country. While there are many reasons for this, it seems likely that a policy of expanding the output of the medical school in Iowa will not necessarily be an effective generator of additional physician manpower for that operating subsystem. Nevertheless, such a policy would represent an increase in the output of physicians for the country as a whole. Perhaps far more effective from the operating subsystem's point of view would be to provide incentives to attract physicians now going elsewhere into Iowa. While this would benefit Iowa, it would not necessarily improve the availability of services of the output of the operating system as a whole.

There are a number of objectives of policy which can be

distinguished from this discussion. The distinction has to be made between policies designed for redistribution of manpower and policies designed at increasing the aggregate supply. While policies of redistribution may be desirable from an aggregate point of view, there is no mechanism within subsystem planning to enable such transfers to take place. The response to physicians being attracted away from low requirement areas to high requirement areas is likely to be a retaliatory response to hold the physicians! Indeed there are ample indications that physicians tend to be attracted to areas with high economic capability for generating incomes. These areas are likely also to be the areas that are in the greatest position to generate incentives to attract more physicians. The areas with the greatest relative shortages of manpower and the greatest deficiencies in health services are also those areas which are less likely to be able to generate kinds of incentives needed to attract physicians away from alternative positions in other suboperating systems. This aggregate redistributive objective among regions may require a level of planning and a choice of policies beyond that which could be expected in a regional subsystem.

The primary purpose of this paper has been to provide a conceptual framework for examining planning and the factors that affect the choice of appropriate policies by the planners. The implications of subsystem planning for policy choices was discussed and applied to regional health subsystems. The argument is that the processes of both establishing appropriate objectives and selecting effective strategies are different when the planning is directed at a region which must interact and share resources with other regions. Nevertheless, the difference is more in degree rather than in kind. The process of selecting and implementing planning policies is a complex one.

Evaluation and Policy Adaptation

The above discussion suggests that the ability to plan effectively will depend primarily on the ability to understand the system which we are trying to affect and to develop planning mechanisms which incorporate that knowledge into the process of policy choice. To be fully effective, such activities should include (or have access to) a process which monitors changes in the operational system and relates them to planning policies. This evaluation process serves as a feedback-learning process and enables the adaptation or addition of policies to stimulate changes consistent with the planners' objectives. Ideally, the information base on which such a process could be built is an essential element of formal planning activities since policy selection, as described here, must be predicated on anticipated system responses. In a formal setting and/or for complex systems, planners' anticipations will often be based on research, both theoretical and empirical. The evaluation process can be viewed as ongoing research designed to make the choice of policies better serve the objectives of the planning. Even in informal planning activities, the incorporation of experience into behavior is highly correlated to success. This argues strongly that evaluation must be an integral part of the planning process.

References

OSTI (Organization for Social and Technical Innovation)
(1969), *Evaluation of State Programs of Educational Services to the Handicapped.* Cambridge, Mass., October.

Tinbergen, Jan
(1952), *On the Theory of Economic Policy.* Amsterdam: North Holland.

Louis B. Barnes

13. Designing Change in Organizational Systems and Structures

In some respects, a business school professor trying to play doctor to the medical care field seems presumptuous. Even though trained in both business and the behavioral sciences, I still sense the rarified atmosphere as I enter the world of medical specializations, patient care, or even hospital administration.

Nevertheless, a combination of systems thinking, consultation experiences, and prolonged discussions with those who know more than I about medical care systems has generated a willingness to comment upon that world. I am now so bold (and possibly foolish) as to think that business practices and problems are relevant to medical systems and structures. Worse yet, my boldness increases as parallel patterns repeatedly appear among business, government, education, and medical care systems. These patterns include a series of ongoing conflicts between specialists and generalists, individualists and group thinkers, task advocates and social-emotional advocates, superiors and subordinates, theorists and practitioners, staff men and line men, clients and consultants.

In each of these conflict areas, I see some cases where aggression becomes debilitating and destructive. Yet other cases move beyond conflict and into a phase of problem-solving cooperation, possibly followed by new but more constructive conflict. The essential problem in these efforts at conflict resolution seems to be whether the conflicting parties can move from a state of differentiated polarization toward and even beyond some form of integration and synthesis. The process of movement involves changes in attitude and behavior. It can be an extraordinarily delicate process, but it is the one I wish to focus upon in this paper.

Man spends much of his time designing ways in which he can both separate and combine his behavior with others. Organizational and professional structures reflect these pressures toward differentiation and integration. We separate and splinter into departments, work groups, special fields, and subspecialties. Each one acquires its own values and dominant norms or ground rules. At the same time, as the differentiation strains increases, we seek integrating mechanisms. We set up coordinators, conferences, interdisciplinary work teams, confrontations, role changes, bosses, and the use of sheer power (e.g. knocking heads together) to knit things together.

The cycle of change suggests that "too much" of either differentiation or integration helps to beget the other. In either case, strain and conflict are likely. Separate entities do not become integrated without strain or conflict. Nor does the "one big happy family" divide easily into separate entities, as any parent can testify. The problem, of course, is to develop a paradoxical system in which both differentiation and integration prevail and in which movement from one to the other is possible without bogging down into either chaos or conflict. Put more practically, a medical specialist is a stronger specialist if he understands and can help his specialization relate to other specializations (Pelz and Andrews 1966). A specialized or differentiated department must somehow be integrated into an overall organizational effort (Blake *et al.*, 1964; Dalton, Barnes, and Zaleznik 1968; Greiner 1967; Lawrence and Lorsch 1967). Likewise, a "group thinker" needs to recognize the value of role differentiations into specialized, though also coordinated activities. The problem intensifies when differentiation or integration become limited ends in themselves rather than means to a deliberately paradoxical system.

The beauty and the binding of a paradoxical system is that "both sides" are valued. The wars between specialist and generalist, staff and line, old and young, structurer and free thinker become valued for the potential in their conflict resolutions rather than condemned for their existence. Above all, what is needed is an organization whose members have capacities for behavior change and social learning, and a culture which encourages its members to use what they learn. In this paper I want to focus upon these two issues: behavioral learning and the developing of a learning culture.

Some Concepts on Behavior and Social Learning

In testimony before Senator Harris' Subcommittee on Government Research, Arthur Brayfield, then editor of the

American Psychologist, identified five concepts as useful to think about when considering behavior change and social learning (Brayfield 1968). Drawn from social research, each concept emphasizes man's conscious thoughts and behavior rather than his underlying motivations. This in itself reflects a growing belief among behavioral scientists that behavior change is focusing on the actual shaping of behavior rather than first trying to provide insight and understanding. The trend suggests that we get better results—and can be more courageous—in focusing on manifest behavior change rather than worrying about a deep understanding of what is unconscious and unrecognized.

Such changes are most effectively encouraged, according to previous research, if one or more of the following five concepts are involved. Expanding upon Brayfield's descriptions, they include

1. *The importance of new assumptions.* A person's assumptions about himself and the world around him are big factors in determining his behavior. If I assume that a particular person is "good," I behave toward him differently than if I assume he is "bad." A patient (or nurse, or technician, or administrator) who assumes that a doctor is to be trusted behaves differently toward the doctor than does one who assumes mistrust. Assuming that the world was round led to far different behavior patterns on the part of man than when he assumed the world to be flat.

2. *Expectations and perceptions.* Related to a person's assumptions are his expectations and perceptions. If I expect or "see" another person or object as threatening, I will behave differently than if I see him or it as rewarding. If I expect to succeed at a task, I will behave differently than if I expect to fail. My "success oriented" behavior will, in turn, provide cues to others which result in behavior modifications on their part. In other words, my expectations can be an important determinant of other people's behavior, even to the point of creating self-fulfilling prophesies. In these, I help to make happen that which I implicitly expect to happen.

3. *Modeling behavior.* There is increasing evidence that the behavior of some people serves as a model for the behavior of others (e.g., parents with children, older siblings with younger siblings, heroes with admirerers). In this way,

the learner observes and tries out behavior patterns he observes in others whom he respects. This experimenting is then modified or intensified as the learner gets responses from the environment.

4. *Selective reinforcement with immediate rewards.* Brayfield calls this "the most powerful tool for the shaping of behavior." Selective reinforcement of approved behavior puts the stamp of approval on a learner's efforts to change. Such "success experiences" provide the incentive one needs to keep repeating a new pattern of behavior. Rewards can take interesting and complex forms, varying all the way from money and love to more subtle cues of approval (e.g., nonverbal expressions, absence of prior pain or punishment, etc.).

5. *Participation in problem solving.* Participation involves a learner in a voyage over which he exercises some control. Rather than feeling that his behavior is controlled entirely by other factors, he exercises influence as well as running the risk of being influenced. Equally important, though, the participation occurs in the solving of problems rather than around strictly social or nonwork interactions.

Thus, new assumptions, expectations and perceptions, modeling behavior, selective reinforcement, and participation in problem solving serve as basic concepts for behavior change. They are applied in and outside of organizations by parents, bosses, therapists, students, and teachers. Summarized as a set of related concepts, we might make the following statement:

Behavior change is encouraged when potential role models provide new role patterns which help disconfirm old assumptions and expectations. As the learner participates in trying to solve old problems using these new behavior patterns, he becomes rewarded, deprived of reward, or punished. If selectively rewarded, he begins to change his expectations and assumptions. The cycle then moves toward the solving of new problems.

As a general statement, the above "makes sense" to me. It fits in with my experience as part of the behavioral science group at the Harvard Business School where one of our foci has been upon studying behavior modification in work groups and organizations (Lawrence and Lorsch, 1967). At the same time, the literature on behavior change in organizations tends to emphasize only one of the above five concepts. Indeed, many of us have been thoroughly schooled in the power of "participative" management. What we have emphasized less, often because the changes seemed nonparticipative, are the powerful change effects of such factors as role models, expectations, assumptions, and selective reinforcements. Any of these change catalysts can occur in an atmosphere of crackling tension, displaced aggression, or raw power. Without participation of problem solving, win-lose conflicts tend to develop in which some people get hurt through power struggles, empire building, opposing forces, and trauma. These win-lose situations also provide the stalemates that frustrate and make power struggles out of organizational change efforts. Two units (either persons, groups, divisions, or levels) become locked in combat so that power gains by one are perceived to be at the expense of the other. The problem is further seen to be one of scarce resources and the relative distribution of power. With these emphases, the situation also appears to be a closed system in which (1) total resources cannot be increased, (2) mutual gains in power are impossible, and (3) traditional boundaries and assumptions appear inflexible.

In one organization, for example, the engineering division felt that its project work was being done by maintenance engineers working in collaboration with production management. In the same organization, research scientists complained that the technical division employees were trying to do "shadow research." In another company, line managers felt that their prerogatives were being grabbed by staff specialists whose knowledge qualified them for the work. None of the parties in these conflicts saw any room for collaboration. In each case, the expectations became win-lose.

The above situations develop in almost any kind of organizational setting. Unit A differentiates itself from Unit B along some real or exaggerated dimension. The issues of relative power and scarce resources form the basis of a mistrust assumption. The mistrust assumption leads to a win-lose expectation, and initial behavior (as well as role modeling for others) takes the form of attacking, defending, or withdrawing. A norm of reciprocity tends to develop and be reinforced which becomes essentially destructive in character. The long-term consequences involve an emphasis on self-oriented needs and further concern for one's relative power in the assumed closed system. Meanwhile, participation in problem solving is still absent.

Disturbing as it may seem, the above pattern fits Brayfield's five concepts for "learning" except for the fifth one, participation in problem solving. Partly for this reason, it could not, as he would wish, lead to "a society—a set of social arrangements—a human environment—that will foster the sense of personal worth and self-esteem required to sustain the human spirit, give meaning to our lives, and provide the energizing force to forge our personal destinies and to ensure the emergence and survival of a humane society" (Brayfield 1968). But the fact remains that many organizational changes are designed and implemented using closed system assumptions. The basic assumption, reinforced through initial experiences, becomes one of mistrust, since power gains by one party are viewed as necessarily at the expense of the other. An oversimplified version of this closed system model, paired with the concepts presented by Brayfield is shown below.

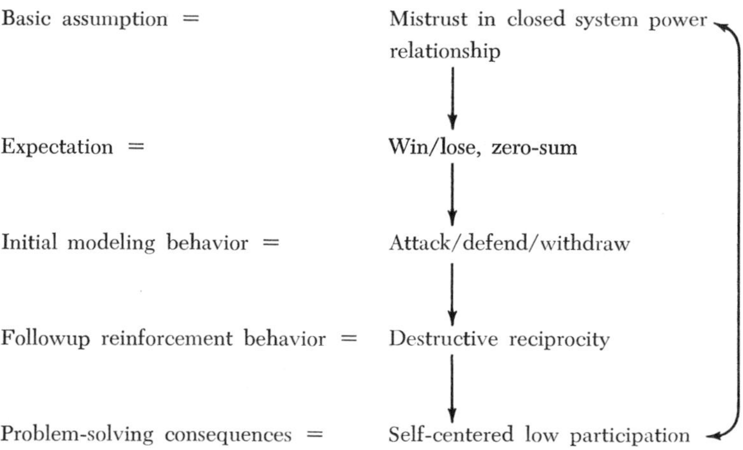

More than a decade of concern with change design and implementation in organizations has left its mark upon me. Although I would guess that over three-quarters of all change designs tend to follow the above pattern, they never have impressed me as optimal from ethical, efficiency, or satisfaction points of view. The case files at the Harvard Business School contain illustrative data which amply support this point, even though, it might be reasonably argued, there *are* times when such closed systems cycles seem inevitable or desirable. But the era of increasing technical complexity makes these situations seem fewer and farther between, since the need for participative problem-solving increases under task-environment uncertainty. The recent research by Lawrence and Lorsch (1967) suggests that increasing uncertainty in an organization's task-environment also increases the needs for both specialization and cooperation. Their study, as well as others, also indicate that, regardless of the task environment, a confrontation style of conflict resolution provides superior problem solving over other styles.

All of these factors support the advantages of an alternative model for organization development, and this is beginning to appear where managers have begun to appreciate the need for a paradoxical system which increases both differentiation and integration. Consequently, it is neither altruism nor nobility which leads managements toward a more open system model of change in which trust tends to challenge mistrust as the basic assumption. It is, instead, a recognition that organizations are arenas in which total power is as crucial to personal success, and more crucial to organizational success, than is relative power. If Units A and B can both gain power over each other or the environment through cooperative interdependence, the win/lose problem is reduced considerably.

Under these conditions, management's map becomes a more open system map in which cooperative power expansion-contraction is more crucial than relative power. Trust becomes a necessary basic assumption compatible with the mutual power expansion. Participative problem-solving expectations then replace the competitive win/lose expectations. Initial modeling takes the form of confrontation/coping behavior rather than attack/defend/withdrawal behavior. The combinations of confrontation and coping behaviors keeps inquiry open while still engaging the stickier issues in problem-solving. Follow-up reinforcement, then, begins to establish reciprocity norms that are basically constructive and cooperative in nature, while the long-term consequences tend to show high participation addressed to multiple needs. An oversimplified diagram of this more open system model is shown in comparison with the closed system model below.

Trust in an open system power relationship	Basic assumption	Mistrust in a closed system power relationship
Mutual problem solving	Expectation	Win/lose, zero-sum
Confrontation/ coping	Initial modeling behavior	Attack/defend/ withdraw
Constructive reciprocity	Followup reinforcement behavior	Destructive reciprocity
Oriented toward multiple needs. High participation	Long-term consequences	Self-centered. Low participation

Developing a Learning Culture

The open system model appears a bit idealistic, but it seems to "work" psychologically and organizationally. By "work," I mean that it describes a number of situations in which employees have reported increased feelings of personal worth and self-esteem while still improving the performance and efficiency of the work situation (Barnes 1960; Blake *et al.*, 1964; *TRW Systems (A) (B) and (C)*). The accomplishment of these multiple human and task goals is no small matter in most organizations, for typically one is gained at the expense of the other as the closed system model suggests. The other extreme, one where human needs for participation are satisfied but without task efficiency, is equally well documented, I suspect, in the implicit failure of the many "human relations" programs which emphasized participation and satisfaction over task accomplishment (Argyris 1962; Fleishman 1953; Strauss 1963). Even today much of the work that goes into T-Group or Sensitivity Training persistently results in group euphoria and the search for such intangibles as self-actualization rather than in an attempt at organizational problem solving. In those situations, the basic assumption of trust is never tested explicitly against "real" organizational problems.

Thus, the open system model walks a fine and delicate line toward optimal consequences. Those of us who have seen it "work" in multigroup organizations sound missionary-like to the skeptic and reactionary to the idealist. Yet while we recognize that the chances of failure outnumber the chances of success, what are the components of success? In addition to adherence to the open system model outlined above, other key qualities can be described using the five concepts addressed earlier.

ASSUMPTIONS AND EXPECTATIONS To form new assumptions that lead to expectations about an idea's potential is to lend that idea new power. As medical research has repeatedly demonstrated, even the placebo furnishes power toward behavior change. At the same time, some assumptions and expectations tend to generate greater payoff than others. By way of review and description, those that seem most useful in designing organizational change are

1. *The "reality" of open as well as closed systems.* For purposes of day-to-day certainty, most of us seem to create a boxed-in world of closed system areas. Useful for some purposes, this assumption becomes a problem when its boundaries are more assumptive than real. Formal lines of organization, status levels, territorial differences, educational backgrounds, and dissimilar experiences are all barriers that lead to self-fulfilling expectations. Employees whose assumptions and expectations include open system possibilities can begin to move toward crossing and lowering the barriers.

2. *The "achievability" of trust assumptions over mistrust assumptions.* We tend to accept the usefulness of greater trust relationships within organizational life, since most of us have experienced the expensive consequences of mutual suspicion, game-playing, political infighting, and empire building. Most of us also see the trust vs. mistrust dilemma as a basic psychological problem much as described by Erik Erikson (1950). It is harder for us to see that trust is also organizationally determined and organizationally achievable. The possibility of mutual power expansion and mutual interdependence makes it easier to assume the achievability of mutual trust within organizations. Expectations then set the stage for mutuality whether it be around superordinate goals, shared problem solving, nonzero-sum negotiations, or joint projects.

3. *The "desirability" of problems as well as solutions.* Just as man seeks certainty in life, so does he paradoxically seek uncertainty in the form of problems. The notion of "problem-

solving" almost furnishes the best of both worlds. It suggests the value of expecting and anticipating solvable problems.

4. *The "usefulness" of interface meetings.* As a result of "groupthink" and "committeeitis" failures, many employees oppose group activities. Indeed, interminable time does seem to be spent in *non*problem-solving sessions whose maps, assumptions, and expectations closely resemble the closed system model. A more open system interface may include any or all units involved in problem-solving and can lead to some bizarre but functionally useful meetings, for example, interdivisional sessions involving 30 to 50 managers divided into problem-solving teams; continuing one-to-one meetings between union president and personnel manager; or "committee on change" meetings between production workers and production managers who jointly assume and plan for the introduction of technological and organizational changes.

5. *The "inevitability" of long-term time requirements.* Deep-rooted organizational change is neither one-shot nor short-term in character. Most organizational training programs, consultants reports, special programs, and top-down orders have suffered from lack of follow-up application. Complex change efforts require expectations of multiphased, long-term commitments involving multiple parts of the organization. These designs for involvement in relevant problem-solving take time, even though the resulting payoff is great.

MODELING BEHAVIOR In some respects, initial modeling behavior by top managers and/or the consultants they hire to help them presents the most crucial stage of change design. The role models are inevitably watched closely for both verbal and nonverbal cues. Their behavior can either change or help to reinforce the expectations of other employees.

From my own point of view, the most impressive description of modeling behavior has been done by Blake and Mouton in their work with the managerial Grid (Blake and Mouton 1964, 1968). Through a series of programmed learning experiences, they provide a "9,9" model of managerial behavior which jointly stresses task concerns and people concerns. They also describe four other basic styles and eight composite styles, but these all become secondarily desirable as the manager tests them against the "9,9" approach, his own experience, and Blake and Mouton's simulated exercises. Indeed, in a cross-cultural study of 1,417 American, 303 British, and 178 Japanese managers exposed to the different managerial styles, over 99 percent of each group chose the "9,9" style as the "most sound" approach to use in operating a company. Some of its behavioral characteristics are (1) open and unobstructed communication . . . forthright identification of personal attitudes . . . confronting of disagreement with others . . . use of critique of past problem-solving efforts in order to learn from experience . . . emphasis on rapid feedback; (2) search for and identification of valid solutions to problems . . . an emphasis on excellence . . . pressure for high quality team work . . . a stressing of individual and team commitment to agreed-upon objectives . . . a continuing quest for knowledge and facts to provide data-based problems and solutions . . . (3) Frequent questioning of organizational practices and culture . . . expectation of study, prework, and data analysis as preparation for problem solving . . . experimental approaches to innovative solutions . . . data-based analyses of experimental approaches.

In effect, Blake and Mouton's "9,9" modeling behavior combines confrontation and coping behavior with standards of excellence in problem-solving. I have seen some managers who seemed to have natural "9,9" characteristics built into their behavior. Others either could not or would not pattern their behavior along these paths. The majority recognize the impressive appeal that "9,9" behavior has for other managers; they aim for it and use consultants and colleagues to let them know when their modeling behavior is falling short of the mark. Some managers seem to recognize instinctively that others have a greater natural ability for "9,9" practices. Consequently, they lean on these others using role complementarity to help them convey a collective modeling behavior. It seems to work.

Selective Reinforcement

I have puzzled at some length over the question of reinforcement in organizational change. Some of it clearly comes in requests for participation. Some of it comes as promotions, new assignments, interesting work, publicity, or colleague compliments. Still other reinforcement comes in the form of problem-solving accomplishment, increased production, accepted change implementations, and other measurable goal achievements. As in the case with other reinforcement situations, immediate or short-term reinforcement tends to have more impact than delayed feedback.

But there is a more fascinating aspect to the reinforcement issue that, for lack of a better term, I shall call "skeptic reinforcement." In almost every organization where I have observed or participated in change design, there were one or more "skeptic" groups. They formed the dialectic "opposition" and, in each case, were invaluable. They raised questions, procrastinated, expressed doubts, remained outside the change effort, and yet they somehow went along for the ride until they either joined up or dropped out. In any given organization, the skeptic groups seem to sandwich themselves above, below, and around the change activists. In one large organization, the president was apathetic while the vice presidents (partly working against his apathy) were the change activists. Below the vice presidents, their subordinates (for example, the plant managers) tended to be outwardly supportive but inactive in taking change initiative. It remained for several division managers to set an open system change model into effect, but the reinforcement they eventually received from the nonactive skeptics tended to be among the most highly valued.

In another organization, a similar pattern prevailed. The regional manager found active field support among his district managers but far less from his own boss or the regional staff. He received reinforcement from regional staff members only after his program began to assist them with their own national staff counterparts and superiors. Once given this skeptic reinforcement, the program began to make marked progress, but the reinforcement was several years in coming. Other examples come to mind also.

Blau and Scott (1962) refer to a phenomenon somewhat similar to this one when they draw a speculative conclusion that the orientations of alternate hierarchical levels would be similar while those of adjacent levels would be different due to the tendency of each level to identify with either superiors or subordinates but not with both. I would go on to speculate that both subordinates and peers use counterarguments to differentiate themselves from managers who advocate change until the possibilities of mutual power expansion become evident. Then a coalition or team is formed, and the skeptic adds his reinforcement to those who have already committed themselves.

PARTICIPATIVE PROBLEM-SOLVING Requests for participation and successful problem-solving were mentioned above as forms of reinforcement. But a participative form of problem-solving has other advantages. It serves as an efficient way to communicate problem concerns and problem parameters. It also includes feedback for correcting false problem parameters and it helps to gain stronger commitment, because change implementers have shared in the problem-solving designs. It may even lead to stronger solutions if participation does not overwhelm problem-solving. This happens when standards of excellence in problem solving are sacrificed for the sake of artificial participation. By artificial, I mean cases where differentiated roles are needed more than widespread involvement but are sacrificed for the sake of integration without differentiation. Needless to say, there are other cases where continuing participation is desirable, but in general the more effective designs tend to value participation for the sake of problem-solving effectiveness rather than for the sake of continuing inclusion. This may sound calloused, but an example for the technical division-production division situation mentioned earlier may illustrate the point.

An interface meeting of over 50 managers from the two divisions was held over a two and a half day period. It soon became apparent that one of the sorest points facing technical division managers was their own perceived low status in the total organization. Their title structure was different, and transfers of engineers and managers into or out of the division was practically nonexistent. The problem could be solved, but decisions could not be made by participation alone in that setting, although a certain catharsis effect was gained from airing of the problem. Instead, the top managers from both divisions subgrouped around the question of what *they* could do to solve this problem. They collectively decided to (1) change the technical division's job title structure so that it was more in line with other divisions; (2) promote and transfer one of the production division's promising younger managers into technical division management; (3) seek other transfer opportunities; and (4) engage in a greater amount of *joint* project work. These decisions were cleared with other company officials and soon implemented.

Although the decision-making was carried out by a subgroup of top managers, the problem identification and parts of the problem-solving were worked out by the larger group of 50 managers. This suggests the usefulness of widespread participation at some levels of problem-solving, but much more restrictive involvement at others. In the above case joint project work was set up using the concept of a matrix organization and temporary assignments of key individuals. The problem-solving structure was established as a temporary system, to be phased out on completion of the project.

Conclusion

The design of change in organization systems and structures described here builds upon the value of conflict resolution in paradoxical systems. Our hypothesis is that a highly valued paradoxical system will tend to sponsor learning and discourage closed system concepts which place an emphasis upon relative power distribution and runs the risk of setting up win/lose expectations. A more open system concept will tend to emphasize total expansion-contraction and places pressure upon designers and participants to solve problems that will then permit such joint power expansion. In any case, the closed or more open concept of power seems to relate to behavior change subsystems involving assumptions, expectations, modeling behavior, selective reinforcement, and participative problem-solving. Each of the subsystems has been linked with social change and human development in past research and practice.

In this chapter, the values held by the writer (as well as the task environments of more and more organizations) point toward the more open system approach to organizational change. In addition to describing a model that seems to describe such changes in large-scale organizations, I have atempted to discuss the assumptions, expectations, modeling behavior, reinforcements, and participative problems-solving that seem to characterize successful organizational change.

References

Argyris, C.
(1962), *Interpersonal Competence and Organizational Effectiveness.* Homewood, Ill.: Irwin-Dorsey.
Barnes, L. B.
(1960), *Organizational Systems and Engineering Groups.* Boston: Harvard University Graduate School of Business Administration.
Blake, R. R., and J. S. Mouton
(1964), *The Managerial Grid.* Houston: Gulf.
——— (1968), *Grid Organization Development.* Houston: Gulf.
———, L. B. Barnes, and L. E. Greiner
(1964), "Breakthrough in Organization Development." *Harvard Business Review, 42,* 133–155.
Blau, P. M., and W. R. Scott
(1962), *Formal Organizations.* San Francisco: Chandler. Pp. 162–163.
Brayfield, A. H.
(1968), "Human Resources Development." *American Psychologist, 23,* 7, 479–482.
Dalton, G. W., L. B. Barnes, and A. Zaleznik
(1968), *The Distribution of Authority in Formal Organizations.* Boston: Harvard University Graduate School of Business Administration.
Erikson, E. H.
(1950), *Childhood and Society.* New York: Norton.
Fleishman, E. A.
(1953), "Leadership Climate, Human Relations Training, and Supervisory Behavior." *Personnel Psychology, 6,* 205–222.
Greiner, L. E.
(1967), "Antecedents of Planned Organizational Change." *Journal of Applied Behavioral Science 3,* 1, 51–85.
Lawrence, P. R.
(1958), *The Changing of Organizational Behavior Patterns.* Boston: Harvard University Graduate School of Business Administration.
———, and J. W. Lorsch
(1967), *Organization and Environment: Managing Differentiation and Integration,* Boston: Harvard University Graduate School of Business Administration.
Pelz, D. C., and F. M. Andrews
(1966), *Scientists in Organizations,* New York: Wiley.
Strauss, G.
(1963), "Some Notes on Power Equalization." In H. J. Leavitt (ed.), *The Social Science of Organization.* Englewood Cliffs: Prentice-Hall.
TRW Systems (A), (B), & (C). Teaching cases, Harvard University Graduate School of Business Administration.

Alan Sheldon,
Frank Baker,
and Curtis P.
McLaughlin

14. Current Issues in Systems and Medical Care

This book may be characterized as having its origin in diversity—a diversity of viewpoints held by the editors and their fellow systems researchers, teachers, and theorists concerning the meaning and proper applications of "systems concepts." In each of the chapters which make up this volume, specific systems issues and professional approaches are dealt with individually. Such differentiation of organization, then, reflects the basic differences which characterize the present stage of development of a "general systems theory," and presents a question of integration. It is the purpose of this chapter to provide an overview of current systems issues as they relate to medical care and thus to attempt to integrate to some degree the variety of topics discussed in the preceding chapters. In this concluding chapter we shall also attempt to indicate to the wary reader some of the many open issues in this developing field.

We shall begin by stating the basic goal of applying systems concepts to medical care, elaborating some of the problems of the health care system, then exploring the variety of systems models and approaches and their attendant problems; and finally, we shall discuss the meta issues—the problems associated with interdisciplinary dialogue and dialectic as, in this instance, they arise among the protagonists involved in the systems area. These protagonists we would identify as the systems theorists, the systems analysts, and the potential consumers of systems theory and analysis, medical planners and practitioners.

Systems in Medical Care: The Basic Goal

Each person participating in the medical care system, whether as professional or patient, has his own conceptual framework which he employs in working with and moving through the network of organizations, individuals, and tech-

The early drafts of the chapters in this book were made available to the participants at the Symposium on Systems and Medical Care, Harvard University, and they served as the basis for the discussion. This chapter is largely the reflections of the editors upon that discussion.

nology making up the medical care complex. Miller's distinction between "conceptual systems" that exist in the mind of the observer and "concrete systems" that are the real, natural objects of scientific study has interesting implications. Depending upon an individual's vantage point and his encounters with the "concrete system" of medical care, he will develop a different "conceptual system" that he will employ to organize his decision-making and future actions. One gets the impression that most highly trained individuals have a view that is like those famous novelty maps of the continental United States which consist almost entirely of the State of Texas surrounded by thin strips of land representing the forty-seven other states. To the surgeon, the hospital may represent the country, and the operating pavilion, the State of Texas. To the parents of the hemophiliac, it may be the blood bank, the orthopedic ward, and the bursar's office. (Patients and their families are indeed highly trained by the system.) Each unique system construct, unless formalized, probably is a Gestalt that is relatively open over time, but the question that the general systems theorist and the practitioner must face is one of integration and control to improve understanding and action.

There is a need for a set of descriptions and analyses which have been rationally arrived at, openly debated, and commonly understood in order to create a more functional relationship over time among the various participants in, and components of, the medical care system. The modifying phrase, "over time," was added to the above sentence specifically to emphasize the importance of having systems constructs that are both open and adaptive.

We might summarize by stating that if the health system is to be responsive and flexible, but also stable; differentiated, but also integrated; technically innovative, but also humane; responsive to the individual situation, but not unmindful of the total picture, then a systems conceptual framework is needed. A systems framework offers at least an *orientation* to complexity, a way of seeing the whole and the parts within it, and how the pieces fit. It further offers some *techniques of analysis* for sorting out relationships, and solving problems, and some organizing *constructs* with which to model real life and understand it better. As Baker observed in his chapter, it is perhaps premature to say that

systems concepts amount to a *theory*, but this is a goal to work toward, and it may soon be attained.

A graphic example of a systems-oriented psychiatrist in action is presented in the following anecdote, which illustrates the power of the nonsegmental approach to illuminate a complex situation, and arrive at a deceptively simple solution. "A Puerto Rican man comes into an internist with a headache. The doctor can't find anything, but he is playing the medical game, which means he takes the history, does a physical, gets the lab tests, etc. Next step is to make the diagnosis; so he called it a typical migraine. He sends the case to a team in our program, and we learn all about the family; that he has a ten-year old boy who is the oldest, constantly in trouble. We get everybody in the same room—that is, the family and representatives of each one of the systems that are involved in the community: the supervisor of welfare, a guidance counsellor from the school. The first thing we run into is that there is a big fight going on between the mother and the father. They have been fighting over who gets the welfare check. She refuses to give it to him, afraid he'll leave her. The boy is afraid he'll have to assume the father role. After we convince the mother to turn over the check to the father, his headaches have disappeared within a week of the session. In two and a half months, the boy is behaving and doing well in school. What was that headache: biological? A psychological or a social problem?"[1]

Issues in Medical Care

There appears to be little doubt that the "health system" is in trouble. Four issues seem to be central: (1) the increasing difficulty of maintaining a spirit of humanism and compassion in the face of technological specialization and volume of services rendered; (2) the problems of planning a care system that is adequate physically and is sufficiently humane in the face of limited resources; (3) the difficulty of articulating increasingly complex sets of skills and subsystems in order to reach any coherent objective; and (4) the obstacles to reaching a sufficiently coherent objective for even specialized adaptive subsystems to be able to guide group and individual behavior effectively.

[1] Dr. Edgar H. Auerswald, in the Symposium discussion.

It is evident that even the definition of the medical care system is becoming more, rather than less, difficult. The image of the doctor as godlike, the sanctity of the "doctor-patient relationship," and the ironclad six functions of the public health department may have been dysfunctional for some purposes, but they had operational clarity. Today, new issues have intervened, which arise from the interaction of essentially three phenomena: the assertion of the rights of consumers (to information, to access, to a degree of control); a growing questioning of the physician's (the establishment's) capacity for the self-regulation of himself or of his enterprises; and the very complexity of those enterprises and the major problems inherent in organizing them. This has led to a series of conflicts—of power (who controls whom and how much), of autonomy (who has what freedoms), and of credibility (who trusts or believes whom). These conflicts are evident and manifest in the fact that in America we are no longer willing to leave the availability and the organization of medical care to be organized by the market mechanism.

Nor are we any longer convinced that professional self-interest, patient interests, and public interests are mutually supporting for a sufficient proportion of the time. Thus, for example, the primary goal of the teaching hospital as a source of educated health professionals is being questioned and its service responsibilities are felt to be more pressing by the public; and even the professionals' criterion of "quality" is being replaced by that of "access."

The problem of credibility is in part a result of the fact that information is being generated about the technology at a rate faster than it is being applied in all but a limited number of applications. Thus there is an increased questioning of the value of research and of the actions of the medical community. Higher educational levels in a sophisticated public and a resultant decrease in blind confidence have led substantial segments of the patient population to assert a right to medical information and, in some cases, to offer alternative judgments. Such information is a determinant of patient behavior, and patient behavior is a determinant of health. Accordingly the physician, who is responsible for the outcome, and yet who is expected to be open and honest, is being placed in an ambiguous position. It happens also that this is occurring at a time when openness and honesty are acquiring values as outcomes, rather than as means, throughout much of our society.

Physician behavior is becoming more and more constrained by the movement of practice from solo to complex institutional arrangements, as Field notes, where new power relationships develop and where authority is fragmented and possibly dissipated, and where goals differ sharply. (The administrator's concern with the economics of bed utilization conflicts with the physician's idea of patient need.) This division of roles and authority has led to results dysfunctional to the health of the patient on enough occasions to begin to alienate patients and to make the physician believe that he must exert more control. Furthermore the multiplicity of institutions and services within institutions which now "process" the patient often leads to incomplete care and, occasionally, to inappropriate care.

A further factor is the rising level of expectations from the medical care system resulting partly from the great successes of recent years with the treatment of communicable diseases and partly from the ballyhoo that has accompanied individual research successes. When these expectations are not fulfilled in the care of the average patient, a "vicious" cybernetic cycle is established. The body politic begins to question the value of research. To counter this, the medical community attempts to publicize its new accomplishments more widely, thereby raising expectations long to be unfulfilled.

The recognition that medicine is a right, not a privilege, of the consumer makes demands on the system in terms of quality and quantity not previously contemplated. This new set of requirements is being brought home more and more forcefully as patient groups begin to organize to achieve their perceived needs. There is little attempt to differentiate between feedback—the capacity of the health system to be more responsive, and power—the right of the public to force action.

The concern with consumers' rights is reflected in the increasing legal liability of the physician for his actions and for those working for him, a trend seen in the legal view of responsibility and warranty applying to all providers of goods and services. This view is especially disquieting because it runs counter to some of the basic assumptions underlying the professional status of the physician.

The rigidity of the current system is seen in the difficulty in using alternative sources and means (semiprofessionals, part-timers) to solve manpower shortages. It is visible also in recruitment, turnover, and retention problems. These shortages, which are exacerbated by a growing population, rising expectations of quality service, and a shift toward comprehensive health programs demanding high staffing ratios, are near critical.

One response to complexity, which has in turn raised new problems, is the formation of an intervening group of persons in government and financial organizations who have achieved responsibility for a new function called *planning*. The formation of a further intervening group within the institutions, responsible for the collection and integration of information and its interpretation for the administrative and planning levels, also represents another indigestible element.

These problems can be interpreted and perhaps mitigated by a look at what is happening in systems terms. The practitioners have interpreted many of these events as a proliferation of constraints which threaten them with a loss of autonomy and of control. This is exemplified by the statement, "Planning threatens the physician as automation threatens the worker." As Baker and Schulberg clearly indicated, a general systems perspective highlights the extremely large number and complexity of systems, subsystems, and intersystems relations involved in the provision of the desired comprehensive medical care. To the extent that an individual is aware of the interrelationships at each interface and chooses (or is forced) to take them into account in his actions, he is indeed losing some freedom of action. The difference, however—and it is an important one—is that the man himself can control these constraints, rather than having them imposed independently and often unexpectedly and in an untimely and unseemly fashion.

There is a question as to whether there is an operational difference. We believe that there is one, and it is more than psychological. The shortest summation of our argument is that old saw that to be forwarned is to be forearmed. Knowledge and understanding of the interfaces means ability through interaction to affect the relationship. In systems terms, the practitioner will exercise control of the process, but this does not mean that he will exercise absolute power or control in the traditional sense. A different kind of control is appropriate to this new situation, one which recognizes that complex interlocking systems require a different perspective and touch, especially since the "obvious" action may well have untoward repercussions in unlikely places. He can, however, become a part of the feedback process with positive or negative effects, stabilizing or unstabilizing effects. The illustration of rising expectations noted above and the response to them of increasing public relations efforts and publicity is an example of an unstabilizing control activity. Another example is the relations of a teaching hospital with its surrounding community. At one time, this community could be ignored. More perceptive practitioners did not choose to do so, but they did not always improve matters by intervening. Their efforts to work with the community might be taken at face value in some settings and be judged—not always inaccurately—as a patronizing attempt to preserve a pool of indigent patients for teaching purposes.

There are a large number of basic questions which relate to this idea of interlocking systems (in or out of equilibrium); in the individual at the (micro-) level of psyche and soma, still a dichotomy, or at the (macro-) level of service where a combination of subsystems compete, collaborate, or fail to treat psychological and physiological problems or to prevent their occurrence. Chin and O'Brien emphasize the interdependency of systems levels in their concept of "feedback dependence."

The system is not, for all its faults, altogether unresponsive to the patient or to the need to shift its views or activities. Thus once Medicare and Medicaid gave the charity patient a free choice of institution, the city hospitals had to shape up. But much of the responsiveness has been reactive, rather than proactive; segmental and inappropriate, rather than considered and in context; or fostering a questionable dependency. This may help to explain the specter of alienation, which is not sufficiently accounted for by the effects of limited accessibility to care and compassion as one might assume, or so it seems from the complaints about the technological performance of and consumer response to the British and Russian care systems.

Perhaps, as we look at the aggregate system, we will reach

the conclusion that is frequently offered, namely, that the goals of the medical care system are improperly defined, either because of fuzziness or overspecification. The two are not mutually exclusive. Someone will have to enumerate a complete set of goals in relatively operational terms to elminate the fuzziness and still make the necessary compromises (trade-offs) to make the objectives internally consistent. At present we have problems with the two objectives of equality of access and quality of care, and the use of the private market system for organizing care. People can and do hold to both firmly, but what we know of economic principles appears to make such a pair of objectives unworkable. It is this area, the display of inconsistencies in one's current system view, that one may produce the greatest fruits of systems studies. There may be more than sheer devil's advocacy to the remarks of those who compare the diagnostician to the motor mechanic, the surgeon to the carpenter, and argue that the replacement of rheumatic heart valve is not a triumph of medicine, but rather a failure since the disease was treatable some time earlier.

Systems Models and Planning

Even though we have discussed the benefits of an improved systems view of medical care from the point of view of both efficiency and humanity, we have intimated that it is a personalized conception. Yet, if we accept the view that its social motivational impact will derive in large part from its commonality, then how is such a view to be arrived at? Who is to be the arbiter, or at least the leader in its definition? Who is to define its goals and obectives? What is to be the general form of the model to be presented? How is it to deal with areas of uncertainty? What will be the level of detail in the specification of components? Their interrelationships? The control mechanisms? What will be legitimate subsystem sets for decision-making? What will be controlled, and what will be coordinated? By whom? What provision will be made for incorporation with nonhealth systems in areas like nutrition, education, population planning, or environmental control? What is to be done in case of resource conflicts with other major systems such as housing and welfare? How is the use of a model to be evaluated over time when the lead time is so long before effects are realized? What is to be considered a controllable element, and what is not? What are to be the purposes to which the systems models are to be put? To what extent should this purpose constrain the complexity of the model?

This list of questions could leave the impression that there never will be a single system construct or model that will govern everything, and that may well be true, at least in a certain sense. Although all models are either descriptive, predictive, or prescriptive, there will be many different forms and variations for individual needs and purposes. Some will be schematic and some quantitative; some static and some dynamic; some probabilistic and some deterministic; and some regional and some national.

It is obvious that we need different models for different purposes; some with which to understand, some with which to prepare for the future, some to guide us to improve, and some to justify the existence of a professional discipline. Indeed it is argued that there never *can* be a unified model —that each discipline is concerned with different levels of analysis that can never be linked logically (Ferdinand 1969). This argument assumes idiosyncrasy for each behavioral science and, therefore, that unity lies in articulation. This articulation, so the logician would have it, violates logical principles and thus theories must of necessity remain incomplete and not comprehensive. We doubt the validity of the preceding argument and the assumptions on which it is based, and shall discuss this topic further below.

There is a strong indication, given the structure of our society, that the models needed (even those that are most aggregative and most descriptive) will be developed and promulgated by professionals in the universities and government under stimuli from grants from the government and pressures from an increasingly alienated public, and perhaps somewhat over the outraged cries of the practitioners. The trend will be to give the user, or individuals who have appropriated the users' mantles, a strong voice in the definition of objectives and policies. Lee and McLaughlin suggest that the current focus on blocks of people is a continuation of a historical trend of the last ten years or so, but there are signs that this approach may break down of its own weight.

The nature of this breakdown represents an interesting case

in the use of systems concepts. It is an article of faith that systems work should be truly interdisciplinary. But how can one get by using only bits and pieces of a multitude of disciplines and then avoid getting burned by an incomplete job due to occasionally using a single disciplinary approach? The pattern of providing care in the United States has been to rely primarily on the market mechanism for the distribution of care to most of the population, and to buy the care for groups of individuals in need, who obviously are outside the market system for medical care. This procedure worked relatively well for seamen, Indians, the blind, and the disabled, until the Medicare and Medicaid legislation was introduced to follow the same route with the other large, but obviously needy, subsets of the population.

Here, however, it appears that what was initially assumed to be a difference in degree accumulated to a difference in kind. The market system responded markedly to the infusion of funds at a time when there was a relatively small increase in the supply of medical services. The market has behaved in a fashion calculated to restore the faith of any classical economist; prices have gone up sharply. A classical economic model of a relatively closed market system might well have predicted this, but the medical system had not been studied in the full context of its behavior as an economic system. We had never determined whether it was or was not stable under the control conditions represented by an introduction of demand of this magnitude. Yet, if one asked an economist what happens to a relatively closed market system under conditions of a substantial increase in effective demand and relatively low supply expansion, he would reply quickly with a prediction of a sharp rise in prices to be followed by an influx of producers from other industries or markets such as nursing homes and hospitals owned by profitmaking corporations. Could not the emphasis on an interdisciplinary focus, borrowing bits from many models, have blinded us to the need to listen to the completely disciplinary and rigorous evaluation of classical economics?

The power of specific, rather than general, models for given circmstances is indubitable. Perhaps the most fruitful role for general systems theory is to provide an overall framework, emphasizing the openness of the system and the connectedness of its parts. Howland and Sheldon suggest in their chapters the utility of adaptive models for understanding the total picture, as well as the smaller frame of the individual and his disease. Howland and Rosenthal each draw attention to the use of the quantitative models for resource allocation at the intermediate level. The quest for a general model should not necessarily end on a logical impediment; that argument is based on the articulation of established theory, and a new level of theory—cutting across established lines—may well still develop.

The more aggregative models, probably the most influential ones, are likely to be quite descriptive. They are likely to focus on the questions of boundary location and identification of system components. Undoubtedly, they will include psychiatric care; curative and preventive medical care; the providers of personnel, materials and facilities; financial institutions, and patients. The extent to which they will include patient family groups, epidemiological vectors, sociological and environmental factors, and planning agencies is open to question. Since open systems wear white hats in this field, they are likely to be adaptive—interacting with some subsystem models but not others.

The most difficult problems to solve will be the establishment of a normative model for organizing services in specific geographic territories and the assignment of varying degrees of control to the competing groups—patients, physicians, administrators, planners, and model builders. The role of historical perspective will be hotly debated also, as will the points raised by Rosenthal concerning the relative responsibilities of planner and decision-maker for making plans and implementing them. In the administrative setting, we may be hampered by the lack of an accepted way of representing control relationships. In the past, control notation and theory have been derived from the work of engineering and physical scientists who handle flows of fluid or electrons. Because of their successes with these materials, we have had a rash of suggestions as to how human relationships might be represented in cybernetic terms, if not controlled the same way. These suggestions have not lived up to their early promise, perhaps due to the aspects of mutuality and dependency in human relationships, which yield very different responses, and a variability in such responses over time. In that regard, Howland's discussion argued that any model should resemble biological processes, including the potential to reorganize in response to external pressures, and to process a number of variables that have a marked range of uncertainty or at least high variability.

It is evident that the process of developing a model will necessarily start with small models, which will be expanded in response to reality and to questions from the practitioners and planners concerning the interim output. The purpose of such models is likely to be predictive; therefore, the first questions are likely to concern the sensitivity of the system to changes in system structure or operating policies. The results should enable the practitioner, the politician, or the planner to foresee effects and interactions and thus to behave in a less reactive, more proactive manner. In that sense, models really do provide control for the user, even though they are neither fully quantitative nor fully predictive. After all, intellectual control derives not from absolute expertise, but from marginally better expertise. Howland has suggested that "doctors have previously been able to function with both intellectual and art types of understandings over relatively small systems. One of the things that they're beginning to feel is pressure from the community: from all kinds of forces. They're not trained to have the manipulative nor the intellectual control over them, because they weren't trained for it and they don't understand them. One of the things that they look to systems theory for is a framework for understanding these processes so that they don't feel this loss of control, and possibly for some techniques for manipulating those processes."

These hopes are unlikely to be fulfilled. At least three key differences exist between the systems understanding that the physician has of own small system, and what he will have to absorb about larger social systems: multiplicity of control, tolerance of uncertainty, and incompleteness of information flow.

Meta Issues

Thus far we have attempted to outline some of the issues preoccupying the health field (as raised by practitioners) and some of the models which might have utility (as proposed by the theorists). Essentially, meta issues are those issues inherent in arriving at the conjunction of theory and practice. Meta isues are the problems of interdisciplinary dialogue, whether occurring in a well-disposed discussion session in elegant surroundings, in the struggles of a behavioral scientist introducing foreign bodies into a medical curriculum, or in the situation of a psychiatrist trying to educate nurses to the value of talking with patients. These meta issues are not unique to systems, or to health, but are important symptoms of a protracted process of mutual examination which leads, hopefully, to a liason (if not marriage) between disciplines.

The first such meta issue has to do with the conflicts underlying language differences, which are rarely talked about, for there is always the problem of what language to speak—whether literally, as terminology, or figuratively. Theorists want to talk abstract models, analysts want to ask questions and talk problems, and practitioners want to talk concrete solutions. As the dialogue continues, it becomes imperative to clarify terms of reference and basic assumptions, for inherent in this dilemma of choice are spiralling complications of priorities and values as the concrete reveals implicit assumptions within it.

The role of the analyst in this morass is to clarify, at each step, these implicit values and assumptions. In so doing, he readily brings ire upon himself, and pain to the beholder, for clarification often polarizes positions and thus reveals carefully masked conflicts. The preceding point explains why organizations tend to talk about laying bare values and assumptions *in theory*, but seldom attempt to follow it to its logical conclusion *in practice*. This fact is discussed by Cyert and March in their book, *The Behavioral Theory of the Firm* (1963), as referred to in McLaughlin's chapter on systems analysis. Herbert Simon, also of the same group at Carnegie-Mellon Institute of Technology, has coined the word "satisficing" to represent the search for a relatively efficient system in lieu of the most efficient system. He believes that many organizations are willing to sacrifice this last step to absolute efficiency for reasons of allowing material and psychological room for people to maneuver and to articulate within the organization. This concept should be more fully incorporated into general systems theory.

There are inherent conflicts, or at least divergences of interest, in any organization, and the organization must accept these conflicts for what they are. This was brought out interestingly in a recent *Wall Street Journal* article concerning the proprietary hospitals which are springing up around the country. These hospitals have been under fire for not carrying a major share of the caseload for disadvantaged people. One such institution has agreed to take any case free of charge, provided that the physician also offers his services free of charge. Thus far they have had no takers. These conflicts may reside within the individual as well as within the organization. M. Halverstam in "The M.D. Should Not Try To Cure Society" (1969) points out that the highly trained physician wishes to treat the more complex and demanding cases and might be willing to turn the minor ones over to nonphysician personnel. Yet the needs of the patient for reassurance and the requirements for preliminary diagnosis call for the physician to spend much or most of his time on such trivial complaints as headache and abdominal pain which may be the result of any one of hundreds of conditions.

A similar dilemma has been brought out in a study of the costs of hospital laboratory analyses.[2] Preliminary results indicate that automation has markedly reduced the cost on a per assay basis. At the same time the number of assays per admission has risen markedly and the billings for laboratory services have skyrocketed; in one hospital, laboratory billings are 500 percent of laboratory costs. One must point to this as an example of the unsystematic relationship between hospital prices and costs. But if one attempts to bring prices back into line, one is faced with the realization that the income will have to be procured somewhere and that room rates will rise accordingly. Thus the cost of medical care in toto may not be changed at all.

A second meta issue is, "Why bother to talk at all?" Is this new thing, systems, simply common sense dressed up? Have we been here before? In essence, how does general systems theory move us toward a better medical care system? What is the value and effectiveness of this new thing? It seems clear that it can make two major contributions to a better health system. The first contribution is through its emphasis on more open and more complex conceptions of the health system, which should lead to a much more sophisticated and thorough analysis. The second contribution is that the

[2] Study directed by Dr. Curtis P. McLaughlin.

analogies and homologies are important in leading potential analysts to new and more appropriate analytical approaches. Beyond these two contributions, it is apparent that the current state of the art of general systems theory does not lead to answers immediately applicable in health settings. An additional inference is that general systems has not yet developed a sufficiently extensive or intensive theory to constitute a particularly pertinent body of knowledge. It is important to note that it seems generally agreed upon, by practitioners as well as analysts and theorists, that general systems theory can and probably will ultimately lead to major contributions.

A point at issue here is, How can one test these ideas and prove their importance to a skeptical audience? We often are dissatisfied with existing concepts, but we have no way of proving that a new concept will be any more effective than the old in the long run. This is one of the sources of friction between the planner and the practitioner. The planner works out a fundamental logic which appears acceptable, and then he must approach the practitioner to try it out. The practitioner, operating in a real-time environment, may accept his logic, but he may have no desire to see it tested in his already harassed organization. "How do you control and study as you make these plans, so that you don't plan that everyone moves one way for five years and then you say that didn't work, now let's go this way."[3] This problem is illustrated in the population control sphere, where, in India, a choice of fertility control technique was made. That way did not work, but now there is precious little information about what will work because certain districts were not set aside for alternative experiments. No one wants to be a guinea pig in something as personally important as health.

Since planned experiments in health care are problematical, it seems a pity that there is no real mechanism in the area of health systems analysis for observing the many natural experiments which take place. Such an approach is not foreign to the research physician, who has always employed serendipity, but the large-scale nature of health systems renders such insightful observations as those of Snow at the Aldgate pump unlikely. Several districts in the above-mentioned study of population control markedly deviated from

[3] Dr. James Miller, in the Symposium discussion.

the standard plan established by the government of India and encountered much better results than the norm. Unfortunately these results are not well documented. Perhaps the development of good mechanisms for identifying and following such natural demonstratons is a major challenge to general systems theory.

A third meta issue lies in the interdisciplinary, or antidisciplinary, nature of general systems. This does not, although some would have it so, mean that it is undisciplined, or that its concepts are so general as to be useless in practice. Implicated in this meta issue is the threat posed by general systems to current disciplines and to well-defined professional identities. The underlying question may be, Do I have to stop being a physician, biologist, or whatever, and if I do, what do I become? This alternative is hardly real, although some people do prefer the "identity" of "systems person" to the more traditional one of psychiatrist or whatever.

What is implied here is that anything which can be brought over from any discipline should be acceptable in proportion to its utility. The utility may be either intellectually or physically productive. Concerns about this meta issue are expressed in such polarized juxtapositions as "rationality versus irrationality"; "efficiency versus inefficiency"; "consistency versus inconsistency"; "power versus persuasion"; "deficiencies versus integration"; "customary versus exceptional"; "local purpose versus general purpose." The only answer is that behavior is generally functional for some purposes and dysfunctional for others at the same time. Up to a certain point in an analysis absolute rationality seems to be functional; beyond a certain point, it cannot be all-inclusive or objective when driven to its absolute logical conclusion. Much the same thing can be said for efficiency. The cost of absolute engineering efficiency is complete loss of flexibility and freedom to operate in a system full of uncertainties and ambiguities. This, however, does not mean that one should not push for efficiencies until he begins to push up against the constraint of loss of flexibility. The problem is that outsiders, dealing in abstracts, are virtually insensitive to perceptions which, in turn, are time variant.

So far then, we have identified three aspects of the meta process: communication, or how do we talk, and about what; value and effectiveness, or show me that it works; and change, or what will it to do me, even if it works. A fourth meta issue lies in the question, "Does it matter if a doctor understands all of the things that Field tells us about all of the changes in the social impact of medicine." In other words, this may all be fine and true, but what good will it do me, and how much of it do I really need to function in my little area? This is a valid and crucial question since one of many priority determinations that the overinformed professional must make is which information to ignore.

Does information at such a level as general as Field's work, or at such an abstract level as the work of Howland or of Sheldon, have any usefulness at the highly specific and concrete level of the interface between doctor or nurse and patient? There are indeed good reasons for possession of this information about the network, which relate to the altered system of power that has been referred to. Rather than to control by direct power, it is essential to understand intellectually and thus be able to alter linkages by a nudge here and a jolt there. In any case, control by direct power is hardly possible any longer because it is nullified by the contrary exertions of other elements in a complex system. Only in this way, through an understanding of these processes and an acquisition of some new techniques for manipulation, can the threat to autonomy and loss of control be countered.

The usefulness of general systems theory lies in its power to serve as a framework for understanding the aforementioned processes. A combination of general systems and systems analysis for developing techniques to manipulate these processes is of great value. To this we could add Howland's model, which shows the major differences from a modeling point of view between levels of the health care system, and identifies the individual as a cybernetic system. Sheldon and Howland both point out that the organizations of intermediate size, such as hospitals, are relatively closed systems with a number of probabilistic elements (see also McLaughlin). They suggest that the full-blown health care system again might be approached best by a cybernetic model.

The relevance of models to the practitioner is also in question, but implicitly he always has a model. This model may as well be explicit, and often it might be amenable to improvement. The development of models, always an uncompleted process, probably goes through in sequence the three phases of being descriptive, predictive, and then prescriptive. One starts out hoping to have a model which at least describes the essential elements of an observed system. From that point, one would prefer to be able to articulate the elements of this system in order to predict the outcomes of certain events or actions. These two phases have as their tests versimilitude and then predictive accuracy. The final phase is one in which alternative policies or actions are tested and evaluated in an attempt to come up with the best one. This exercise can be useful only if the first two phases have been completed satisfactorily.

In both the first and third phases, we can see the importance of a general systems orientation which leads one to move upward or downward from the level of the hierarchy on which he is focusing. One moves up and down to check out the versimilitude of the model in relationship to these other levels and also to evaluate the recommended results in terms of their ramifications upon the other levels of the hierarchy.

Conclusion

Perhaps the best way to conclude is with a brief discussion of boundaries. Traditional disciplines demarcate their fields so that they can isolate processes relevant to their interests, but thereby they possibly omit important relationships. Boundaries are erected in operating situations to define financially or legally an organizations' identity and goals. So it is with the individual, who says, "I am this," or "I need to know only this or do only this." General systems theory encourages us to extend our boundaries and make them rubber; to fix them for this purpose, and move them for that; to recognize that a boundary lets in and puts out; includes and excludes.

This essay, indeed this book, is an attempt to present some ideas that which excite us, with the hope that it will expand the boundaries of the reader.

References

Cyert, R. M., and J. G. March
(1963), *The Behavioral Theory of the Firm.* Englewood Cliffs: Prentice-Hall.

Ferdinand, T. N.
(1969), "On the Impossibility of a Complete General Theory of Behavior." *American Sociologist 4,* 4, 330–332.
Halverstam, M.
(1969), "The M.D. Should Not Try to Cure Society." *New York Times,* Magazine Section, November 9, P. 32.

Index

Name Index

Abdellah, F. G., 135, 141
Ackoff, R. L., 1, 4, 22, 28, 42, 62, 233, 264, 287
Aesculapius, 76
Affel, H. A., Jr., 28, 42, 230, 233, 264
Alexander, Christopher, 213, 228
Allen, S. I., 40, 42
Allport, F. H., 12, 22
Allport, Gordon, 12, 22
Anderson, O., 160, 161, 164, 180
Anderson, S., 35, 48
Andrews, F. M., 315, 328
Andrews, L. P., 266
Angyal, A., 9, 23, 86, 122
Apter, M. J., 49, 59
Arbib, M., 49, 59
Argyris, C., 321, 328
Arrow, K. J., 30, 42
Ashby, W. R., 1, 2, 23, 49, 53, 59, 279, 288
Asimow, M., 31, 42
Attinger, E. O., 22, 25, 58, 59
Auerswald, Edgar H., 331
Avant, O. W., 42, 47

Babbage, Charles, 231
Badgley, Robin F., 147, 163, 169, 180
Baehr, G., 137, 140
Bailey, N. T. J., 34, 38, 42, 48, 263, 264
Baker, F., 21–25, 62, 183, 187, 194, 195, 204, 206
Baker, Norman R., 240, 264
Bales, R. F., 12, 13, 25
Balintfy, J. L., 38, 40, 42, 242, 263, 266, 275, 288
Balitsky, K. P., 115, 123
Bamforth, K. W., 19, 26
Barker, R. G., 15, 23
Barnard, Chester, 82, 83
Barnett, G. O., 40, 42, 43
Barnes, Louis B., 315, 321, 328
Bartlett, M. K., 99, 122
Bartlett, M. S., 35, 42, 263, 264
Baruch, J. J., 40, 42
Battersby, Albert, 218, 229
Battit, G. E., 99, 122
Bauer, R. A., 20, 23, 247, 264
Baumol, W. J., 256, 264
Beer, S., 57, 59
Bellman, R., 233, 264
Bennis, W. G., 212, 217, 229
Bernard, C., 277, 288
Berrien, F. K., 3, 16, 23
Berry, R. E., 255
Bertalanffy, Ludwig von, 1–5, 9, 12, 18, 19, 23, 184, 205, 211, 229
Biderman, A., 235, 264
Biggs, Herman, 132
Blackett, P. M. S., 270, 288
Blake, R. R., 315, 321, 323, 324, 328
Blanco-White, M. J., 38, 43
Blau, P. M., 325, 328
Blum, H. L., 20, 21, 23
Blumberg, M. S., 29, 43
Boguslaw, R., 249, 264
Boguslaw, W., 4, 23
Bolman, W. M., 16, 23
Boulding, K. E., 1, 2, 5, 23, 227, 229, 235, 264
Brayfield, Arthur, 315–319, 328
Brehm, J. W., 108, 122
Brewster, A. W., 30, 43, 270, 288
Broglie, M. Louis de, 50
Brown, F., 116, 122
Bruce, R. A., 36, 43
Brunner, N., 283, 289
Buckley, Walter, 3, 10–13, 23
Burch, P. R. J., 94, 122
Burdick, D. S., 266
Burgess, J., 57, 59

Caceres, C. A., 36, 43
Cameron, S., 49, 61
Candib, L. M., 135, 142
Cannon, W., 277, 279, 287, 288
Carr, John, 310
Castleman, P. A., 40, 42
Caws, P., 4, 23
Chapman, A. L., 127, 141
Chapman, B. L., 49, 59
Chapman, R. L., 288
Chase, R. A., 49, 59
Chen, E., 112, 122
Cherkasky, M., 164, 180
Chin, Robert, 207, 211, 217, 229, 335
Chu, K., 266
Clark, W. E., 40, 47
Cleveland, S. L., 13, 14, 24
Cobb, S., 112, 122
Cohart, E., 41, 43

Cohen, A. R., 108, 122
Connor, R. J., 39, 43
Copeland, William E., 283
Covert, R. P., 38, 48
Cowan, J. D., 54, 59
Crile, G., Jr., 113, 122
Crystal, R. A., 30, 43, 270, 288
Cumming, E., 200, 205
Cushing, 76
Cyert, R. M., 248, 264, 341, 346

Dalton, G. W., 315, 328
David, A., 50, 59
Davies, J. O. F., 41, 43
Davis, B. J., 90, 92, 123
Davis, M. M., Jr., 126, 141
Demarche, D. F., 191, 205
Densen, P. M., 41, 43
Dickson, W. J., 17, 25
Donabedian, A., 39, 43, 249, 264
Dorfman, R., 29, 32, 43, 273, 288
Drossness, D. L., 41, 43, 46
Dubos, R., 85–89, 95, 117, 122
Duncan, O. P., 15, 23

Easton, David, 3, 23
Ebert, R. H., 174, 178, 180, 249, 264
Eddison, R. T., 33, 43
Edgecumbe, R. H., 38, 43, 245, 264
Egbert, L. D., 99, 122
Ehrenwald, J., 112, 122
Eicker, W., 57, 59
Emerson, Haven, 126, 131–135, 140, 141
Emery, F. E., 19, 23
Emery, S. W., 183, 188, 189, 205
Engel, G. L., 86, 91, 92, 95, 97, 98, 122
Engel, Joseph H., 231
Engle, R. L., 90–94, 123
Engle, R. L., Jr., 36, 46
Erikson, Erik, 322, 328
Etzioni, A., 191, 205

Fagen, R. E., 4, 8, 24, 211, 229
Falk, I. S., 173, 180
Falliers, C. J., 52, 59
Fein, R., 42
Feldstein, M. S., 29, 38, 39, 42, 43 255, 263, 264
Feldstein, P. J., 42, 44, 46
Ferdinand, T. N., 337, 347
Fetter, R. B., 38, 42, 44, 47, 252, 263, 265, 267
Field, Mark G., 96, 333, 345
Fisher, S., 13, 14, 24
Fitzpatrick, T. B., 39, 46
Flagle, C. D., 28, 30, 36, 40–45, 244, 245, 247, 263, 265, 273, 275, 288
Fleishman, E. A., 321, 328
Foley, A. R., 199, 205
Forrester, J. W., 34, 44
Fox, Renee, 143, 181
Freeman, J., 31, 38, 47, 263, 267
Freud, S., 67
Froh, R. B., 136, 141
Fry, John, 33, 41, 44, 252, 263, 265
Fuchs, V. R., 146, 153, 180

Gann, D. S., 34, 44, 263, 265
Garfinkel, D., 34, 44
George, F. H., 49, 59
Gerard, Ralph W., 2
Gesser, A., 35, 48
Gibson, Count D., Jr., 137, 141
Gilmore, J. S., 232, 244, 265
Goldman, S., 55, 60, 94, 123
Goldstein, 12
Gonzalez, R. F., 261, 266
Goode, H. H., 28, 44
Gorry, G. A., 36, 44
Gould, W. S., 232, 244, 265
Gray, W., 6, 9, 24
Greenberg, B. G., 266
Greene, W. A., 116, 123
Greenes, R. A., 41, 44
Greenwood, F., 42, 44
Greiner, L. E., 315, 328
Gresham, 234
Grinker, Roy R., 3, 24
Grodins, F. S., 49, 60
Gross, B. M., 20, 24, 190, 205
Gross, M., 40, 44
Guest, R. M., 8, 24

Haldeman, J. C., 135, 141
Haley, T. J., 102, 123
Hall, A. D., 4, 24, 28, 44, 211, 229
Halverstam, M., 342, 347
Hamlin, R. H., 194, 205
Handyside, A. J., 38, 45
Hansell, N., 120, 123
Hare, E. H., 112, 123
Harrington, J. J., 28, 35, 45, 263, 265
Harris, Senator, 315
Harris, S. E., 29, 45
Harvey, N. A., 34, 45, 50, 52–56, 60, 263, 265
Havens, A. E., 31, 33, 48

Hawthorne, 17
Hein, Piet, 262
Helpern, M., 169, 180
Henderson, L. J., 17, 24
Herodotus, 96
Hersh, E. M., 115, 123
Hilleboe, H. E., 204, 205
Hinkle, L. E., 86, 87, 123
Hippocrates, 76, 165, 179
Hitch, C. J., 269, 271–276, 288
Homans, G. C., 76
Hooper, D., 97, 125
Hopkins, C. E., 29, 47, 125
Horvath, F., 50, 60
Horvath, W. J., 2, 22, 24, 25, 39, 42, 45, 127, 141, 236, 247, 248, 263, 265
Howard, R., 242, 265
Howland, D., 21, 24, 39, 45, 271, 274, 278, 280, 288, 338–340, 345
Huggins, W. H., 28, 44
Hutton, G., 19, 24
Hylton, L. F., 194, 198, 206

Iker, H., 116, 125
Israel, S., 95, 123
Iversen, O. H., 54, 60

Jackson, Henry M., 270
Jackson, R. R. P., 252, 265
Jacobs, A. R., 41, 45, 136, 141
Jacobs, G., 53, 54, 60
James, G., 41, 43
Jensen, R. T., 169, 180
Johns, R. E., 191, 205
Jonas, A., 115, 123
Jydstrup, R. A., 40, 44

Kafka, Franz, 171
Kahn, R. L., 17, 24, 50, 60
Kaplan, S. R., 200, 206
Katz, D., 17, 24, 50, 60
Kavet, J., 38, 45, 254
Kavetsky, R. E., 115, 123
Kelley, J. G., 14, 15, 24
Kelly, David M., 254
Kendall, D. G., 35, 45, 263, 265
Kendrick, C. R., 42, 44
Kennedy, K. L., 288
Kershner, R. B., 233, 265
Kety, Seymour, 143
Kiesler, F., 200, 205
Kimball, A. W., 279, 289
Kimball, G., 271, 289
Kirkpatrick, C. A., 241, 266
Kissen, D. M., 116, 123
Kissick, W. L., 29, 45, 127, 141, 151, 180
Klarman, H. E., 29, 30, 42, 45, 135, 141, 262, 265
Kment, H., 49, 60
Koestler, Arthur, 89, 94
Kohli, D. A., 52, 61, 121, 125
Koivumaki, Judith, 143
Kuhn, T. S., 237, 265

Lange, O., 49, 60
Langner, T. S., 87, 124
Laqueur, H. P., 16, 24, 50, 60
Larrabee, J., 283, 289
Lawrence, P. R., 18, 24, 106, 124, 315, 317, 320, 328
Leavell, H. R., 132, 141
Lechat, M. F., 30, 36, 45, 263, 265
Ledley, R. S., 36, 45
Lee, Sidney S., 32, 39, 337
Leopold, R. L., 198, 205
Lerner, M., 160, 161, 164, 180
LeShan, L., 115, 116, 124
LeTourneau, C. U., 40, 45, 50, 60
Levin, R. I., 241, 266
Levine, S., 191, 193, 205, 248, 266
Lincoln, T. L., 36, 46, 263, 266
Lipkin, M., 36, 46
Lipschutz, A., 113, 114, 124
Litchfield, E. H., 233, 266
Litwak, E., 194, 198, 206
Long, M., 39, 46
Long, M. F., 29, 46
Long, N. E., 187, 198, 206
Lorsch, J. W., 18, 24, 106, 124, 315, 317, 320, 328
Lortie, D. C., 248, 266
Lubin, J. W., 41, 43, 46
Lucero, R. J., 102, 124
Lusted, L. B., 36, 45

Machin, K. E., 34, 46, 263, 266
Machol, R. F., 28, 44
Mackworth, N. H., 271, 289
Maelzer, D. A., 15, 24
Magraw, R. M., 149, 157, 163, 181
Makover, H. B., 136, 142
Mansfield, E., 128, 141
March, J. G., 248, 264, 341, 346
Marmorston, J., 115, 124, 125
Marples, D. L., 140, 141
Maron, M. E., 49, 60
Marschak, T. A., 232, 266
Marsh, R., 155, 181
Maruyama, M., 50, 60, 93, 105, 114, 118, 124

Mase, Darrel J., 163
McDonough, J. J., 249, 250, 266
McDowell, W., 39, 45, 278, 288
McEwan, W. J., 192, 206
McIntosh, C. S., 267
McKean, R. N., 30, 46, 271–273, 288
McKeown, T., 137, 141
McLachlin, G., 41, 46
McLaughlin, C. P., 32, 39, 41, 45, 62, 255, 337, 341, 342, 345
McMillan, C., 261, 266
McNamara, Robert, 272
McNerny, W. J., 136, 141
McPeak, W., 177, 180
Mechanic, D., 124
Meissner, W. W., 112, 124
Mendelsohn, Everett, 143
Menninger, K. A., 50, 60
Menzies, I. E. P., 99, 124
Messinger, H. B., 127, 141
Mesthene, Emmanuel G., 143
Michael, D. N., 128
Michael, S. T., 87, 94, 124
Millendorfer, H., 58, 59
Miller, E. J., 10, 19, 24, 185, 187, 206
Miller, James G., 3–11, 25, 143, 181, 190, 206, 217, 229, 330, 343
Miller, R. L., 17, 26
Mills, D. L., 37, 48, 248, 267
Mills, Wilbur, 135
Morgenstern, O., 2, 26
Morris, D., 38, 45
Morris, W. T., 240, 241, 266
Morse, P. M., 33, 46, 271
Mountin, Joseph W., 132, 133
Moustafa, A. T., 29, 47
Mouton, J. S., 323, 324, 328
Mullendorfer, H., 22, 25
Muses, C. A., 50, 60

Naylor, T. S., 242, 266
Nightingale, Florence, 135

O'Brien, G. M., 195, 205, 335
Odum, E. P., 15, 25
Oppenheim, J. J., 115, 123
Osler, 76
OSTI (Organization for Social and Technical Innovation), 290, 313
Overall, J. E., 36, 46

Packer, A. H., 41, 46, 235, 266
Page, T. L., 266
Pareto, V., 17
Parker, R. D., 36, 46, 263, 266
Parsons, T., 12, 13, 25, 143, 181
Paul, B., 191, 205
Payne, A. M. M., 95, 124
Peachey, R., 111, 124
Peck, H. B., 200, 206
Pelletier, R. J., 267
Pelz, D. C., 315, 328
Perrow, C., 31, 46
Pervin, L. A., 14, 25
Peterson, O. L., 36, 46, 249, 266
Pett, L. B., 247, 266
Phillips, D. L., 105, 124
Pierce, L., 283
Pierce, J. R., 279, 289
Pike, M. C., 38, 43
Pines, M., 164, 180
Polak, O. R., 111, 124
Pondy, L. R., 187, 206
Potter, V. R., 54, 60, 114, 124
Priban, E., 52, 60
Priban, I., 104, 124
Price, D. K., 31, 46, 135, 141

Quade, E. S., 271, 289

Rapaport, Anatol, 2, 25
Rapoport, A., 49, 61
Rappoport, A. E., 50, 61
Reed, I. M., 41, 43, 46
Reidel, D. C., 39, 46, 136, 141
Reiser, Stanley, 143
Reusch, J., 25
Reynolds, J. A., 40, 47
Rice, A. K., 10, 18, 19, 24, 25, 187, 196, 206
Rice, C. E., 21, 25
Rice, D. P., 30, 46
Richards, D. W., 104, 105, 124
Rilke, A. E., 36, 43
Rivett, P., 28, 42
Roberts, Ed, 236
Roemer, M. I., 29, 47, 193, 206
Roethlisberger, F. J., 17, 25
Rogers, E. S., 127, 141
Roman, M., 200, 206
Rosenbloom, R. S., 251, 266
Rosenfeld, L. S., 136, 142
Rosenthal, Gerald, 42, 339
Rosner, M. M., 56, 61
Rossiter, C. E., 40, 47
Roy, R. H., 28, 44
Rubel, R. A., 36, 47
Ruesch, J., 13, 25
Russell, J. M., 136, 142
Rutstein, D. D., 159, 167, 178, 181

Ryan, J. J., 232, 244, 265
Ryan, W., 200, 206

Samis, H. V., Jr., 54, 61
Sanders, D. S., 199, 205
Saunders, B. S., 29, 47, 235, 266
Saxberg, B. O., 249, 267
Scheff, T. J., 36, 47, 263, 267
Schlaifer, R., 36, 47
Schmale, A., 116, 125
Schneider, J. B., 41, 47
Schulberg, H. C., 21–25, 95, 125, 187, 194, 195, 205, 206, 334
Scott, W. G., 57, 61
Scott, W. R., 248, 267, 325, 328
Scott, W. S., 17, 25
Seiler, J. A., 18, 26
Shannon, C., 2, 26, 53, 61
Shaw, G. K., 112, 123
Sheldon, Alan, 34, 62, 95, 97, 125, 127, 338
Shils, E. A., 12, 25
Sidel, V. W., 41, 44
Siebold, G., 50, 61
Sigerist, Henry, 84, 90, 96, 125
Sigmond, R. M., 173, 181, 196, 198, 206
Silver, A. N., 282, 286, 289
Simon, H. A., 36, 47, 341
Slobodkin, L. B., 230, 232
Slocum, J. W., Jr., 249, 267
Smalley, H., 31, 38, 47, 263, 267
Smelser, N. J., 12, 25
Smith, Adam, 82
Smith, H. E., 248, 267
Smith, H. L., 39, 47
Smith, W. F., 30, 47
Snider, R. S., 102, 123
Snow, 343
Sofer, C., 19, 26
Somers, A. R., 135, 142, 163, 181
Somers, H. M., 135, 142
Sommer, R., 15, 26
Soricelli, D. A., 40, 47
Souder, J. J., 40, 47
Spain, R. S., 266
Spiker, E. D., 42, 47
Stanley-Jones, D., 49, 54, 61
Steele, J. D., 38, 48
Stein, M. R., 21, 26
Stephenson, R., 267
Stern, E., 125
Stewart, W. H., 167, 181
Stoeckle, J. D., 135, 142
Strauss, G., 321, 328
Sullivan, D. F., 29, 47
Swazey, Judith, 143
Szasz, T. E., 85, 125
Szego, G. C., 244

Tagiuri, R., 102, 125, 249, 267
Taubenhaus, M., 127, 142
Taylor, Frederick, 231, 267
Teeling-Smith, G., 95, 123
Terreberry, Shirley, 189, 206
Terris, M., 132, 142
Thomas, W. H., 38, 40, 47
Thompson, J. D., 38, 42, 44, 47, 192, 206, 252, 263, 265, 267
Thompson, J. W., 101, 125
Tinbergen, 296, 313
Toronto, A. F., 36, 47, 48, 267
Towne, Henry, 231
Trist, E. H., 18, 26
Trist, E. L., 19, 23, 26, 183, 188, 189, 205
Tsao, R. F., 36, 37, 48, 263, 267
Turkevich, N. M., 115, 123
Turner, C. D., 34, 48
Turner, R. J., 99, 125

U.S. Congress, 270, 289

Veasey, L. G., 267
Vickers, G., 50, 61
Vitosky, H. M., 120, 123
Vollmer, H. M., 37, 48, 248, 267
von Neumann, J., 2, 26

Waaler, H., 35, 48
Warner, H. R., 36, 48, 263, 267
Warner, W. K., 31, 33, 48
Warren, R. L., 189, 197, 206
Watt, K. E. F., 35, 48
Wayne, E. J., 36, 48
Weaver, W., 2, 26, 53, 61
Weiner, J. M., 115, 125
Weisbrod, B. A., 29, 48
Welch, C. E., 99, 122
Welch, J. D., 38, 48
Whatmore, G. B., 52, 61, 121, 125
White, K. L., 127, 142, 152, 158, 174, 181, 235, 267
White, P. E., 191–195, 205, 206, 248, 266
Whitehead, Alfred North, 82
Whitmeyer, Frederick, 255
Whitson, C. W., 38, 48
Wiener, N., 2, 26, 49, 61, 271, 278, 279, 288, 289
Wilinsky, C. F., 133, 142
Williams, E. M., 36, 46

Williams, N. J., 38, 48
Wilson, E. A., 193, 206
Winslow, C. E.-A., 132, 133, 142
Wiseman, J., 29, 48
Wodarczyk, M., 120, 123
Wohlstetter, 31
Wolf, S., 101, 125
Wolfe, H., 39, 40, 48
Wolfe, Samuel, 147, 163, 169, 180
Wolff, H. E., 86, 87, 123
Worstell, G. L., 41, 46
Wylie, L. G., 41, 46

Yarnell, S. R., 36, 43
Yerushalmy, J., 36, 48
Young, O. R., 4, 26, 211, 217, 229
Young, J. P., 38, 39, 48, 275, 288
Yovits, M. C., 49, 61

Zaleznik, A., 315
Zeman, J., 49, 61
Zweber, J. E., 17, 26

Subject Index

Absenteeism, 146
Academic disciplines, 62
Adaptation, 53, 87
 adjustment processes in, 67
 chronic disease as form of, 109, 110
 and the patient, 278
 and systems, 278–283
Adaptive models, 339
Agencies, 183, 186, 188, 189, 199, 200
 activities of, 195
 authority structure, 194
 communication, 196
 competition, 223
 complexity of, 193
 consultation programs, 200
 goals, 197
 interdependency. *See* Interdependency, organization
 psychiatric, 200
 referrals, 214, 220
 relations, 213–215, 220
 relationships of, 191, 202
 specialization, 194
 supraorganizational, 198
 as systems, 211–213
 types of, 194
Aggregative models, 339
Air Ministry, 271, 287
Analogy, 65
Analysis
 benefit-cost, 29–34, 68, 249, 250, 254
 cost-effectiveness, 30–34, 249, 250, 253, 254
 systems, 27–42, 138–140, 230–263
Analyst, role of, 341
Analytic systems, 11
Automation, 50
 and society, 147

Barrier score 13, 14
Behavior
 assumptions and, 316
 change in, 314–327
 expectations and perceptions, 316
 modeling, 316, 323, 324
 reinforcement in, 317
Benefit-cost analysis, 29–34, 68, 249, 250, 254
Bingham Associates, 136
Biology, 2, 11
Blocks of people, 133, 134, 138–140
Body image, 13, 14
Boundaries, 13, 18, 70, 185–188, 190, 213, 214, 346
 biochemical, 13
 boundary crossings, 225
 boundary roles, 187, 195
 boundary spanning, 186–188, 195, 219
 controls, 185, 186, 204
 definition of, 225
 modifications, 225
 of medical care system, 143
 organ systems, 13
 permeability, 185, 186
 physical, 13
 psychological, 13
 regulation of, 10
Breakdown of system, 221
Bureaucratization, 31

Cancer, as example of model, 112–117
Care-giving systems, 182, 186, 197, 200, 214, 215, 219, 221, 222, 225
 and client system, 213, 215, 219
 community health, 190–192
 mental health, 190, 199
Centralized communications resource, 222, 223
Change, 227, 228. *See also* Organizational change
Change agent, 208

City Community Services Organization, 213
Closed system, 5–7, 17, 18, 33, 34, 184
Coercive policies, 299, 301, 302
Community, 15, 21
Community health, 41, 126, 132–135, 137
Community mental health, 182, 183, 198, 200
center, 195, 200–204
role of, 199, 200
system models, 199–204
comprehensive health services model, 200, 201
human services model, 200–204
medical model, 199–204
psychiatric medical practice model, 199–201
Competition, agency, 223
Component, 8, 66
Comprehensive health planning, 182, 183, 186, 198, 199, 201, 204
Comprehensive state planning, 136, 137
Computers, 35–37, 40, 232, 233
simulation, 34, 35, 38
Monte Carlo, 35
Conceptual systems, 11, 330
Concrete systems, 11, 330
Conflict, 67, 220, 314
resolution, 314, 327
win-lose, 318
Constituencies, 203
input, 185, 187–189, 193, 203
input and output, definition of, 189, 190
output, 185, 188, 189, 193, 203
Construct, medical care, 126–240
Control, 32, 302
Control mechanisms, lack of, 217
Control notation, 339
Control theory, 339
Coordinating agencies, models for, 199–204
Cost
benefit analysis, 29–34, 68, 249, 250, 254
and effectiveness, 272, 273
of health services, 154
Cost-effectiveness analysis, 30–34, 249–250, 253–254
Crossings, boundary, 225. *See also* Boundaries
Custodial care, 197
Cybernetics, 5, 9, 34, 35
and biology, 49
definitions of, 49
in human relationships, 339
and medical care, 99
and medicine, 50–55
models, 278–283, 345
and psychiatry, 50

Decentralization, 71
Decision-making, 197, 220, 330
Diagnosis, 35–37, 40, 263
Differentiation, 8, 9, 18, 314
and conflict, 315, 320
of health system, 155
Disease
classification of, 92–96, 119
cybernetic models, 52–55
diagnosis of, 90–96
germ theory of, 85, 88, 89
and normality, 87
primitive ideas of, 84
psychological and social factors in, 87, 115–117
response to by individual, 283–286
response to by society, 149–156
Doctor-patient relationship, new issues, 332
Duplication
of effort, 217
of services, 221

Echelon, 65
Ecology, 14, 15, 35, 263
Economic models, 338
Economics, 27, 41, 42, 290–313
Economies, 20
Ecosystem, 15, 100
Efficiency, 253
Elements
common, 211
noncontinuous, 211
nonoverlapping, 211
as parts of sets, 208–210, 212
Entropy, 7
Environment, 8, 14, 21, 22
causal texture of, 188
community, 188, 189, 203
and disease, 93, 94, 101
ideal types of, 188, 189
disturbed-reactive, 188
placid-clustered, 188
placid-randomized, 188
turbulent field, 188
Epidemiology, 35, 37, 242, 263
Equicausality, 9

Equifinality, 9, 20
Equilibrium, 6, 225–227
Feedback, 9, 10, 34, 201, 204, 221, 222, 227, 263, 335
adaptive, 22
deletion, 114
dependence, 227, 335
and disease, 96
lack of, 217
linkage, 103, 104, 121
loop, 104–107
and medical care system, 99–122
negative, 22, 51, 52, 54, 55
positive, 10, 51, 52, 55
and system effectiveness, 287

General models, 339
General practitioner
and family, 170
as gatekeeper, 169
as integrator, 171
need for, 167
specialization and, 157, 158
and triage officer, 170
General systems theory, 27, 65, 68, 184, 204, 230, 263
contributions to a health system, 342, 343
interdisciplinary nature of, 344
role of, 338
General Systems Yearbook, 2–3
Goals
in medical care, 336
models, 183, 184
multiple, 196–199, 203
Groups, 15
family, 16, 17
psychotherapy, 16, 17
small, 16
social, 15, 16

Health organizations, 183, 185, 186, 189, 203
environment of, 184, 188, 202, 203
as open systems, 183, 186
social service, 185
Health planner, 27, 29, 136, 137
Health-related organizations, definition of, 194
Health system, 204, 330. *See also* Medical care system
central issues, 331
Health workers
specialization of, 157–164
types of, 1, 152, 153
in U.S., number of, 161

Holistic approaches, 33, 34, 127
Homeostasis, 51
homeostat, 53
and organism, 101
and patient, 277, 278, 283–286
Hospitals, 37–40, 42, 135–138, 255–261, 263
proprietary, 342
teaching, 332, 335
Human relations programs, 321
sensitivity training, 321
T Groups, 321
Human Resources Group, 120

Iceberg effect, 95
Illness behavior, 99
Independence, 225, 226
Industrial engineering, 27, 31, 38, 232
Information
of cell, 93
and critical subsystem, 70
flow, 186
general, 62, 68, 81
processing, 11, 62
systems, 40, 246
theory, 55
Information referral center. *See* Centralized communication resource
Input, 7, 11, 18, 66, 100–108, 273
consequences of deviation in, 108–112
to health system, 143
mechanisms, 219, 221
Integration, 8, 9, 18, 314, 315
Interagency coordination, 193–199
Interdependence, 225–227
conjunctive, 266
disjunctive, 226
Interdependency, organization, 192, 193. *See also* Organizational networks
competition, 192, 193
cooperation, 192, 193
bargaining, cooptation, coalition, 192, 193
coordination, 193–199, 204
barriers to, 193–199
beliefs and attitudes, 195
deficient communication, 196
lack of goal priorities, 196
Interface, 224
Interlocking systems, 335
International relations, 20
Interorganizational networks, 183, 189, 191, 198, 202–204. *See*

Interorganizational networks (continued)
also Interdependency, organization
component interdependence, 191–193
conflict, 187, 193, 197
exchange relations, 193
interorganizational bridges, 195
Interorganizational systems. *See* Interorganizational networks
Intersystem
communication, 220–222
general properties, 211, 224
linkages, 218, 219, 221, 224. *See also* Boundaries, spanning
Intersystem model, 207, 208, 215, 224
advantages of, 208, 224, 226, 228
Intersystemic relations, 216, 217
tensions in, 217, 220, 221, 223

Learning
assumptions, 322, 323
behavioral, 315
concepts in, 316
culture, 315
open system and, 321
Linear programming, 34, 244, 255–261, 263
Living systems, 209

Magnetic fields, and psychology, 102
Management
businesslike, 245, 246
new techniques of, 319, 320
participative, 318
Manpower, shortages, 334
Marker chains, 38, 40, 242, 244, 263
Market mechanism, 338
Market system, 338
closed, 338
Mathematical models, 32, 34, 251
Mechanism, market, 338
Mechanism-vitalism controversy, 49
Medicaid, 335, 338
Medical care, 6, 15, 19–22
construct, 126–140
goals. *See* Goals
issues in, 331–336
quality of, 39, 249
research in, 21
Medical care systems, 183, 202, 329–331
as abstracted system, 72
delivery of care, 72
depersonalization, 156
differentiation, 96, 97, 151–180
as feedback device, 100–102
fragmentation, 167
institutionalization, 174
management and planning, 268–273
models, 55–59, 273–289
as open system, 143
role of hospital, 164
and society, 143, 144
Medical science, 34, 263
Medicare, 335, 338
Medicine
cybernetic, 51–55
primitive ideas, 84
scientific, 85
Mental health care, 21, 22
Mental hospitals, 185, 197
Meta issues, 341–344
definition of, 340, 341
Midlife crisis, 102
Models, 63, 336–340
adaptive, 339
aggregative, 339
characteristics of, 337
cybernetics, 345
developing of, 340, 345, 346
of disease, 112–117
economic, 338
general, 339
mathematical, 32, 34, 63, 251
normative, 339
prescription, 275, 276
purposes of, 337
quantitative, 339
systems, 336–340
Monitoring, 10
Morphogenesis, 10, 11, 52
Morphostasis, 10, 11
M.P.H. degree, 132
Mutual causal systems, 52, 93, 106
and cancer, 114

National planning, 29–34
Network analysis, 218
Normality, 87
Normative models
problems of, 339

Open systems, 5–7, 10, 12, 17, 18, 183, 184, 186, 190, 204
Operating systems, 290–313
Operations research, 27–42, 230–263, 270–273

Organismic disease theory, 52, 53, 85–98
Organization, 127–130, 138–140, 248, 249
Organizational change
closed system approach, 319
open system approach, 320, 321
selective reinforcement, 324–326
Organizational domain, definition of, 193
Organizational goals. *See also* Goals
environmental conditioning of, 193
Organizational strategies, 188, 189
Organizational systems, 17–20
Oscillation, 101
Output, 7, 18, 66, 100, 273
maintenance functions, 214
mechanisms, 219, 221
transactions, 220

Patients
doctors and, 332
progressive care, 127, 135, 136
as a system, 208
Personality, 12–14
Persuasive policies, 299–301
Physician. *See also* General practitioner
and patient, 332
in primitive society, 88–90, 96, 97
role of, 149, 150
as systems manager, 120, 121, 165
Planner, 343
health, 27, 29, 136, 137
Planning, 290–313, 334, 336
increased significance of, 174
and medical care system, 118–122
methods for, 268–273
national, 29–34
operational, 275, 276
strategic, 276
Planning - programming - budgeting systems (PPBS), 268. *See also* PPBS
Policies
coercive, 299, 301, 302
persuasive, 299–301
prohibitive, 299
restrictive, 299, 300
stimulative, 299, 301
Policy selection, 296–312
Population, 15
control, 343, 344
Power, 67
cooperative, 318
and health personnel, 153, 154
and scarce resources, 318
Practitioner, 343
Prevention
chronic disease, 127
primary, secondary, tertiary, 202, 203
Primary care, 168, 169
Primary task, 18, 19
Probability theory, 34, 38, 39, 41, 263
Problem
cybernetic models, 279
solving and participation, 317, 320–327
types of handling, 107, 108
Professionalization, 37, 38, 245, 248, 249
PERT (Program Evaluation and Review Technique), 241, 263
PPBS (Program-Planning-Budgeting System), 249, 250
Programming, linear, 34, 244, 255–261, 263
Progressive patient care, 127, 135, 136
Prohibitive policies, 299
Psychiatry, 127
Psychotherapy, 16, 17
Public health services, 76, 126–140

Quality of care, 39, 249
Quantitative models, 339
Queuing theory, 38, 39, 252

Regional Medical Program, 136, 137
Regionalization, 136, 239, 308, 309, 311
Regulation
cybernetic models, 280–287
of medical care systems, 56, 57
of psychophysiological processes, 54
of systems, 51, 54
Rehabilitation, 126, 127
Research operations, 27–42, 230–263, 270–273
Resource allocation, 29–34, 302–306
in health services, 151, 173–176, 268
Restrictive policies, 299, 300
Roles
evolution of professional, 174
institutionalization of, 144
motivation and, 145
socialization in, 145
specialization, 156–164

Satisficing, definition of, 341
Scheduling appointments, 38, 41, 251, 252, 263
Secretary of Health, Education, and Welfare, 30, 249, 250
Semilattices, 209
Senior Citizens Multipurpose Center, 213–215, 217
Sensor-receptor functions, 218, 219
Sets, 208–210
Simulation, 34, 35, 38, 242, 244
computer, 63
with model, 273, 286
Social indicators, 247
Social system, 144
and health system, 146, 147
roles in, 146
understanding of, 340
Somatic mutation, 94
Steady state. *See* Equilibrium
Stimulative policies, 299, 301
Strain, 67
Stress, 67, 88
Structural-functional approach, in health system, 143–180
Subsystems, 7, 8
agencies as, 190, 198
of community mental health system, 191, 204
critical, 66, 70
differentiated, 186
information processing, 71–80
matter-energy processing, 71–76
of medical care system, 73–79
operating, 187
process, 8
structure, 8
types, 70, 71
Suprasystems, 8, 66, 68, 190, 219, 221
Surgeon General, 29, 129, 130, 249, 250
System
abstracted, 62–64
analysis, 27–42, 138–140, 230–263
basic concepts, 4–11
boundaries. *See* Boundaries
break, 227
breakdown of, 221
change in, 320–327
client, 214
closed, 5–7, 17, 18, 33, 34, 184
component, 81
conceptual, 62–64, 330
concrete, 330
cultural, 13
definition of, 4, 17, 209–211, 224
degree of systemness, 210
differentiation, 81
General Systems Yearbook, 2, 3
general theory, 1–4, 27, 65, 68, 184, 204, 230, 263
health, 330
history, 1–3
improvement, 218
individual, 11–13
information, 40, 246
interlocking, 335
levels of, 5–7, 81, 100, 111
animal, 5
cybernetic, 5
dynamic, 5
genetic-societal, 5
human, 5
open, 5
social, 5
static, 5
transcendental, 5
medical care. *See* Medical care systems
models, 336–340
open, 5–7, 10, 12, 17, 18, 143, 183, 184, 186, 190, 204
definition of, 184
theory, 190
operating, 290–313
organizational, 17–20
political, 214, 217
simulation of, 286
social, 5, 13, 15, 16, 340
societal, 214
transcendental, 5
veridical, 11
Systems games, 17

Tavistock Institute of Human Relations 18, 19
Technology, and medical care, 148, 150–154, 172, 173
Theory
control, 339
germ, of disease, 85, 88, 89
general systems. *See* General systems theory
information, 55
medical care, 72
open system, 190
probability, 34, 38, 39, 41, 263
Title XIX, Medicare, 134
Transducer functions, 214
Transducing agents, 222
Treatment selection, 36, 37, 40

Trust, 322
in conflict, 318, 319
in organizational life, 322
of medical system, 152, 153

U.S. Congress, 135–137
U.S. Public Health Service, 127–130